Systemic disease for dental students

Systemic Disease for Dental Students

T. J. Bayley FRCP

Consultant Physician,
Broadgreen Hospital, Liverpool

and

S. J. Leinster BSc FRCS(Ed.)

Senior Lecturer in Surgery
University of Liverpool

WRIGHT·PSG

1984   Bristol   London   Boston

Published by:
John Wright & Sons Ltd,
823–825 Bath Road,
Bristol BS4 5NU, England.

John Wright PSG Inc.,
545 Great Road, Littleton,
Massachusetts 01460,
USA.

*British Library Cataloguing in
Publication Data*
Bayley, T.J.
　　Systemic disease for dental students.
　　1. Mouth–Diseases　　2. Teeth–Diseases
　　3. Oral manifestations of general disease
　　I. Title　　II. Leinster, S.J.
　　617'.522　　RC815

ISBN 0 7236 0638 8

Library of Congress
Catalog Card Number: 83-50883

Typeset by Activity,
Salisbury, Wiltshire

Printed in Great Britain by
John Wright & Sons
(Printing) Ltd.
The Stonebridge Press,
Bristol BS4 5NU

Preface

The necessity of teaching medicine and surgery to dental students has long been accepted and does not need justification. The dentist needs to recognize and understand all basic pathological conditions; must be able to recognize and elicit physical signs of disease in head, neck and hands; should be able to elicit an adequate medical history and so recognize patients who are at high risk of complications of dental surgery or general anaesthesia; and must know how to manage emergencies that occur in the dental chair.

The Trustees of the Nuffield Foundation sponsored a conference of medical teachers of dental students at Cumberland Lodge in Windsor Great Park on the 13th and 14th October, 1981, during the course of which it was perceived that a syllabus was necessary to help students to know what was expected of them. This book contains most of that suggested syllabus and emphasizes the relevance of each field to dentistry. The use of 'practice points' in the text is intended to aid revision, and to highlight the matters which are most important and relevant to dentistry.

It is a great pleasure to acknowledge the patient and tolerant help of our secretaries, Mrs Joan Bowstead, who produced the majority of the typescript, and Miss Maureen Edwards; also Mrs Joan Atkinson who gave valuable help with the typing in the early stages. Dr John Gillman, of John Wright P.S.G., has been an important source of encouragement to both of us, as was Dr Donald Derrick, during those times when the book was 'becalmed'. Mr Ken Biggs produced the clear and artistic illustrations.

T.J.B.
S.J.L.

v

Contents

The medical history   1

Diagnosis of medical disease and disorder largely depends on the taking of an accurate history. Although the dentist will not need to take a detailed medical history from his patient, it is important that he should be aware of points in the past history, certain symptoms and signs and current drug prescription, since these may alter or modify management of the dental problem. Few patients appreciate that some previous illnesses and non-dental symptoms may have important significance for the dentist, and few are told by their doctor to report their history and current drug prescriptions when undergoing treatment of an oral problem.

Previous illness

Rheumatic fever and St Vitus' dance are unusual illnesses in modern clinical practice, but history of either, even thirty or more years previously, should alert the dentist to the possibility that a patient may have valvular disease requiring prophylactic antibiotic cover. A history of a heart murmur in childhood, a ban on games at school or a history that the patient had investigation of or surgical treatment for a congenital heart lesion also suggest the need for prophylaxis, after discussion with the patient's doctor (*see* Chapter 3).

If the patient is receiving treatment for pulmonary tuberculosis it is important to enquire whether the disease is inactive, particularly if inhalation anaesthesia is contemplated. Similarly, any recent (6 months) in-patient or out-patient hospital treatment needs enquiry as to what the nature of the illness was and how it was treated, since the medical condition may have oral manifestations, may modify dental management and, if drug treatment is being continued, may have some importance in deciding any prescription for the oral problem (*see* Chapter 16).

Present state of health

Enquiries must be made about current treatment and attendance at a hospital out-patient clinic. Information about possible medical disorders can be obtained by a simple (yes/no) check list of symptoms, which may also provide a useful guide as to whether the patient is fit for general anaesthesia.

A story of effort-induced chest pain, rapid palpitations and persistent ankle swelling should alert the dentist to the possibility of cardiac disease which will influence management, may require antibacterial prophylaxis and which may be the cause of facial pain (*see* Chapter 3).

Breathlessness with cough and sputum each day, plus wheezing with exertion, and at night or during certain seasons, suggest lung disorders. Spitting blood (haemoptysis) is also an important symptom of lung disorders which can be mistaken by the patient for oral bleeding. Respiratory disease has important influence on the decision concerning general anaesthesia and the necessity to use a pharyngeal pack to avoid accidental inhalation of amalgam or small pieces of broken teeth (*see* Chapter 5).

Since many gastro-intestinal diseases have oral manifestation a story of diarrhoea with blood, heartburn, acid regurgitation, vomiting and food-related abdominal pain should alert the dentist to the possibility that an oral lesion may be an indicator of alimentary tract disorder (*see* Chapter 6).

A history of jaundice in the past month or heavy alcohol consumption may have importance in the dental management of a patient. Jaundice may be due to hepatitis B virus which is present in saliva in large concentration – with the risk that the dentist himself or his assistants may acquire the infection. Jaundice also implies failure of the liver to excrete or metabolize drugs as well as bilirubin, particularly short-acting barbiturates used for general anaesthesia. A history of heavy alcohol consumption also influences the decision concerning general anaesthesia and use of intravenous benzodiazepines, since some of these patients become violent and excited during induction (*see* Chapter 7).

Dryness of the mouth with unusual thirst and an increase in urine volume may indicate uncontrolled diabetes mellitus or renal disease, both important disorders which may be associated with oral problems including ulcer and infection. In the diabetic patient there is the additional question of management during dental treatment if general anaesthesia is necessary (*see* Chapter 9).

A history of fits is important, the patient being more likely to have a seizure during the emotional or painful stress of oral treatment. Some anticonvulsants may cause gingival hypertrophy, particularly phenytoin, which may also cause oral ulceration. A history of headaches with vomiting and visual disturbance may suggest migraine or cerebral tumour, both of which may be associated with non-dental facial pain (*see* Chapter 11).

Rheumatoid arthritis has importance for the dentist for several reasons, principally because of temporo-mandibular joint involvement but also because of the association with dry mouth and absence of tears of Sjögren's syndrome, with a high incidence of dental caries; and because of involvement of the cervical spine with the important risks of sudden movements of the neck during general anaesthesia. In addition juvenile chronic polyarthritis may lead to mandibular growth disturbance (*see* Chapter 12).

Drug usage

It is important that the dentist should know what drugs the patient is receiving on a regular basis. In the case of corticosteroids it is relevant, if the patient is to have general anaesthesia, if these drugs have been pre-scribed in the preceding twelve months. Many drugs used to treat internal disease may result in oral lesions, affecting the hard or soft tissues of the oral cavity, or disturb oral flora. Other drugs may influence manage-ment of dental problems because of the risk of bleeding (anticoagulants), or because of possible interaction with drugs likely to be used by the dentist, such as those used to induce general anaesthesia (*see* Chapter 16).

A history of hypersensitivity to drugs or allergic reactions during treatment should make the dentist cautious about prescribing drugs, particularly antibiotics. Most patients who are allergic to penicillin are aware that they should not receive drugs of this group, but few tell their dentist about such complications.

Table 1.1 Short check list for medical history

1. Previous health: Have you had any of the following?

Rheumatic fever	Asthma	Jaundice
Congenital heart disease	Cough and sputum	Diabetes
A heart murmur	Pulmonary tuberculosis	Epilepsy
Raised blood pressure	Arthritis	Psychiatric illness
Angina or a 'heart attack'	Anaemia	Sinus trouble

2. Have you been in hospital in the past two years?
   Have you been under the care of your doctor in the last year?
   Have you been prescribed any medicine or drug in the last year?
   Are you allergic to any drugs, such as penicillin?
   Have you ever had excessive bleeding after surgery requiring special treatment? or blood transfusion?
   Are you pregnant?

3. Present health: Do you have any of the following symptoms or diseases?

Effort chest pain	Allergy
Breathlessness with effort or lying	Hay fever, hives or skin rash
Ankle swelling	Fainting attacks
Fast palpitations	Excessive thirst and dryness of mouth
Painful swelling of joints	Migraine
Indigestion or stomach ulcers	Venereal disease

4. Drug therapy: Are you taking any of the following drugs?

Antibiotics or sulphonamides	Tranquillizers
Anticoagulants (blood thinning)	Antidepressants
Medicine for raised blood pressure	Aspirin
Steroids	Insulin or antidiabetic drugs
Antihistamines	Oral contraceptive or hormones

5. Personal habits:
   Are you a smoker? How many per day?
   Do you drink alcohol? How many glasses (pints) per day?

Family history

Family history is of importance to the dentist in the patient who claims to bleed heavily after dental extraction, particularly the male. Some patients may proffer the information that other members of their family suffer from illness which is hereditary or congenital, but few such disorders have any relevance to oral problems and their management.

Some illnesses do cluster in families. This, obviously, applies to infectious diseases such as pulmonary tuberculosis and hepatitis B. A similar history may be elicited for rheumatoid arthritis, pernicious anaemia, thyroid and rheumatic heart disease.

Taking a history of medical disorders is time consuming and can easily be achieved by asking the patient to look at a check list of the points which are important to diagnosis and management of oral problems. The use of such a check list is common practice in many dental hospitals and departments (*see Table* 1.1).

Physical signs

Symptoms usually appear before striking physical signs of disease are evident and, for this reason, an accurate history is the first and most important part of the clinical method. However, the ability to elicit and interpret physical signs is an important additional clinical skill, of help in the recognition of medical disorders which are of relevance to the dentist and likely to have some influence on management of the patient's oral problem.

Although the patient may be fully clothed and seated it is possible by noting the general aspect of the patient, his respiration, emotional state, the pulse, the appearance of the hands, eyes, mouth and neck to gain important information about the patient's general medical health and how dental treatment should be altered, if at all. A long and detailed examination is not required, although an accurate description of lumps, ulcers, lymph nodes and signs of inflammation should be made, particularly if this information is to be communicated to other members of the health team, such as the patient's general medical practitioner. Most of the physical signs that are seen in practice are either obvious on first appearance of the patient or by a glance at the part visible – so-called 'spot diagnosis'.

General appearance

The general aspect of the patient, including the emotional state, should always be noted. The patient's facial appearance may immediately suggest a medical disorder, particularly such endocrine disorders as hypothyroidism ('peaches and cream' complexion with hair loss, involving the eyebrows) and acromegaly (prognathism with coarse features and prominent frontal bones).

It is important to distinguish the anxious patient from the one who has hyperthyroidism, the latter showing other features of endocrine disorder such as goitre (enlargement of the thyroid gland), ocular abnormalities and profuse sweating with heat intolerance.

The skin colour is often a helpful observation. The recognition of cyanosis, jaundice and pallor suggestive of anaemia gives important clues to the possibility of serious medical disorder. Pigmentation, whether non-racial (such as that associated with Addison's disease) or ethnic, is also of importance. The black patient may have the sickle cell trait and investigation of this possibility should always be done if the patient is being considered for general anaesthesia.

Cyanosis is a bluish colour of the skin and mucous membranes due to an increased amount of reduced haemoglobin in the capillaries (*see* Chapters 3 and 5). It may affect the lips, face, nose, tongue and buccal mucosa (central), or the hands and feet, unilateral or bilateral (peripheral). The cyanosed limb is usually cold, due to slow circulation of blood, but in central cyanosis the extremities are warm. Central cyanosis reflects reduced arterial oxygen content (hypoxaemia), but failure to detect this sign does not preclude hypoxia, particularly in respiratory disorders such as asthma. Imperfect oxygenation of blood due to pulmonary diseases and mixing of venous and arterial blood in the heart are the important causes of central cyanosis. Peripheral cyanosis reflects excessive reduction of oxyhaemoglobin in the capillaries, caused by slowing of the circulation, both arterial (as in Raynaud's phenomenon) and venous (obstruction by thrombus or, simply, dependence and immobility of the extremity).

◀ Cyanosis of the tongue and lips is a feature of severe respiratory disorder or congenital heart disease with R to L shunting

Yellowness of the skin and mucosa, *jaundice*, is due to excess of bile pigments in the body tissues and fluids. Jaundice may occur because of over-production of pigments (haemolytic); reduced capacity of the liver to excrete (hepatic); or to reabsorption from blocked bile ducts (obstructive). Haemolytic jaundice is usually mild and may not be detected. Obstructive jaundice is accompanied by intense itching, due to bile salt retention, with excoriations due to scratching.

◀ Jaundice may be most obvious from the appearance of the buccal mucosa

A pale skin does not always signify anaemia; thick and opaque skin and reduced capillary blood flow, as in shock, syncope or reduced arterial blood supply also cause pallor. Anaemia is better judged, although never with great accuracy, from the mucosa of the mouth and conjunctivae.

◄ Skin pallor is not always a good indicator of anaemia, especially in the 'shocked patient'

The general development and nutrition can usually be assessed in the clothed patient, whether the appearances are those expected of someone of the same age and sex, whether underweight or obese and whether, in a teenager, the sexual characteristics have developed.

It is informative to watch the patient walk, not only to assess the gait, which may suggest orthopaedic, neurological disability or muscle disease, but also as a means of assessing exercise tolerance, particularly if the patient has had to climb stairs. Cyanosis and an increase in respiratory rate (tachypnoea) may only become obvious with effort. High pitched wheezing may also be provoked by mild exercise in some patients with bronchial asthma, which can also be noted when the subject is seated or lying. Wheezing is due to narrowing of the smaller air passages; lower-pitched noises, exaggerated by breathing through the mouth (stridor), are due to narrowing of the larynx, trachea or one of the major bronchi. Stridor occurs with narrowing, by goitre, enlarged lymph nodes, tumour or a foreign body inhaled from the mouth. The development of stridor during a dental procedure, particularly under general anaesthesia, is an important sign of respiratory obstruction.

◄ High pitched respiratory wheezing is a feature of small airways obstruction, stridor a feature of major airways narrowing

Examination of the face

Observation of the shape and movements of the face can provide helpful information about some medical disorders.

Generalized swelling of the face is usually due to fluid retention, with puffiness of the lower eyelids, particularly in the morning after lying flat in bed. Acute nephritis, nephrosis and obstruction of the superior vena cava by tumour (usually metastatic mediastinal lymph nodes from carcinoma of bronchus) are the usual causes of facial oedema.

◄ Facial oedema occurs in some patients with renal disorders because, unlike those with cardiac disorders, they are able to lie flat

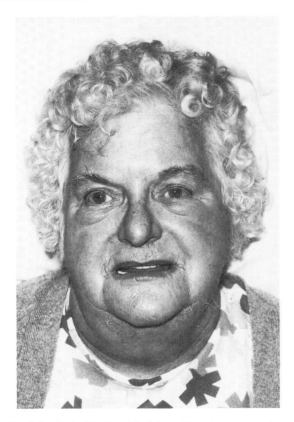

Fig. 2.1. Periorbital and facial swelling due to superior mediastinal obstruction caused by enlarged lymph nodes secondary to carcinoma of bronchus.

Localized swelling of the face can be due to bone lesions (Paget's disease and tumours) or soft tissue lesions, particularly salivary gland enlargement. The parotid, submandibular and sublingual glands can be enlarged and this may be unilateral or bilateral, due to inflammation or tumour. It is usually easy to distinguish which gland is involved, but in generalized enlargement, such as mumps, the parotid and submandibular glands seem to merge.

If the lesion is unilateral the duct of the parotid gland should be inspected for redness, oedema and pus, suggestive of stone formation. Benign tumours are localized to one part of the gland, particularly the lower

Table 2.1. Salivary gland swelling

Salivary gland swelling

- Involving more than one gland
  - Dry mouth, dry eyes
    - Yes (Sjögren's syndrome)
    - No → With ocular features (red eye)
      - Yes (sarcoidosis)
      - No → Painful with systemic features
        - Yes (Mumps)
        - No
          - Generalized lymphadenopathy (Mikulicz's disease)
          - Alcoholic liver disease

- Involving one gland
  - Abnormal duct
    - Yes (sialolithiasis)
    - No → tender
      - Yes (Mumps sialodinitis — bacterial, ascending)
      - No → Nodular
        - Yes
          - Mixed parotid tumour
          - adenolymphoma
          - adenocystic carcinoma
          - muco-epidermoid tumours
        - No → painful with facial nerve involvement
          - Yes adenocarcinoma
          - No squamous carcinoma

Table 2.2.   Differential diagnosis of parotid swelling

Swelling of the parotid itself
    parotitis
    mixed salivary tumour etc.
    carcinoma

Swelling of other structures in vicinity
    sebaceous cyst
    lipoma
    enlarged pre-auricular
      lymph nodes
    neuroma of facial nerve
    adamantinoma of mandible

Examination should —
    1. Inspect the parotid duct
    2. Test the facial nerve
    3. Inspect the fauces
    4. Palpate the regional lymph nodes

pole over the angle of the jaw, although there may, occasionally, be deep prolongation into the fauces. Some benign lesions of the parotid show fluctuance on pressure, due to cyst formation. The facial nerve, which runs through the gland, can be damaged by carcinoma of the parotid.

Abnormalities of facial movement may be obvious on inspection of the patient. Facial paralysis is an important sign for the dentist to elicit, particularly if he has attempted an inferior dental nerve block (*see* Chapter 11). Facial tics — repetitive, purposeless and irregular movements which can be mimicked by the patient — are not due to organic disease. Abnormal facial movements, of which the patient is unaware and which he cannot mimic, can be seen in Parkinsonism, Huntington's chorea, multiple sclerosis, partial epileptic seizures and treatment with some drugs (levodopa).

Examination of the eyes

The eye may be affected by generalized disorder, such as diabetes, as well as specific diseases. Abnormalities may be noted in the cornea, such as scarring following

Table 2.3. Mucocutaneous syndromes affecting the eye and
buccal mucosa

Stevens–Johnson syndrome	— drug-induced related to infections
Reiter's syndrome	— including arthritis and urethritis oral ulceration (rarely erosion of hard palate) iritis
Benign mucous membrane pemphigoid	— particularly gingival
Systemic lupus erythematosus	— oral ulceration, systemic features
Behçet's syndrome	— aphthae, vascular lesions, perineal ulcers

previous ulceration and leading to visual impairment.
The sclera (the white of the eye) is sometimes the site
of bleeding in haemorrhagic diseases although small
bruises are usually due to trauma or occur without
cause. Jaundice is easily detected by inspecting the eye.
The sclera can be involved in systemic disorders such as
rheumatoid disease, usually as a generalized red
appearance (episcleritis), which is painful but, occasionally, rheumatoid nodules resulting in areas of
thinning (scleromalacia), having the appearance of
dark areas in the white sclera. Some mucocutaneous
disorders may affect the eye and buccal mucosa (*see
Table* 2.3).

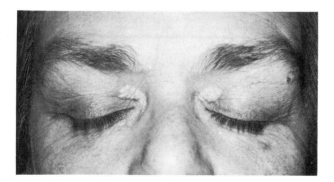

Fig. 2.2. Xanthelasma. Creamy white plaques at inner
canthus of both eyes in a patient with ischaemic heart disease.

Table 2.4. Pupillary abnormalities

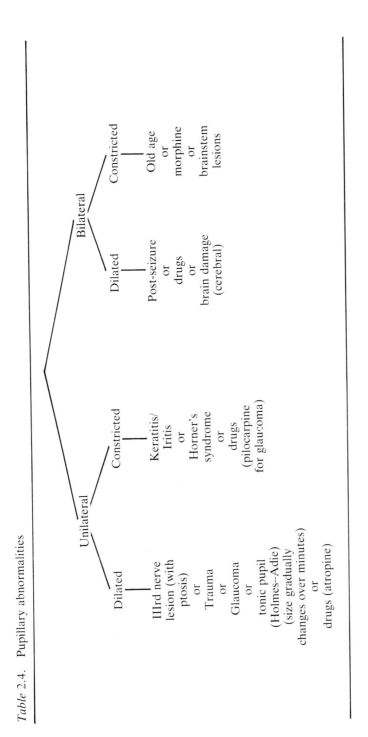

Table 2.5. The painful red eye

	Acute conjunctivitis	*Acute iritis*	*Acute glaucoma*	*Acute keratitis*
Pain	grittiness	Moderate/ severe	severe, radiating to maxilla	moderate plus grittiness
Discharge	purulent	none	none	purulent
Photophobia	mild	severe	moderate	mild/moderate
Cornea	clear	precipitates	oedematous	cloudy, ulcer may be seen
Pupil	normal	constricted later irregular	dilated, oval fixed	usually constricted

An obvious abnormality of eyelid movement is drooping of the upper lid (ptosis). Ptosis rarely interferes with vision but may be associated with external ocular muscle paralysis as part of the underlying disease, causing double vision (e.g. myasthenia gravis). Rodent ulcer (basal cell carcinoma of the skin) and simple papillomas may occur on the eyelids as well as xanthelasma, plaques of creamy, fat deposits at the medial end of upper and lower lids which are often symmetrical, and which may be the marker of disturbance of lipoprotein metabolism, causing premature vascular disease. Swelling of the lids due to stye or widespread inflammation (blepharitis) may be a feature of generalized skin disorder such as seborrhoeic dermatitis.

Squints and abnormalities of eye movement occur either with neuromuscular damage (paralytic squint) or associated with poor sight from any cause (concomitant or congenital squint). Paralysis of ocular movements may be associated with pupillary changes, usually dilatation (mydriasis). Unilateral small pupil (meiosis) is usually due to sympathetic damage (caused by lesions in the neck or cervical cord) and associated with ptosis (Horner's syndrome).

The painful, red eye is a common ocular problem which has importance for the dentist. It is usually unilateral, rarely bilateral (*see Table* 2.5). A painful red

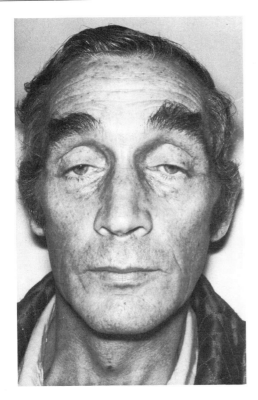

Fig. 2.3. Bilateral ptosis (congenital).

eye can be due to inflammation of the outer layers of the eye (acute conjunctivitis), inflammation of the inner eye (iritis), a combination of conjunctivitis and iritis presenting as corneal ulcer (acute keratitis) and a sudden rise of pressure in the eyeball due to blockage in drainage of the aqueous (acute glaucoma).

Acute conjunctivitis is a bacterial infection (usual organisms being *Staphylococcus*, *Haemophilus*, *Pneumococcus* and, rarely, *Gonococcus*) causing grittiness rather than pain in the eyelids, with a purulent discharge. It affects the whole conjunctiva, unlike acute iritis which shows redness only around the cornea. The pupil in acute iritis is contracted and irregular because of adhesions of the iris to the lens. As well as pain, which may be severe enough to keep the patient awake, iritis also causes blurring of vision.

Acute glaucoma is very painful, often associated with nausea and vomiting. The pupil is dilated and unresponsive. Vision may be reduced to a bare perception of light. Both iritis and glaucoma require urgent treatment to preserve sight.

The signs and symptoms of acute keratitis are those of the underlying conjuctivitis and iritis, the corneal ulcer appearing as a cloudy opacity.

Any cause of the acute 'red eye' can produce referred pain in the face, but it is usually obvious on careful examination that the ocular lesion is responsible. Conversely, some cases of iritis improve following removal of impacted teeth. Oedema of the lower lid may occur with apical abscess, particularly of the upper canines. Infection can sometimes spread to the orbit subperiosteally or via the antrum.

◄ Ocular pain may be referred to the face although examination of the eye usually shows abnormality likely to be the cause of the symptoms

Examination of the neck

Swellings and pulsations in the neck are easily visible in the clothed patient and the dentist should be able to describe such physical signs and know of the likely causes.

The method for description of a swelling or lump is standard and should include the site, size and shape, consistency, and relationships to skin or deeper structures (*see Table* 2.6).

Swellings in the midline are usually in the thyroid gland or thyroglossal tract along which the developing gland migrates from the tongue. Thyroglossal cysts may occur anywhere from the tongue to the cricoid cartilage. Occasionally dermoid tumours may present as midline swellings.

Swellings in the lateral aspect of the neck may arise from lymphatic tissues, remnants of the embryonic branchial arch, blood vessels, the pharynx (pharyngeal pouch), the salivary glands or from infections such as Ludwig's angina, actinomycosis and space infections emanating from sublingual, submandibular and pharyngeal areas.

Lymphatic swellings in the neck are usually due to infection or neoplastic disease, rarely to congenital abnormalities such as cystic hygroma (*see* Chapter 13).

Table 2.6. Examination of lumps in the neck

Anatomical site — midline

anterior to $\Big\}$ sternomastoid

posterior to

Size — whether constant or varying
Shape
Consistency — firm, soft or fluctuant
Attachment to skin and deeper structures
Movement with swallowing, effects of sternomastoid
       contraction (lump superficial or
       deep?)
Over-lying skin — red, thick or puckered
Temperature compared with surrounding skin
Tenderness
Size and consistency of draining lymph nodes

Lymph node swellings are frequently multiple, can be unilateral or bilateral and found either in the anterior triangle (anterior to the sternomastoid muscle) or the posterior triangle. Lymphadenopathy due to infection and secondary carcinoma frequently becomes confluent. Lymph nodes infiltrated by lymphoma (Hodgkin's disease) remain discrete and rubbery in consistency. Tenderness and reddening of the overlying skin may occur with inflammatory conditions and, in rare instances (tuberculosis), the skin may break down to form a sinus.

Branchial cysts present in the anterior triangle of the neck, arising beneath the upper border of the sternomastoid muscle, and are both fluctuant with pressure and transilluminate with a pencil torch. Pharyngeal pouch also presents with a soft swelling in the anterior triangle of the neck, varying in size and not transilluminable.

Vascular swellings are recognized by their pulsatility and relationship to the carotid artery. Lipoma (fatty tumours) and sebaceous cyst also occur in the neck, the former having a soft, lobulated structure. Sebaceous cysts are discrete and non-tender (except when secondarily infected), being attached to the skin in which a small hole (punctum) may be recognized.

Pulsation in the neck may be venous or arterial. The venous pulse is impalpable and varies with the position

◀ Palpable pulsation in the neck is arterial

Table 2.7. Swelling in the neck

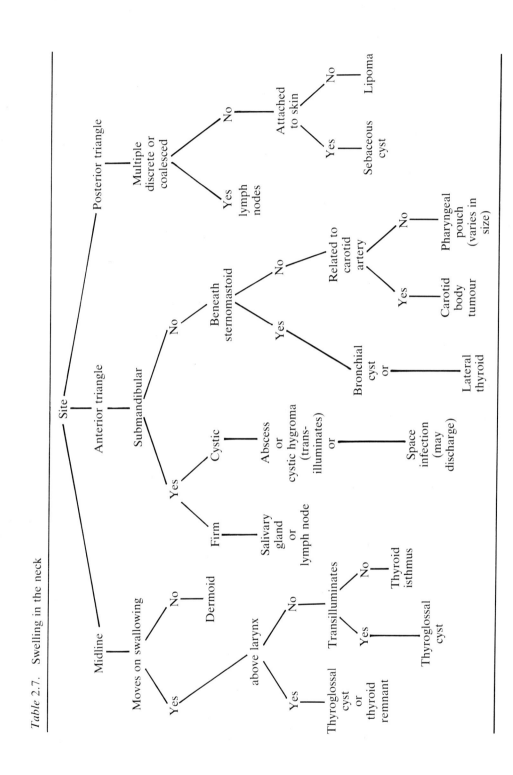

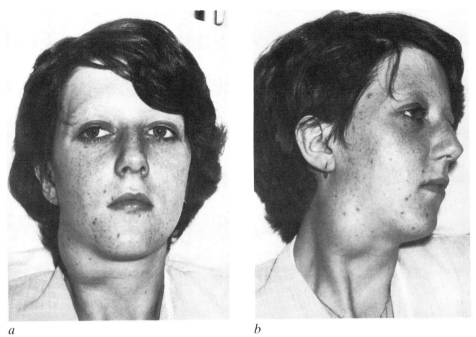

a   *b*

Fig. 2.4. Swelling of R. side of neck due to branchial cyst. Note that the mass arises anterior to and beneath the sternomastoid muscle.

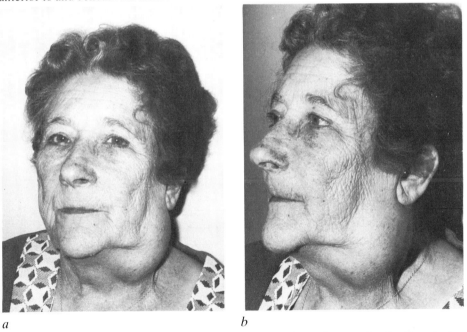

a   *b*

Fig. 2.5. Aneurysm of L. carotid artery. The swelling in the neck was pulsatile. Note that the swelling extends anterior and posterior to the sternomastoid muscle.

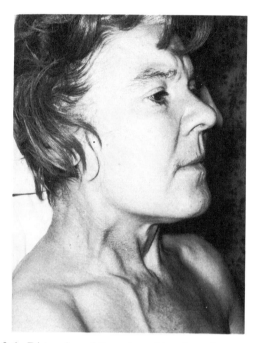

Fig. 2.6. Distension of the external jugular vein caused by superior mediastinal obstruction due to metastatic lymph node enlargement.

of the patient, except when there is superior mediastinal obstruction in which the veins are grossly distended but do not pulsate. Marked arterial pulsation occurs in hypertension, aortic valve regurgitation and with a hyperdynamic circulation, as in severe anaemia or hyperthyroidism. Marked venous pulsation in a patient lying at 45 degrees or more from the horizontal reflects raised pressure in the right atrium, a diagnostic feature of congestive and right heart failure. Venous pressure shows fluctuation with respiration, falling during inspiration, a variation exaggerated in patients with airways obstruction.

◀ Venous distension in the neck which does not vary with posture and is not pulsatile is due to superior mediastinal obstruction and may be associated with tracheal compression

Examination of the hands

Observation of a patient's hands can provide important evidence of medical disorders that are of relevance to the dentist. The size and shape, palms, nails, abnormal movements, skin appearances, joints and musculature should be noted.

The large, 'spade-like' hands of the patient with acromegaly is often an obvious feature, particularly in the female or non-manual worker. Long thin fingers (arachnodactyly) can be a feature of Marfan's syndrome. Tapering, with reduction in the size of the terminal phalanges is a feature of scleroderma, the skin showing thickening and attachment to underlying bone.

Palmar erythema occurs both with liver disease (hepatic cirrhosis, of whatever aetiology, and metastatic carcinoma) and with rheumatoid arthritis. Skin lesions rarely occur on the palms, although contact dermatitis and the secondary stage of syphilis can present in this way. Thickening of the palmar fascia with flexion contraction of the small and ring fingers, which is usually bilateral (Dupuytren's contracture), usually occurs in manual workers, but can be a manifestation of alcoholic liver disease. Pallor of the palmar creases is not a reliable indicator of anaemia, but pigmentation is an important sign of Addison's disease (*see* Chapter 9). Yellow deposits of fat in the creases may be a feature of disturbances of lipoprotein metabolism predisposing to ischaemic heart disease.

◄ Palmar erythema may be due to hepatic disease, or be associated with rheumatoid arthritis and may occasionally be unexplained

Table 2.8.   Digital clubbing

Pulmonary causes
    carcinoma of bronchus
    bronchiectasis and other chronic
      suppurative disorders
    fibrosing alveolitis

Cardiac causes
    infective endocarditis
    cyanotic congenital heart disease

Hepatic cirrhosis

Coeliac disease

Inflammatory bowel disease

Unilateral
    subclavian artery stenosis

Idiopathic   ?congenital

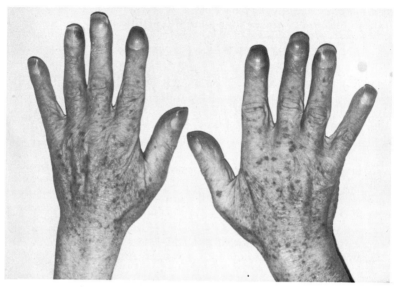

a

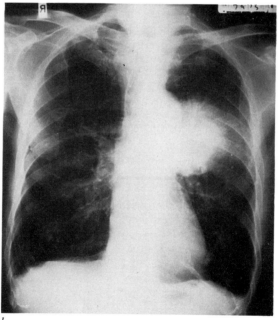

b

Fig. 2.7. Digital clubbing due to carcinoma of bronchus. Chest radiograph from same patient showing large mass in L. lung.

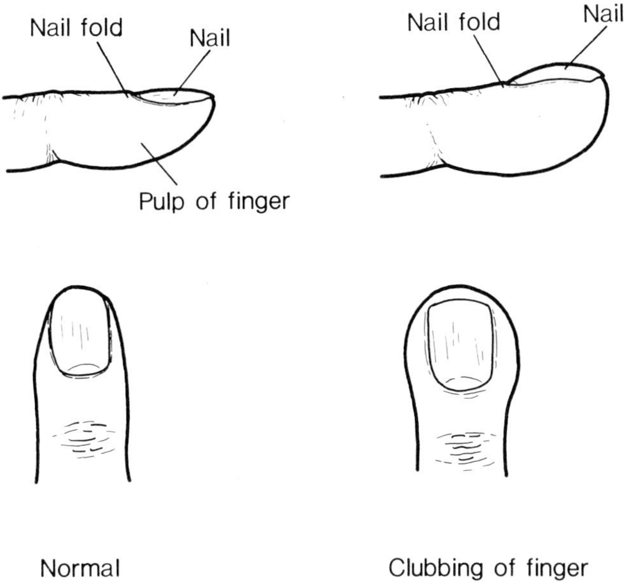

Fig. 2.8. Digital clubbing. Note loss of normal angle between nail and nail fold.

Abnormalities of the nails can reflect systemic disorder. Clubbing, in which the terminal phalanx is enlarged like the head of a match, with loss of the angle between nail and nail fold, is often the first sign of pulmonary lesions, such as carcinoma of bronchus. Other pulmonary disorders may be associated with clubbing which can also be a physical sign of cardiac lesions, hepatic cirrhosis, coeliac disease, and inflammatory bowel disease. In a few patients there may be no explanation for clubbing, in spite of extensive investigation.

Brittle nails are common, especially in the female, usually without associated systemic disorder. Spoon-shaped nails (koilonychia) are also brittle and can be associated with iron deficiency anaemia, but sometimes occur without obvious cause. Splitting of the nails (onycholysis) may be a feature of hyperthyroidism. Splinter haemorrhages may occur in a variety of conditions, including infective endocarditis, but in most cases there is no cause other than trauma. Telangiectasia may present with lesions under the nail and in the

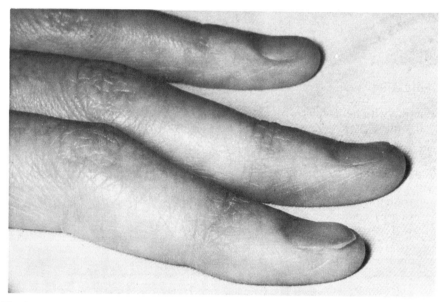

Fig. 2.9. Koilonychia with iron deficiency anaemia. Note the spoon-shaped appearance of the index (nearest) finger.

pulp, but are larger than splinter haemorrhages and associated with similar vascular abnormalities in the mucocutaneous junctions. Rheumatoid arthritis and systemic lupus may cause digital gangrene presenting with black lesions in the periungual tissues. Fungal infections cause gross deformity and hyperplasia of the nails, occasionally associated with vascular problems, including Raynaud's phenomenon. Psoriasis of the nails causes pitting and occurs with arthropathy (*see* Chapter 12).

Abnormal movements of the hands and fingers may be of little significance, especially in the anxious young patient, but they can be due to neurological diseases, such as Parkinsonism and multiple sclerosis, due to drugs (phenothiazines) or to hyperthyroidism. The abnormal movement may be present at rest (static), with arms outstretched (positional) or provoked by voluntary movements (intention tremor). The causes of involuntary movements are discussed in Chapter 11.

Diseases of the joints often occur in the hands, notably the swelling and partial dislocation of rheumatoid disease, and the hard nodes related to the distal interphalangeal joints with osteoarthrosis. Other forms of arthropathy affect the hands, including psoriasis, and are discussed in Chapter 12.

Wasting of the muscles of the hands occurs both with joint disease, due to disuse because of pain, and in association with neurological lesions. Wasting of thenar (thumb) muscles is a feature of median nerve lesions (often due to compression at the wrist — carpal tunnel syndrome — a feature of hypothyroidism and acromegaly). Wasting of the hypothenar (little finger) muscles occurs with ulnar nerve lesions (the nerve being frequently damaged at the elbow by trauma or joint disease) and associated with flexion of the ring and little fingers (*main-en-griffe*). Wasting of all groups of muscles is usually due to nerve root or cord lesions, such as motor neurone disease and syringomyelia.

◀ Wasting of the intrinsic muscles of the hands in the absence of joint disease suggests a neuromuscular cause

Examination of the mouth and fauces

Several medical disorders present with lesions of the tongue, buccal mucosa, gingivae, palate and teeth.

The loss of papillae on the tongue is a sign of iron, vitamin B_{12} and B_6, deficiency. Hypertrophy of the papillae in patches with intervening atrophy gives an appearance termed the 'geographical tongue', the surface being divided into irregular zones by zigzag white lines; it is of no clinical significance. Scarring of the tongue may follow previous trauma, particularly in the epileptic, or may follow ulceration. Macroglossia and apparent hypersalivation occurs with acromegaly, congenital hypothyroidism, amyloid disease and Down's syndrome. In the latter the tongue is deeply grooved — the 'scrotal' appearance.

Malignant ulcer and tumour may occur anywhere in the oral cavity (*see Table* 2.9). The site, size, shape and appearance of any lesion should be carefully described (*see Table* 2.10). The lesion should, if possible, be palpated to detect thickening of surrounding tissues (induration), to determine whether the lesion is fixed to deeper structures, such as bone, whether it is tender and if movement produces pain in the distribution of the trigeminal nerve. Lingual movements, such as

◀ Depapillation of the tongue suggests vitamin or iron deficiency

Table 2.9.   Oral tumours

Dental origin (odontogenic)

Osseous origin (osteogenic)
    primary
    secondary — usually carcinoma

Bone lesions not of osseous origin
    fibroma
    inclusions of salivary
      tissue

Salivary tumours and other swellings of the glands

Epithelial lesions
    benign (papilloma)
    malignant (squamous carcinoma)
      presenting as ulceration
        or warty appearance
        or nodular thickening
        or leucoplakia with
          fissuring

Extension of malignant tumours (e.g. from antrum)

---

protrusion, may be affected. Dysphagia, hoarseness and regional lymph node enlargement should be noted.

Tongue movements may be affected by tumours and neurological disorders. Difficulty in protrusion, tremor, wasting and irregular contraction of the tongue (fibrillation) may be seen.

Scarring, moistness, colour (pallor or cyanosis), pigmentation, ulceration and bleeding of the mucosa may be features of systemic disorder. Dryness of the mucosa may be temporary in the anxious or dehydrated

Table 2.10.   Examination of oral ulcer/tumour

Describe its size
    site
    shape and appearance (flat, warty, its edges and base)

Describe the surrounding tissues (by palpation)
    fixation to deeper structures (particularly bone)

Examine lingual movements (particularly protrusion)

Examine the regional lymph nodes

Enquire of symptoms such as dysphagia and hoarseness

Table 2.11.   Xerostomia

Salivary gland or duct disease
    sialolithiasis
    sialoadenitis (postoperative)
    Sjögren's syndrome
    damage by irradiation (for rodent ulcer)

Emotion and anxiety

Drugs
    atropine and anti-Parkinsonian drugs
    antidepressants
    antihistamines
    phenothiazines
    hypotensives (clonidine, ganglion-blocking agents)

Dehydration
    vomiting
    diabetes mellitus

General disorders
    chronic renal failure

patient but may be due to salivary gland or duct disease and systemic disorders such as diabetes mellitus and insipidus and chronic renal failure (*see Table* 2.10). There may be associated caries, periodontal disease and infections, such as candidiasis.

Over-production of saliva (ptyalism) occurs with Parkinsonism and some psychiatric disorders. Some drugs cause sialorrhoea, including the cholinergic drugs used to treat myasthenia gravis. Apparent over-production occurs with macroglossia as well as with neurological lesions that cause facial and lingual paralysis and disorders of pharyngeal function.

◄ Hypersalivation may be real, such as occurs with Parkinsonism and drugs for myasthenia, or apparent, as occurs with macroglossia and true dysphagia of any cause

Melanin pigmentation of the mucous membranes is frequent in Negroes, as well as in patients with Addison's disease, pregnancy, malabsorption and vitamin deficiency, such as pellagra.

Gingival hypertrophy occurs with systemic disorders such as leukaemia, and with drug therapy, particularly phenytoin. Bleeding tendencies are obvious from inspection of the gums and abnormal pigmentation on the gum margin occurs with lead poisoning (blue) and bismuth (brown), usually in patients with excess tartar deposition.

Palatal swelling is usually due to enlargement of lymphatic tissues, due either to infection (quinsy) or neoplastic disease, such as lymphoma. Petechiae appear on the palate in bleeding disorders and infections such as glandular fever. Vesicles can occur with herpes (zoster and simplex) and aphthous ulcers are occasionally seen on the palate. Loss of palatal movement and gagging is a feature of bulbar and pseudo-bulbar palsy. Paralysis of one half of the palate is associated with movement of the uvula towards the normal side when the patient gags or says 'ah'. In bilateral weakness the palate does not move and fluid may regurgitate through the nose during attempts to swallow.

Ankle swelling (*see Table* 2.12)

Swelling of the ankles can be an important sign of disease. Swelling due to fluid retention is confirmed by pressure over the ankle, which produces pitting that persists for a few seconds.

Oedema of the ankles occurs with a variety of disorders, not all of which are due to serious disease. Ankle swelling occurs in the immobile subject, particularly the elderly and the patient suffering from orthopaedic or neurological disability involving the lower limbs. Oedema due to heart disease can be

Table 2.12.   Ankle oedema

Generalized fluid retention
    congestive cardiac failure (venous pressure raised)
    renal disorder (acute nephritis and nephrosis)
    hepatic disease (usually with ascites)

Venous/lymphatic obstruction
    by thrombus
        tumour
        pelvic lesions

Immobility and neurological disorders (probably venous in origin)

Physiological
    some females (premenstrually)

recognized because of an increase in jugular venous pressure, and 'renal oedema' by the history of facial swelling after over-night recumbency. Oedema associated with liver disease is often accompanied by ascites (abdominal swelling due to fluid) and other stigmas such as jaundice, spider naevi and Dupuytren's contracture. Obstruction of the femoral vein by thrombus or pressure from pelvic tumours causes unilateral oedema, which also occurs with blockage of lymphatic drainage vessels by tumour. Venous obstruction can be recognized by the cyanosed appearance of the limb below the level of obstruction, due to slowing of capillary circulation.

Pulse

Abnormalities of the pulse are described in Chapter 3. The rate should be observed as well as the rhythm, whether it is regular or irregular and, if the latter, whether the irregularity is related to respiration (slowing during expiration being a normal finding in the younger subject, called 'sinus arrhythmia') or is random. The pulse volume can be assessed, being large in systemic hypertension but small in aortic stenosis and extensive myocardial disease. An estimate of blood pressure may be made by how easily the pulse can be compressed by the palpating finger. The thickness of the vessel wall can also be assessed; normally the wall is barely palpable but may be greatly thickened by vascular diseases, such as atherosclerosis. The character of the pulse should also be noted, a sustained wave being a feature of aortic stenosis, a jerky but large volume being typical of aortic regurgitation, anaemia and hyperthyroidism.

Although, by tradition, the pulse is palpated at the wrist the carotid, facial and temporal arteries can be equally useful in assessing the patient during general anaesthesia.

◀ Palpating the pulse, the rate, regularity and the ability to compress the wave should be noted

Cardiac diseases   3

Cardiac diseases are important in relation to dental practice for many reasons including the risk that oral treatment may result in bacterial endocarditis, the radiation of the pain of coronary insufficiency to the lower face and mandible, and the hazards of general anaesthesia and local anaesthesia with adrenaline in such patients.

Symptoms of cardiac disease

Although there are many different pathological varieties of heart disease they present with similar symptoms. Breathlessness and chest pain are the most common symptoms of cardiac disorder; palpitations, swelling of the ankles, faints and undue fatigue are the other less common and less specific complaints.

Breathlessness is a symptom of both cardiac and respiratory disease, as well as anaemia and renal failure. The breathlessness of cardiac disease is due to failure of the left side of the heart, and the history of its provocation and progression will usually distinguish the cause. Dyspnoea due to heart failure is initially only with effort, but is progressive, so that the exertion needed to cause symptoms becomes less. The progression may occur over a few weeks, months or even years until the patient finds that he cannot sleep lying flat because of breathlessness, having to use more pillows, a stage called 'orthopnoea'. Even with extra pillows the patient may find that he suddenly wakes at night with severe breathlessness so that he must get out of bed to obtain relief. This symptom, paroxysmal nocturnal dyspnoea, can sometimes be the first manifestation of cardiac disease, without preceding breathlessness on exertion: it may also be reproduced by the dentist if the patient with cardiac disease is operated on when lying flat.

Angina is the symptom of myocardial ischaemia and is usually associated with coronary artery atheroma, but may also occur with disease of the aortic valve, severe anaemia, rapid heart rates and any disease that causes failure of the left ventricle. The pain is usually provoked by effort but may be related to food, smoking or emotion: at times the pain comes on when the patient lies flat, angina decubitus, or it may wake him at night. The pain is felt in the centre of the chest and is variously described as 'crushing', 'like a band', or 'like a heavy weight', but not 'sharp' or 'knife-like'. The pain radiates upwards to the throat and is often associated with a choking sensation; there is also radiation to the arms, more often the left arm, to the back in some instances and to the mandible and lower face. Variants of angina occur in which the pain occurs only in the face and mandible, in this instance the patient thinking that the pain is of dental origin, often forgetting the provocation. Angina is of short duration, usually a few seconds or minutes, and rarely longer than 20 minutes. Pain which lasts several hours is a feature of myocardial infarction.

Swelling of the ankles is usually due to fluid retention of many possible causes. The oedema of cardiac disease is entirely in the lower half of the body, never occurs in the face, and persists even after rest in bed. It differs from the fluid retention of renal disease which does occur in the face because the patient can lie flat, and from oedema due to posture or venous obstruction in the legs, which clears with recumbency.

'Palpitations' may have many meanings for patients. The usual description is that the heart 'stops' or 'turns over' and is the sensation that some feel with an extra cardiac beat, usually of ventricular origin, which is not a feature of heart disease. Some patients use the term to describe heart beating, with effort or emotion, which is normal and not a feature of cardiac disease. The sudden onset of rapid heart beating, associated with breathlessness and sometimes with angina, is the description of paroxysmal tachycardia, which occurs in many forms of heart disease.

◀ Breathlessness can be provoked by lying flat patients with cardiac disease

◀ Variant forms of angina may begin and remain in the mandible

◀ Facial oedema occurs in renal disease and respiratory failure but not in cardiac disease

Signs of cardiac disease

Palpation of the pulse at the wrist may give some clue to the presence of cardiac disease. The rate, regularity, force or volume may be abnormal in many forms of heart disease.

The normal resting heart rate is between 72 and 80 beats per minute, although the rate may vary over short periods of time in response to emotion or pain. Slowing of the heart (bradycardia) is a feature of ageing, a pulse of 60 per minute being normal in a man of 65, but also occurs in the young athlete and in adolescents, without any evidence of cardiac disease. Bradycardia may occur with disease of either the sinoatrial node, or the conduction system, particularly in the bundle of His. Bradycardia due to heart disease is usually less than 50 per minute and often slower than 40, but may slow to such levels with acute hypoxaemia or during treatment with beta-adrenergic receptor blockers.

The heart accelerates in physiological circumstances such as emotion and exertion. Tachycardia also occurs without heart disease pro rata any increase in metabolism, such as hyperthyroidism or with fever. Sinus tachycardia may be as fast as 120 per minute although the rate varies over the matter of a few minutes, even at rest. When the cause is intrinsic or is a secondary cardiac disorder, such as hyperthyroidism, the rate is persistently fast over long periods, even at rest. Rates faster than 120 per minute, particularly if sustained and constant, are always an indication both that there is an abnormal pacemaker and that there is underlying heart disorder. Drugs may cause cardiac acceleration: adrenaline and atropine because of autonomic effects and analgesics and sedatives in therapeutic doses, probably because of an associated fall in blood pressure.

Irregularity of the pulse may occur without cardiac disease. The variation with respiration in younger subjects, speeding with inspiration and slowing during expiration (sinus arrhythmia) is normal. Extra beats, either from atria or ventricles, are commonly observed in patients with normal hearts and may feel to the patient, and observer, as if the heart stops briefly and restarts. Although there is usually no cause for extrasystoles they may occur in smokers after virus

Table 3.1.   Causes of atrial fibrillation

Rheumatic mitral valve disease
Ischaemic heart disease
Thyrotoxic heart disease
Hypertensive heart disease
Pulmonary disease — usually vascular, rarely bronchitis

---

illnesses, in subjects who are sensitive to caffeine in coffee and in patients taking digoxin, when they may be a sign of drug intoxication.

A persistent but *irregular irregularity of the pulse* is usually the sign of atrial fibrillation, almost invariably due to underlying cardiac disease. Acceleration of the heart with mild exertion exaggerates the irregularity of the pulse in atrial fibrillation, unlike extrasystoles which usually disappear. Most patients with atrial fibrillation are unaware of the abnormality, only experiencing palpitations when the disturbance of rhythm is of sudden onset. Atrial fibrillation occurs with any form of cardiac disease but most frequently with rheumatic mitral valve disease and ischaemic heart disease (*see Table* 3.1).

◄ Irregularity of the pulse due to atrial fibrillation is exaggerated by mild exercise

Variations in pulse volume are sometimes difficult to detect but, usually, a small volume pulse indicates low blood pressure or reduced cardiac output, following cardiac infarction and with narrowing (stenosis) of the aortic and mitral valves. A pulse of large volume may be found with a raised blood pressure, with an increase in cardiac output, as in hyperthyroidism, with aortic valve incompetence or hardening of the aorta (atheroma) in the elderly.

Swelling of the ankles and lower legs, which pits on pressure, is due to fluid retention in the extracellular spaces, called *oedema*. Oedema also occurs with liver disease, renal disease and malnutrition with severe protein deficiency. Oedema occurs with venous obstruction and when the return of blood from the legs is reduced, as in prolonged inactivity and with orthopaedic problems such as arthritis of the knees. Drugs, particularly steroids, may cause oedema because of generalized fluid retention, which occurs in the face as well as the legs, as in renal disease.

Cyanosis of the oral soft tissues is visible in some patients with cardiac disease. Central cyanosis, of the lips, indicates the presence of congenital heart disease with right-to-left shunts or severe lung disorder with impaired oxygenation. Peripheral cyanosis, of the hands or feet only, may occur without cardiac or pulmonary disease, being due to either stagnation of venous blood or to poor arterial supply.

An *increase of venous pressure in the neck* is also a sign of heart disease, reflecting an increase in pressure on the right side of the heart due to heart failure. When a normal subject lies flat the jugular veins can be seen because these vessels are at the same level as the right atrium and distend with blood. At 45 degrees to horizontal the veins are not visible except with heart failure or obstruction to venous return in the superior mediastinum. Pulsatile distension of the jugular veins indicates that the cause is cardiac. Non-pulsatile increase in pressure occurs with obstruction.

◀ Pulsatile distension of the neck veins at 45° is due to cardiac failure

Cardiac function in health and disease

Cardiac output, the volume of blood ejected by the left side of the heart each minute, varies with physical activity and with changes in metabolism, such as occurs physiologically in pregnancy, and in disease such as hyperthyroidism. The increase is achieved by tachycardia without any reduction in stroke volume, the amount of blood ejected each beat. The mechanisms responsible for physiological increases in cardiac output are complex, being partly due to the autonomic nervous system effects on heart rate and the force of contraction of heart muscle. Five-fold increases in cardiac output occur during moderate-to-severe exercise such as bicycling or running.

In cardiac disease the mechanisms that in normal subjects cause the increase in output with exertion are needed to maintain function at rest. The force of contraction of the heart is maintained by an increase in pressure in the chambers which causes enlargement of the heart (or dilatation) and thickening of cardiac muscle (hypertrophy). These compensatory mechanisms have an upper limit, beyond which further increases in intracardiac pressures do not increase cardiac output. Beyond this point the symptoms and signs of heart failure appear.

Most common cardiac diseases affect the left heart chambers, and the right heart secondarily and later in the natural history. The symptoms are therefore initially those of left heart failure: dyspnoea with exertion, orthopnoea and nocturnal breathlessness. Later the signs and symptoms of right heart failure appear: oedema of the legs and an increase of pressure in the jugular veins, also termed 'congestive cardiac failure'.

Disturbances of cardiac rhythm

The heart rate varies with exertion and emotion due to changes in the normal pacemaker, the sinoatrial node, which lies to the right atrium at the point of entry of the superior vena cava, and is under the influences of the

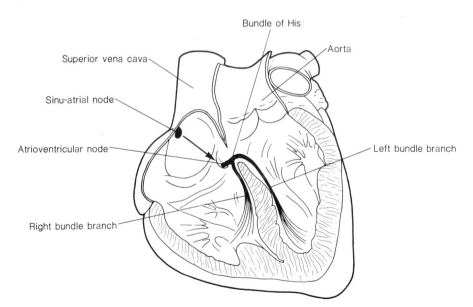

Fig. 3.1. Conduction system of the heart. Impulse spreads from the sino-atrial node to the atrioventricular and, via the bundle of His, to the ventricles through the bundle branches.

Table 3.2.   Tachycardia

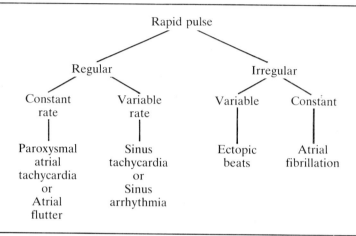

autonomic nervous system. Any part of the heart muscle is capable of taking on a pacemaker function, and will control the heart rate if faster than the inherent rhythm of the sinoatrial node.

Abnormal pacemakers are usually in the atria and less often in the right or left ventricle, the interventricular septum or the atrioventricular node, the latter being the natural pacemaker that succeeds the failing sinoatrial node. An abnormal pacemaker may have a very rapid rate, in excess of 300 per minute in the case of atrial flutter, or there may be many pacemakers, as in atrial fibrillation, which summate to produce an atrial rate in excess of 500/min. In flutter and fibrillation the conduction of the electrical impulse to the ventricles is delayed, so that the effective heart rate (the rate of ventricular contraction) is only half or less that of the abnormal pacemaker.

Supraventricular (atrial) rhythm disturbances occur in any form of heart disease but may also occur in apparently normal hearts, usually paroxysmal, lasting for less than 24 hours (*see Table* 3.2). When tachycardia is sustained, the patient is unaware of the irregularity and often unaware of the rapid rate. Palpitations are the presenting symptom of paroxysmal tachycardia along with breathlessness and chest pain. The provocative factor for paroxysmal supraventricular tachycardia is often difficult to identify, although the use of sympathomimetic drugs may precipitate or exaggerate any dysrhythmia and should be used with caution in combination with local anaesthetics in the patient at risk. Digoxin and beta-adrenoreceptor blocking agents may control sustained or paroxysmal supraventricular tachycardias. Paroxysmal supraventricular tachycardia can be controlled by increase in vagal nerve tone induced by carotid sinus pressure. Although this is not recommended in dental practice some patients, who have frequent troublesome paroxysms, learn manœuvres of this kind that abort an attack.

Disturbances of ventricular rhythm, with the exception of premature beats (extrasystoles), are uncommon except in the early stages following myocardial infarction. The extrasystole is the commonest rhythm disturbance detected in clinical practice and is usually asymptomatic, occurring in many people with normal hearts, sometimes provoked by smoking, alcohol or virus illness such as influenza. The irregularity of the pulse caused by extrasystoles disappears with mild exertion, which distinguishes this irregularity from atrial fibrillation. Drug therapy is never prescribed for extrasystoles except in patients with known heart disease in whom there is the risk that the ectopic beat may provoke dangerous dysrhythmias such as ventricular tachycardia.

Damage to the natural pacemakers and the conduction system causes slowing of the heart, which may cause symptoms such as fatigue and faintness and sometimes transient loss of consciousness — syncope. Physiological bradycardia occurring in young people, trained athletes and in the elderly, does not cause symptoms (*see Table* 3.3). Cardiac slowing due to heart

Table 3.3.   Causes of bradycardia

Athletes in training

Teenagers

Sinoatrial or atrioventricular block

Drugs — beta-adrenergic blocking agents
           digoxin in excess

disease results either from damage to the sinoatrial node, a slower pacemaker (atrioventricular node) taking over control of heart rate, or to the conduction system in the bundle of His, the ventricles acting as their own pacemaker, permanently or intermittently. Any cardiac disease that causes bradycardia may be complicated by episodes of cardiac standstill of a few seconds' duration, in which the patient feels faint and, if it is prolonged (8 or more seconds), loses consciousness. These episodes (Stokes–Adams attacks) vary in frequency from several each day to less than one per year. Stokes–Adams attacks are always an indication for the implantation of a permanent electronic pacemaker, although sympathomimetic drugs are used in less urgent circumstances.

Rheumatic fever and chronic rheumatic carditis

Acute rheumatic fever is an affective disorder involving the heart muscle and valves, the joints and other connective tissues; in approximately 20% the brain is affected. Although the cause is not definitely known it is thought that the damage to target organs is caused by immune complexes formed following infection, usually of the tonsils, but also of the skin and other organs, with beta-haemolytic *Streptococcus* (Lancefield Group A). About 90% of cases occur between the ages of 8 and 15, especially in temperate climates and in those living in bad housing and overcrowded conditions, the lack of which may account for the diminishing occurrence in the British Isles.

An attack of rheumatic fever usually follows 7–21 days after a streptococcal throat infection, beginning with fever, pain and swelling of one or more large joints, which after a day or two settles, subsequently appearing in another, and so flits from joint to joint. Rashes also appear during the illness as well as nodules over the bony prominences (the shins, elbows and spine). In about 20% of patients, more often girls, involuntary movements of the limbs and grimacing of the face occur, associated with muscle weakness and emotional changes, these symptoms (chorea) being due to brain lesions, which nearly always recover completely, although cardiac damage may follow. Evidence of cardiac involvement, tachycardia, heart murmurs and congestive failure occurs in half the patients with rheumatic fever, although chronic rheumatic carditis is found in later life in many who have had an insidious form of the disease.

Chronic rheumatic carditis

Over half the children who have acute rheumatic fever subsequently develop valvular heart disease, but only half of those who have chronic rheumatic carditis give a history of acute rheumatism. The interval between the acute attack and appearance of symptoms due to valve damage is variable — from one or two years to forty or more — so that the age at which rheumatic heart disease is diagnosed may be between 20 and 70 years. Symptoms usually appear at the age of 30–40 years, and in the female may be related to pregnancy. Symptoms are usually due to the onset of atrial fibrillation.

The mitral valve is the most commonly affected (three-quarters of all cases) and the only one damaged in nearly half. The aortic valve is involved in fewer than half the patients and the pulmonary and tricuspid valves are rarely directly affected.

◀ Half the patients who have acute rheumatic fever subsequently develop heart disease, but only half those who have mitral valve disease have a history of acute rheumatism

Rheumatic mitral valve disease

Mitral stenosis consists of narrowing due to fusion of the two valve cusps with subsequent, gradual obstruction to the passage of blood from left atrium to ventricle. Consequently, pressure rises in the left atrium and is transmitted backwards to the pulmonary veins and capillaries, to the pulmonary arteries and, ultimately, to the right heart chambers (*see Table* 3.4). Some patients have incompetent as well as stenosed mitral valves, blood leaking back to the left atrium during ventricular systole, which also causes a rise in atrial pressure, often with considerable dilatation of the chamber, and transmission backwards to the pulmonary circulation.

The symptoms of mitral valve disease are due to pulmonary congestion which leads to 'stiffness' of the

Table 3.4. Development of heart failure in mitral valve disease

---

Pressure rise in left atrium
↓
Rise in pressure in pulmonary veins
↓
Rise in pressure in pulmonary capillaries
↓
Pulmonary arterial hypertension
↓
Right ventricular and congestive heart failure

---

lung. The commonest presentation is progressive breathlessness. Dyspnoea is initially with effort and later becomes orthopnoea. Occasionally acute pulmonary congestion occurs induced by excitement, unusual exertion, or during the third trimester of pregnancy. Many patients have chronic cough with clear sputum, unrelated to smoking or the winter months; the sputum may sometimes contain streaks of blood and haemoptysis may be heavy at times.

Sooner or later, most patients with mitral valve disease develop congestive heart failure, the onset being insidious after many years of effort dyspnoea and often precipitated by the onset of atrial fibrillation, by intercurrent bronchitis, pregnancy or infective endocarditis.

Some patients with mitral valve disease have no symptoms, lead a normal life, have uncomplicated pregnancies and so do not require surgical or medical treatment. The majority of patients, however, develop atrial fibrillation and require digoxin and diuretics to control this and congestive failure. When medical measures alone are not able to control the condition assessment by means of right and left heart catheterization is carried out, to measure intracardiac pressures and define the state of the valve by injections of radio opaque dyes into the left ventricle. This information helps to decide whether and in what form surgery would be beneficial. Simple splitting of the valve (mitral valvotomy) may be performed or it may be excised and replaced with a prosthesis.

Two important complications of mitral valve disease

◀ The age at onset of symptoms in mitral valve disease is very variable, but may occur after the age of 55, and usually progresses slowly

Table 3.5. Complications of mitral valve disease

Pulmonary oedema
Atrial fibrillation
Systemic arterial embolism
Infective endocarditis
Bronchitis

---

seriously affect the patient's prognosis and have important implications for the dentist. Thrombus may develop in the left atrial appendage, particularly with atrial fibrillation, and pieces may break off, passing into the systemic circulation where they cause obstruction of the major arteries (embolism). Embolization of the cerebral vessels causes a stroke; of the femoral artery loss of blood supply to a leg and subsequent gangrene; of a renal artery kidney infarction; of the mesenteric artery bowel ischaemia and, potentially, gangrene. Patients who have embolic episodes are treated with anticoagulants, and many physicians believe that embolism can be prevented by anticoagulation in any patients with mitral valve disease and atrial fibrillation. Both groups have special problems for the dentist (*see* Chapter 8).

The second important complication is infective endocarditis, although this is uncommon in the heart with atrial fibrillation.

Not all patients with mitral valve lesion have chronic rheumatic heart disease. Mitral incompetence may result from dilatation of the valve ring due to enlargement of the left ventricular cavity; or the valve may become incompetent due to damage of the chordae tendineae following myocardial infarction. Congenital abnormalities of the valve may also result in incompetence. The symptoms and complications are similar to rheumatic valvular disease, except that infective endocarditis is less common.

Aortic valve disease

Aortic valve disease may be a consequence of rheumatic endocarditis, congenital disorders and ather-

Table 3.6.   Causes of aortic valve disease

Rheumatic endocarditis
Congenital — often associated with coarctation
Atheroma
Aortic disease — Marfan's syndrome
Dilatation of heart

oma in the older patient (*see Table* 3.6). Whatever the cause the symptoms are similar and are due to strain on the left ventricle and ischaemia of heart muscle. The usual presentation is dyspnoea with effort, progressing rapidly over a period of a few months, unlike the gradual deterioration of mitral valve disease, with attacks of acute left ventricular failure and progression to congestive heart failure over a period of two years or less. Aortic stenosis may cause fainting on effort and angina, the narrowed valve reducing the cardiac output response to the increased demands of exercise.

Many patients with aortic valve disease are asymptomatic and this group constitutes a problem for the dentist; infective endocarditis following dental treatment being a risk because prophylaxis with antibiotics is not given. Aortic stenosis may not be diagnosed in life and may be the cause of sudden death associated with severe effort, such as playing games.

◀ Sudden death in previously asymptomatic young adults is often due to aortic stenosis

Aortic regurgitation (incompetence) is rarely as dramatic in presentation as valvular stenosis, and the progression of symptoms is more gradual. Aortic incompetence may be due to dilatation of the valve ring: as part left ventricular enlargement; congenital abnormalities of the cusps; and syphilitic aortitis involving the valve ring.

Symptomatic aortic valve disease is treated by operation. Replacement of the valve with a prosthesis is a highly successful operation in most cases. The risk of infective endocarditis on the aortic valve following dental extraction is greater than for the other three; the patient's heart being in sinus rhythm, and prophylaxis may not be thought necessary.

◀ Asymptomatic aortic valve disease is a likely site for infection due to bacteraemia following dental treatment

Congenital heart disease

Congenital heart disease of all kinds occurs once in

every 200 live births and in 2 per 1000 children of school age, some of whom are at risk of developing infective endocarditis following dental treatment.

The heart reaches a fully differentiated form by the end of the 2nd month of gestation and it is before this time that environmental factors, infections such as rubella, and drugs such as thalidomide may cause cardiac malformations. Genetic factors seem to play only a minor part in determining CHD; chromosome abnormalities are rare; but there is a high incidence in some families.

The most commonly encountered malformations are septal defects, persistence of the ductus arteriosus, the tetrad of Fallot, stenosis of the pulmonary valve and coarctation of the thoracic or abdominal aorta.

Communications occur between the atria, the ventricles and between the aorta and pulmonary artery. Blood flows across the defect from high pressure zone to low, from the left heart to right, through the lungs and back to the heart. Eventually cardiac failure may occur because of overloading of the involved ventricle or, for reasons unknown, the shunt damages the

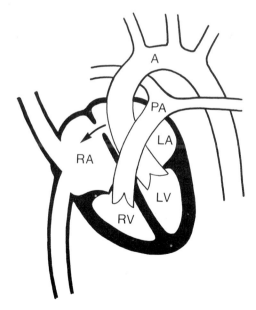

Fig. 3.2. Atrial septal defect. Low pressure in both atrial chambers but direction of flow is from left to right.

pulmonary arteries, causing increase in resistance to blood flow through the lungs. Right heart pressures may rise to a level at which flow is reversed across the defect, from right to left, a situation called 'Eisenmenger's syndrome'.

In patients with *atrial septal defect* blood is shunted through a hole between left and right atrium and thence to the right ventricle. The commonest defect is one due to failure of development of the septum secundum which does not reach the valves; less common is the defect due to failure of development of the septum primum, often associated with abnormalities of the mitral valve. Secundum defects are compatible with normal life until the age of 45–55, and small holes may never cause symptoms. Because of the associated valve abnormalities and its position, the primum defect has higher morbidity and mortality. Infective endocarditis only occurs with the primum variety.

◀ Infective endocarditis only occurs on the primum type of atrial septal defect

Ventricular septal defects vary in size and some small ones are compatible with a full, normal life. There is a

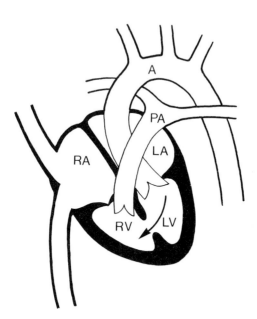

Fig. 3.3. Ventricular septal defect. Pressure is higher in left ventricle, until pulmonary arterial (PA) pressure rises, and flow is reversed, from right to left.

risk of infective endocarditis, even with small defects, about one-third of all patients having an episode during their lives.

A quarter of all defects close spontaneously during childhood. The larger defects have a poorer prognosis and, untreated, the life expectancy is about 35 years, death being due to cardiac failure and changes in the lung blood vessels. Blood is shunted through the defect from left to right ventricle, the size of the shunt varying with the size of the defect. Eventually, unless there is spontaneous closure, the resistance to blood flow through the lung increases, right ventricular pressure rises and flow through the defect is reversed.

◀ A quarter of ventricular septal defects close spontaneously

Surgical closure of these defects may be performed in two stages; in infancy a band is put on the pulmonary artery to limit the shunt, definitive closure being performed later in childhood; by a procedure which carries a risk of complete heart block because of damage to the bundle of His by sutures.

Before birth blood flows from the pulmonary to systemic circulation through the *ductus arteriosus*

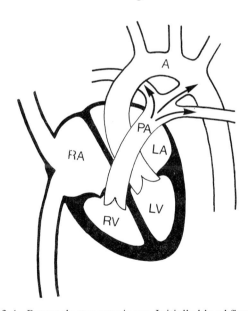

Fig. 3.4. Patent ductus arteriosus. Initially blood flows from aorta (A) to pulmonary artery (PA), but then later (as diagram) the flow is reversed.

connecting the pulmonary artery and aorta. After birth, when the lungs are inflated, the ductus is obliterated within hours or days, but if the fetus is hypoxic or there has been maternal rubella closure does not occur. Blood flows from aorta to pulmonary artery in patients with persistent ductus until pulmonary arterial pressure rises due to changes in the lung blood vessels and flow is then increased. With a small ductus the main risk to life is infective endocarditis, which occurs in 1 patient in 10. The large ductus has a poor life expectancy because of left ventricular failure, reversal of the shunt and endocarditis. Division of the ductus is performed in all cases because of the risk of endocarditis. The operation may sometimes be curative if infection proves difficult to control with antibiotics.

The most common form of cyanotic congenital heart disease is *Fallot's tetrad*, which consists of a large ventricular septal defect, pulmonary stenosis and a right-to-left shunt through the defect directly into the aorta. The child is usually cyanosed, particularly with exercise, and may have syncopal attacks. Squatting, sitting on the heels after effort, is a common feature, the child finding that this relieves dyspnoea. Unless treated surgically most patients die in childhood, although occasionally they can survive to middle age. Because of hypoxaemia, polycythaemia develops which increases blood viscosity and predisposes to vascular obstruction, presenting in the brain particularly as stroke. Infective endocarditis may occur on either the pulmonary valve or the septal defect. Ideal management of these patients is to correct both valve and septal abnormalities in late childhood.

Pulmonary valve stenosis is the most frequent congenital valvular abnormality, accounting for 10% of all congenital heart disease. It may occur alone or in association with atrial septal defect. The child typically has a rounded face and may have either peripheral or central cyanosis. Symptoms vary with the degree of stenosis and consist of fatigue, dyspnoea, angina and syncope. Unless corrected surgically most patients with pulmonary stenosis die in the third decade from right heart failure, serious cardiac dysrhythmias or infective endocarditis.

Coarctation is a congenital narrowing of the aorta, which in over 90% is immediately distal to the origin of

◄ Pulmonary stenosis is the most common congenital valvular abnormality

the left subclavian artery, and commonly associated with a bicuspid aortic valve which may be incompetent. Most patients have no symptoms, the diagnosis being made on routine examination or when the patient is being investigated for a raised systemic blood pressure, but some present with left heart failure or intracranial haemorrhage from rupture of associated congenital aneurysms of the cerebral arteries.

◀ Aortic valve abnormalities are commonly associated with coarctation of the aorta

Most patients do not survive beyond the age of 40, dying as the result of rupture of the aorta, the effects of the raised blood pressure or infective endocarditis, which may occur on the narrowed segment, but usually on the aortic valve. Operation to resect the coarctation and reconstitute the aorta is performed in all patients in the early teens unless cardiac failure in infancy necessitates earlier surgery.

Infective endocarditis

Bacteria, viruses and fungi may invade a heart valve, an area of damaged endocardium, the site of turbulent blood flow through a congenital heart defect, or a prosthesis (*see Table* 3.7). At sites of turbulence due to valve damage, flow through a septal defect, across a prosthesis or in relation to damaged heart muscle, following cardiac infarction, there is fibrin deposition which is readily invaded by organisms in the blood. Any organisms entering the bloodstream are quickly killed by normal body defences except when they

Table 3.7. Cardiac lesions at risk of infective endocarditis

Mitral incompetence (especially mild cases)
Aortic incompetence
Small ventricular septal defects
Persistent ductus arteriosus
Bicuspid aortic valve (congenital)
Pulmonary valvular stenosis
Coarctation of aorta
Prosthetic aortic valves
Endocardial ('mural') thrombus

become enmeshed in damaged endothelium where they survive and proliferate.

Organisms may enter the body in many circumstances, but in dental practice the most important mode of infection is that which follows dental extraction and extensive conservative treatment including scaling. Chewing food may cause a significant bacteraemia in 80–90% of people with apparently normal teeth, lasting for half an hour. The organism involved, *Streptococcus viridans*, is of low virulence and a normal oral commensal. When settled on damaged endothelium the accumulation of platelets and fibrin forms large friable vegetations in which the bacteria are protected from the normal defence mechanisms and, except in high plasma concentration, from antibiotics in the bloodstream. Since valves and prostheses have no direct blood supply, the elimination of infection depends on diffusion of antibiotics through layers of fibrin and platelets to the organisms at the base of the vegetation.

◄ The incidence of infective endocarditis is 1 per 500 dental extractions in those at risk

Although the most important invading bacteria in dental practice is *S. viridans*, the organisms that cause infective endocarditis have changed in recent years, possibly related to the introduction of prosthetic heart valves, the increase in the number of drug addicts using the intravenous route and the increasing use of immunosuppressive therapy. However, 80% of 'medical' endocarditis is caused by viridans streptococci although in patients over the age of 65 this falls to 50%. 'Surgical' endocarditis may occur early or late after cardiac operations, the organisms commonly found being *Staph. epidermidis*, *Staph. aureus*, or even *candida*. Endocarditis in the narcotic usually follows the intravenous injection of water from sources such as the tap or lavatory pan, the commonest organism being *Staph. aureus* as well as unusual pathogens such as serratia. Infection with *Coxiella burnetii* and chlamydia may also occur in patients with heart disorder, which may prove difficult to diagnose because routine blood cultures will be negative. Infection with these organisms can only be recognized by using serological tests.

Most infections are of insidious onset, at an interval of 1–3 months following dental manipulation. The presenting features are vague, consisting of malaise, anorexia, weight loss and night sweats. The possibility of the disease has always to be kept in mind in cases of unexplained fever, particularly in those at risk, rather than wait for the classic triad of heart disorder, signs of infection and embolism before making the diagnosis. Embolism in the spleen, kidney or small bowel may present as abdominal pain. Hemiplegia or loss of vision occurs following embolization of the cerebral vessels. Progressive symptoms of heart failure appear in the later stages following valve destruction.

◄ The classic triad of heart disorder, signs of infection and embolism should suggest infective endocarditis, but early diagnosis depends on suspecting the condition in any case of unexplained fever

The signs of the disease are a low grade fever, anaemia and a brownish skin discoloration. Haemorrhages appear in the nail beds and finger clubbing appears within 6 weeks of the onset of symptoms in more than half the cases. Small, tender, red swellings of the pads of the fingers, toes and sometimes on the palms (Osler's nodes) may be signs of endocarditis, as may frank haematuria. The other signs found on examination are those of heart failure, changes in the cardiac murmurs, splenic enlargement and evidence of emboli.

The diagnosis is made by isolating the organism from the patient's blood, a positive blood culture being obtained in most cases provided that there has not been a recent course of antibiotics. In the latter case diagnosis rests on the suspicion of infection, although choice of effective antibiotic therapy is difficult.

Treatment of *S. viridans* infections with benzylpenicillin, provided that there is no evidence of hypersensitivity to this antibiotic, combined with gentamicin, is usually effective. Penicillin is given intravenously for at least two weeks, usually by a bolus injection through the side arm of an intravenous needle or subclavian venous catheter. After two weeks oral therapy with amoxycillin (1 g 6-hourly) may be given in those patients where the infection has been quickly brought under control, and there have been no embolic complications. Erythromycin is sometimes given in the last few days of treatment if penicillin has been the only drug used throughout the course of treatment, and is a useful alternative in patients who are penicillin hypersensitive. If dental treatment is necessary during the course of penicillin therapy for viridans endocarditis, vancomycin may be given to cover bacteraemia. Some physicians believe that oral amoxycillin, combined with probenecid, achieves adequate blood levels and is an effective and simple means of treatment.

◄ In the treatment of infective endocarditis antibiotics are given intravenously for two weeks, then orally for at least two further weeks

Table 3.8. Prevention of infective endocarditis

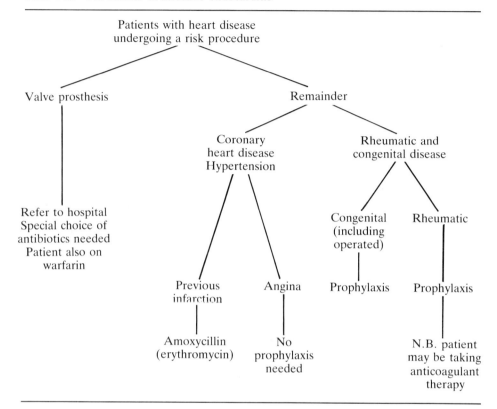

Duration of antibiotic treatment depends on the response to treatment, but in many instances may be for a minimum of 4 weeks. Most relapses are due to inadequate dosage, or inappropriate route and duration of the chosen antibiotic therapy. Relapse is usually treated with vancomycin, at least until sensitivities of the organism are known, and may require surgery to close a persistent ductus or replace an infected prosthetic valve.

Prophylactic antibiotics should be given to cover the transient bacteraemia that occurs with dental extraction, scaling, those root filling procedures with risk of forcing infected material through the apex, as well as instrumentation of the respiratory and genito-urinary tracts, in all patients having cardiac lesions likely to become the site of endocarditis (*see Table* 3.8).

◄ Prophylaxis should be given to those at risk of infective endocarditis, even for minor procedures such as scaling

Operative correction of some congenital abnormalities greatly reduces the risk of endocarditis but it is safest to regard such patients as in need of prophylaxis. The patient with a prosthetic valve seems even more prone to infection and a second antibiotic may be needed to provide adequate cover.

Except in patients who are penicillin-sensitive, prophylaxis consists of amoxycillin as a 3 g sachet 1 hour before the procedure and possibly 8 hours later. Erythromycin is the alternative antibiotic when the patient is hypersensitive to penicillin, 2 g being given 1–2 hours before treatment and 500 mg 6 and 12 hours afterwards. Where the patient requires a general anaesthetic intramuscular amoxycillin (1 g) 1 hour before the procedure is appropriate prophylaxis. Intravenous erythromycin (1 g) at the time of induction of anaesthesia is a suitable alternative in the patient known to be allergic to penicillins.

Some physicians request dental clearance after an attack of endocarditis, usually 3 months or more after the end of antibiotic treatment, at which time the oral flora will have recovered its sensitivity to penicillin. Viridans endocarditis has, however, occurred in patients at risk even after dental clearance, although this is rare.

Ischaemic heart disease

When coronary blood flow is insufficient for the needs of cardiac muscle patients may develop the symptoms of cardiac pain or heart failure. Cardiac ischaemia is usually due to coronary artery disease (atheroma), but may occur in other conditions with reduced coronary blood flow, such as aortic valve disease, syphilitic aortitis and paroxysmal tachycardia. In severe anaemia, when the oxygen-carrying capacity of the blood is greatly reduced, angina may occur with only minimal coronary atheroma. Angina also occurs with apparently normal coronary arteries and has been shown to be due to vessel spasm.

The cause of coronary atheroma is not known, although it becomes more obvious in those over the age of 30, particularly males, smokers, women who have an

Table 3.9.   Natural history of coronary heart disease

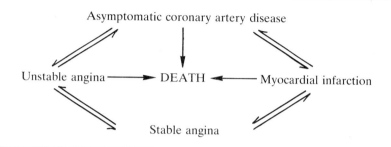

early menopause, in diabetics and in those with hypothyroidism, in patients with unusually high levels of serum cholesterol and, possibly, in some populations with diets that contain large quantities of saturated fats.

The clinical feature of coronary artery disease is angina that may progress after months or years to myocardial infarction. Some patients, however, are asymptomatic despite extensive disease; some present with myocardial infarction without preceding angina; and some with heart failure without ischaemic pain. A large number present as sudden death.

Angina, occurs with varying frequency, from one attack per month, or even six months, to several per day; once angina begins there is a 14% risk of myocardial infarction within 6 months, and 5% per annum risk of infarction thereafter, so that the average life expectancy is 10 years from onset of symptoms (*see Table* 3.9). The two important problems of angina for the dentist are the radiation of the pain to the mandibular and maxillary areas, which may be being mistaken by the patient and his doctor as being dental pain, and the provocation of angina by the stress, pain and emotion of dental treatment. Angina may also be provoked by lying flat, a variant called 'angina decubitus'.

Angina is usually relieved by rest or, when provoked by lying flat by sitting up, and by chewing glyceryl trinitrate tablets. Drugs that block the adrenergic nerve supply to the heart are frequently prescribed for patients with angina, unless the pain occurs infrequently or is stable and easily predicted and prevented by

◄ Angina is an important cause of non-dental facial pain

trinitrin. Many beta-blockers cause marked bradycardia but rarely faintness on standing and few other major side effects other than bronchospasm in some patients. Coronary and peripheral vasodilators that interfere with calcium ion movements in the heart and blood vessels are used as an alternative to beta-blockers.

Coronary artery surgery may be beneficial for angina that cannot be controlled by drug therapy, particularly when arteriography (X-ray contrast medium injection into the arteries) shows obstruction of the major arteries. The relief of pain following surgery is often dramatic in those with involvement of all three coronary vessels.

The most important complication of coronary artery disease is myocardial infarction, in which an area of heart muscle becomes necrotic as a result of reduction in coronary flow to the affected part. Myocardial infarction is not invariably associated with thrombus in the supplying vessel. Most patients with cardiac infarction have an episode of cardiac pain lasting longer than angina, by definition greater than 20 minutes, often without provocation and associated with sweating, faintness, nausea and vomiting. Pain is not invariable, particularly in the older patient, and infarction may be 'silent' or present with complications such as heart failure and systemic arterial embolism, causing stroke or femoral artery occlusion.

Most deaths occur within 6 hours of the onset of symptoms, usually from ventricular dysrhythmias; late deaths being due to 'shock' and heart failure. Other late complications include arterial embolism, pulmonary embolism due to venous thrombosis in the legs and ventricular aneurysm. Embolic disease is treated with anticoagulant therapy which is continued for some weeks after the event. Thrombus develops in the ventricle overlying the area of myocardial infarction, because the endocardium is abnormal and because the underlying myocardium is dead with reduced contractility. Mural thrombi are a potential site for infection during transient bacteraemia, so that the same antibiotic prophylaxis should be used as in patients with valvular and congenital heart disease before dental manipulations.

Following myocardial infarction the patient may

◄ Thrombus may develop in the ventricle overlying a myocardial infarction, with a risk of infection and systemic embolism

have a symptom-free interval lasting from a few weeks to several years. Reinfarction may occur at any time and there is no effective prevention, though there are claims that anti-platelet drugs such as aspirin may do this. The only measure that has been proved to be effective is that the patient stops smoking. Sudden death may occur at any time after infarction, particularly in the first 6 months, and it is believed that this is due to ventricular dysrhythmias, which may be prevented by beta-adrenoreceptor blocking agents. Because of this risk the use of sympathomimetic drugs, such as adrenaline, in combination with local anaesthetics should be avoided in patients undergoing dental treatment who have a previous history of cardiac infarction. Anti-platelet drugs, which may prevent episodes of ventricular dysrhythmias also increase the bleeding tendency following dental extraction, and care must be taken to ensure haemostasis in patients taking them.

◀ Sympathomimetic amines should be avoided in any patient known to have coronary heart disease

Systemic hypertension

It is not possible to set precise upper limits for normal blood pressure, particularly as the level rises with increasing age in normal subjects. Nevertheless, in large communities at least 12% of the population in the sixth decade (50–59 years) have a pressure that is higher than expected. There is, however, an important difference between 'high blood pressure' and 'hypertension', the latter term being used when there is evidence of secondary cardiac or blood vessel damage.

Prolonged elevation of blood pressure results in hypertrophy of the left ventricle, a self-limiting response to the increased work of pumping against a

Table 3.10. Target organs for damage by raised blood pressure

Heart
Brain
Kidneys
Blood vessels

high resistance. Raised arterial pressure also damages blood vessels of all sizes, particularly the arterioles and the aorta, the former resulting in complications such as cerebral haemorrhage and infarction and renal failure; the latter resulting in dilatation (aneurysm) and episodes of tearing (dissection) of the aorta (*see Table* 3.10).

Most patients with raised arterial pressure have no symptoms and the abnormality is only discovered during routine or insurance examination, and in those with nose bleeding or headaches. Discovery of raised blood pressure when stroke or other complications have occurred is the usual way in which the diagnosis is made. The best results of treatment are, however, obtained in the asymptomatic group, particularly in the prevention of vascular and renal disease.

Most patients with raised blood pressure have no secondary cause for the abnormality, only one in ten have renal disease such as chronic nephritis or arterial disease (*see Table* 3.11). Coarctation of the aorta is an important cause in teenagers. Some pregnant women have transient blood pressure elevation, called 'toxaemia'. In rare instances hypertension may be secondary to endocrine disease such as excess production of corticosteroids from the adrenal gland (Cushing's syndrome), excess aldosterone production (Conn's syndrome) and functioning tumours of the adrenal medulla, causing excess noradrenaline and adrenaline release (phaeochromocytoma). Secondary hypertension may be very severe, with rapid development of arterial and renal damage, unlike the slow development of such complications in the primary form (so-called 'essential hypertension'). This accelerated development of hypertensive disease is sometimes labelled 'malignant hypertension'.

Table 3.11.   Causes of hypertension (per 1000)

Renal disease ('nephritis')	50
Renal artery disease	45
Adrenal disease	8
Coarctation of aorta	6
Essential hypertension	891

Table 3.12.   Hypotensive drug-induced oral disease

Xerostomia
    clonidine
    ganglion blocking drugs

Salivary gland swelling
    methyldopa
    ganglion blockers

Salivary gland pain
    clonidine
    guanethidine

Lichenoid reactions (tongue)
    methyldopa
    labetalol
    oxprenolol

Trigeminal paraesthesiae
    hydralazine
    propanolol
    labetalol

Although drug therapy to lower blood pressure, or surgical treatment of renal disease or endocrine disorders, may have beneficial effects in preventing or delaying such complications as stroke and renal failure, angina and myocardial infarction are not dramatically reduced and remain the commonest cause of death in treated patients. A wide variety of drugs is available to lower blood pressure, some of them with important interactions with narcotics, such as that of debrisoquine with pethidine causing profound hypotension. The dentist must, therefore, enquire about drug treatment of hypertension and modify his prescriptions to avoid interactions. Some drugs, notably ganglion blockers and clonidine, cause dry mouth and/or enlargement of the salivary glands, which may be painful (*see Table* 3.12). Some cause lichenoid reactions in the mouth, such as methyldopa, which can cause oral ulceration as part of a lupoid reaction (*see* Chapter 16). Others such as beta-blocking agents and vasodilators cause paraesthesiae in the face and jaw.

Patients with hypertension cause other problems for the dentist for reasons apart from the side effects of drugs and their interactions with narcotics and anaesthetic agents. Angina is a common symptom of raised blood pressure and is an important cause of non-dental facial pain. Stroke resulting in facial weakness may predispose to caries on the side of the lesion and malfitting dentures. Renal failure in both essential and secondary hypertension may cause xerostomia, oral ulceration, a bleeding tendency, and predispose to candida and other infections.

Problems of cardiac disorder in dental practice

In summary, the patient with cardiac disease may cause several problems to the dentist, notably the risk of endocarditis that follows extraction, root filling procedures and even minor procedures such as scaling. There is a risk of provocation of cardia dysrhythmias by the use of adrenaline with local anaesthetics. Angina may also pose a problem in that the pain can be mistaken for that of dental disease. Syncope occurs with some forms of cardiac disease, such as aortic stenosis or rhythm disturbance, and may be the cause of loss of consciousness in the dental chair. Finally, the patient with cardiac disease is a poor risk for general anaesthesia, because of the circulatory problems and the interaction of drugs, notably the hypotensive drugs with narcotics and anaesthetic agents.

Peripheral vascular disease   4

The vascular system can be regarded as a system of plumbing. This chapter is concerned with the peripheral vascular system which is an arbitrary division to exclude the vessels supplying the heart and central nervous system. The division is not hard and fast and many peripheral vascular surgeons will operate on the carotid arteries which are the main supply of the brain. However, the intracranial arteries are the province of the neurosurgeon and the coronary arteries are the province of the cardiac surgeon.

Like any system of plumbing the pipes may become blocked or they may burst. It is helpful to keep this simplistic concept in mind when considering the problems arising in the vascular system. Again like other plumbing systems the problems increase with the age.

By common acceptance peripheral vascular disease refers to the arterial side of the circulation rather than the venous.

Aetiology of peripheral vascular disease

The commonest problem to affect the vascular system is atherosclerosis. The major component of this disease process is the laying down of atheroma in the intima of major blood vessels, thus gradually narrowing and eventually occluding them. The exact mechanism by which atheroma is produced is still controversial. The material is lipid and contains large quantities of cholesterol. Diet had been implicated in the aetiology of atheroma. Certainly, if rabbits are fed with high

◀ Atheroma is the major cause of peripheral vascular disease

cholesterol diets they develop atheroma, which is not a naturally occurring phenomenon in the animals.

In humans the dietary level of saturated fat seems more important than that of cholesterol. Some nutritionists believe that refined carbohydrate (e.g. white sugar) is more important in the production of atheroma than dietary fat.

One factor that is universally agreed to be of major importance in producing atheroma is cigarette smoking. It is very rare for a non-smoker to develop peripheral vascular disease whereas it is common for smokers to do so. Cigar and pipe smokers are also at risk, but less so. The likelihood of developing vascular disease increases directly with the number of cigarettes smoked.

◀ Smoking is the most important factor in the production of peripheral vascular atheroma

A second feature of the process of atherosclerosis is increasing loss of elasticity in the wall of the artery. The loss of elasticity results in lengthening and tortuosity of the vessels which is a characteristic feature of peripheral vascular disease. Eventually the artery wall becomes calcified.

Other disease may be associated with or accelerate the development of atherosclerosis. The commonest disease association is diabetes mellitus. In addition to predisposing to atheroma, which occurs in diabetics at an earlier age than in the general population, diabetes also produces symptoms of vascular disease due to specific effects on the smaller vessels, particularly in the lower limb. Ulceration is also made more likely because of the neuropathy produced by diabetes.

◀ Diabetics are at increased risk of peripheral vascular disease

Blood vessels may also be blocked by the process of embolization. Most commonly such emboli consist of thrombus (blood clot) and on the arterial side the usual source is the heart. Thrombus may form in the heart because of inefficient emptying due to atrial fibrillation or may form on the wall of the ventricle following a myocardial infarction (mural thrombus). In either case, it may break free and travel in the bloodstream to impact in, and block, a major artery (commonly the femoral). Other sources of emboli are aneurysms (which contain clot) or plaques of atheroma.

Peripheral vascular disease may also arise as a result of blood disorders. These may give rise to an increased tendency to clotting, thus blocking the vessels, or may lead to increased viscosity in the blood which leads to diminished blood flow and may exacerbate a poor blood supply due to atheromatous narrowing.

The collagen disorders (q.v.) may also give rise to occlusion of blood vessels, and ischaemia of the limbs. This is particularly associated with scleroderma, disseminated lupus erythematosus and polyarteritis. In these conditions the vessels are prone to go into spasm. This initially produces temporary ischaemia but may progress to more permanent damage and loss of digits. A characteristic sequence of events occurs in the reversible stage. The digits first become white, then blue and then, as the spasm wears off and the blood returns, red. These changes are known as 'Raynaud's phenomenon' and are often precipitated by cold or wet. Similar changes may occur in the absence of any detectable disease and are then described as 'Raynaud's disease'. This principally affects young women.

The weakness of the wall produced by atherosclerosis may produce dilatation of the vessel, eventually forming an aneurysm. The most commonly affected vessel is the aorta but aneurysms may occur in any vessel. Usually the aneurysm is filled with clot leaving an irregular channel through the middle through which the blood flows. Emboli may arise from this thrombus or the channel may become occluded. More commonly the aneurysm may leak, an event described as rupture of the aneurysm.

Less common diseases of the blood vessels may give rise to damage to the middle coat of the vessel — the media. This process gives rise to degeneration of the medial layer with the formation of clefts. The commonest presentation of this disorder is dissection of the aorta. In this process a tear occurs in the intima and blood enters the media and tracks along the aorta lifting the intima. The process normally occurs in the region of the origin of the aorta and as the dissection progresses the vessels arising from the aorta are sequentially occluded. Occlusion of the renal vessels may be the event leading to death.

Symptoms of vascular disease

Peripheral vascular disease may present as an acute

problem or a chronic problem. Chronic vascular disease is very much more common. The symptoms are progressive.

Chronic vascular insufficiency

The earliest symptom of vascular insufficiency is pain on exercise. This is very typical in presentation. The pain is known as 'intermittent claudication' (from the Latin *claudicare* – to limp), as it usually affects the lower limb.

◀ Intermittent claudication is usually the first symptom of peripheral vascular disease

The characteristic of intermittent claudication is severe pain in the calf brought on by walking. The pain is so severe that the patient must stop walking and rest. After a period of rest the pain disappears and the patient can again walk the same distance before being forced to stop again. The claudication distance for a given patient at a given time is remarkably constant but if the patient continues to smoke the claudication distance will gradually become shorter. It is rare for a patient to complain until he claudicates at less than 400 yards. When the claudication develops at 20–50 yards the patient will be grossly restricted in his activities and may find it necessary to give up work. With time, blood vessels may open up to give new channels bypassing the blockage (collateral circulation). When this occurs the symptoms may improve or disappear completely.

A more serious symptom is rest pain. This is very severe, persistent and disabling. As the name implies, it is present even at rest. This is a sign of incipient tissue death or gangrene. If there is to be any chance of preventing loss of the limb urgent treatment must be carried out.

◀ Rest pain is a serious symptom. It implies severe ischaemia likely to proceed to gangrene

Pregangrene may proceed to frank gangrene. The tissues of the limb die. Gangrene is divided into wet gangrene, which is infected and as a result tends to spread, and dry gangrene in which there is no infection. In such cases the affected part of the limb becomes black and shrivelled and is said to 'mummify'. Eventually demarcation occurs and the mummified area drops off, leaving a granulating area which will slowly heal.

Trauma in a limb with a poor blood supply may give

rise to ulceration. This is often sited over bony prominences such as the heel or external malleolus. The poor sensation in diabetics makes them particularly prone to ulcer formation.

Acute vascular insufficiency

Acute vascular insufficiency is usually due to embolism. Characteristically, the pain is of sudden onset and is associated with sudden loss of function. If walking the patient may stumble and then find he is unable to use his leg. As with chronic disease, the lower limb is much more frequently affected than the upper limb. The affected limb is pale and has lost sensation. No pulses can be palpated. Treatment is a matter of urgency if the limb is not to be lost. In less severe cases, collateral circulation may develop leading to a slow improvement in symptoms.

◀ Embolization resulting in acute ischaemia must be treated urgently

Aneurysm

Aneurysms may be symptomless and found coincidentally; they may present as a pulsatile swelling noticed by the patient or they may present with complications.

Chance finding is the commonest presentation of aortic aneurysm followed by symptoms produced by rupture. In the latter, the patient usually complains of severe back pain or epigastric pain and often collapses. He will be found to have a rapid pulse and low blood pressure and a pulsatile swelling will be palpable in the abdomen. Superficial examination often leads to the patient being sent to hospital as a case of myocardial infarction. With urgent operation the mortality rate from ruptured aneurysm is around 50%. Without operation it is universally fatal. The commonest complication of aneurysm of smaller vessels (such as femoral or popliteal) is ischaemia of the distal limb resulting from emboli breaking off from within the lumen.

◀ Untreated aneurysms may rupture giving rise to sudden serious collapse. The operative mortality of repairing a ruptured aneurysm is high

Investigations

The definitive investigation in peripheral vascular disease of arteriography. This involves puncture of the vessel and the injection of a radio-opaque medium to outline the vascular channels. Because it is invasive it is usually undertaken only if surgery is contemplated.

◀ Arteriography is carried out before surgery in order to plan the treatment

The simplest route for arteriography is femoral. It may be carried out under local anaesthesia or general anaesthesia. A catheter is inserted and can then be passed up into the aorta. Contrast medium is injected and the image formed observed on an image intensifier. A series of pictures showing progress of the contrast down the blood vessel is taken.

Other routes which may be used if the femorals are too diseased are the transaxillary (cannulating the axillary artery) or the translumbar (cannulating the aorta directly – now less frequently used).

The arteriograms may show a simple stenosis of a vessel due to atheroma. This is uncommon. More commonly multiple stenoses will be present although only one of them may be significant in producing symptoms. When rest pain and pregangrene are present, there is usually complete occlusion of at least one of the vessels in the limb.

The presence of other contributing diseases must be excluded. A full blood count with platelet count will detect the presence of blood dyscrasias. A urinary sugar and blood glucose estimation will detect diabetes mellitus. If doubt exists more detailed tests of glucose metabolism may be necessary (*see* Chapter 9). A range of antibody tests should be carried out to exclude the collagen disorders.

In the investigation of aneurysms scanning ultrasound is the most useful tool. This allows measurement of the aneurysm in all planes and also measurement of the internal diameter of the blood channel. Arteriography is not useful in delineating aneurysms as the lesion is filled with clot and appears on the radiograph as a normal calibre vessel.

◀ Ultrasound is useful in delineating aneurysms

Computerized axial tomography (CAT) may also be used in outlining the aneurysm but it is expensive and is not yet widely available. Many radiologists consider that the information obtained from the ultrasound scan is more useful.

Treatment

As with all surgical conditions treatment can be divided into conservative and operative. The major criterion for deciding between the two is the viability of the limb. If the limb is unlikely to survive then operative treatment is undertaken. It may also be necessary if the symptoms become so severe as to interfere markedly with the patient's life.

Conservative management

The most important conservative manœuvre is to persuade the patient to give up smoking. The patient who has presented with intermittent claudication will certainly stop deteriorating if he stops smoking and will almost certainly improve. Combined with advice on smoking should be advice on exercise. The patient should be encouraged to walk within the limits of his pain as this will promote the development of collateral circulation.

◄ Patients with peripheral vascular disease must stop smoking

Vasodilator drugs are commonly prescribed. These are of limited value. An ischaemic limb already has maximum vasodilatation from the build-up of metabolites in the limb. Little improvement will therefore result as no nett increase in blood flow into the limb will be achieved. What may occur is redistribution of the total blood flow with an increase in flow to the skin at the expense of muscle. This may be of some value in attempting to achieve healing of ulcers.

◄ Drug treatments are of limited value in peripheral vascular disease

Drugs are now available which lower the viscosity of the blood. The flow of blood through the tissues at a given blood pressure is directly proportional to the radius of the vessel and inversely proportional to the viscosity of the blood. Thus, by lowering the blood viscosity flow can be increased without altering the size of the vessels. Such drugs are under evaluation for long term use in chronic vascular insufficiency. In acute vascular insufficiency dextran, which lowers blood viscosity, is of some use in delaying or avoiding the need for operation. It is often used in conjunction with a vasodilator to improve blood flow to the superficial tissues. It has to be administered as an intravenous infusion and is therefore unsuitable for longterm use. Heparin may be used as an anticoagulant in the acute situation to prevent extension of the blockage and to improve patency of collateral vessels. This too must be given intravenously.

Diabetes mellitus should be controlled by a suitable regimen (q.v.) and any infection that is present should be treated with an appropriate antibiotic (determined if possible by culturing the organism and determining its sensitivity pattern.) If the problem is caused, or exacerbated by increased platelet activity leading to an increased tendency for the blood to clot the symptoms will be helped by an agent with antiplatelet activity such as low dose aspirin or dipyridamole.

Operative treatment

If there is a blockage in a pipe, that blockage can either be removed or bypassed in order to restore flow in the system. This applies to the vascular system.

1. Embolectomy

When acute ischaemia occurs as a result of an embolus, embolectomy is carried out. If necessary this can be performed under local anaesthesia. The usual route is to open the femoral artery and clot is then removed from wherever it has lodged using a Fogarty balloon catheter. The catheter is passed beyond the blockage and then the balloon is inflated and the catheter withdrawn. The vessel is repaired and the wound closed. It is usual to anticoagulate the patient with heparin following this procedure to prevent recurrent embolization or the formation of thrombus in the artery which is, inevitably, damaged during embolectomy.

2. Endarterectomy

In this operation atheromatous narrowings are removed from the vessel after opening it. The operation is more successful in large vessels such as the aorta or the iliac vessels. It is not often performed today having been superseded by grafting operations, which have more dependable longterm results.

3. Grafting operations

These are the most commonly performed vascular

procedures. The grafts may replace the diseased vessel or may bypass the diseased segment. In the aorta and the iliac region synthetic grafts give excellent results. The usual material used is Dacron, which is woven or knitted into a tube. Below the groin, because the vessels are narrower, the synthetic grafts do less well. The long saphenous vein is often reversed and used as a bypass graft for the femoral artery. (Reversal is necessary because of the presence of valves in the vein. Less commonly the valves may be destroyed by passing an instrument up the vein which can then be attached to the artery without removing it from the leg and turning it round.)

When the saphenous vein is unsuitable or has previously been damaged, substitutes have to be found. Newer synthetics have been used but are no better than Dacron. A promising approach is the use of a specially prepared umbilical vein graft which has been tanned to remove its antigenic properties and stop its rejection by the body. The operations are denoted by the names of the proximal and distal vessels involved, e.g. 'Aorto-iliac replacement' graft; 'Femoro-popliteal bypass' graft.

Aortic aneurysms are replaced by a graft to remove the risk of rupture.

Graft survival depends on rate of flow through the graft. Large vessel grafts have a better chance of surviving than distal grafts. For this reason operations below the groin are usually only performed as 'limb salvage procedures' where the limb is about to die. Often in such cases, even if the graft eventually fails, the limb continues to survive because time has been gained for the collaterals to open. A narrowing of a vessel upstream from a graft will slow the flow and increases the likelihood of graft failure. It is also more likely to be causing the symptoms than the more distal block. For these reasons it is common practice to deal with the proximal lesion first unless both are dealt with at the same operation.

4. *Transluminal angioplasty*

A recent development in arterial surgery has been the use of a special inflatable balloon to dilate narrow segments of arteries. Under radiological control the

◄ The most widely used operative technique is replacement or bypassing of diseased vessels with natural or synthetic grafts

balloon catheter is introduced into the vessels through a needle in the femoral artery. It is guided into the strictured area and then the balloon is inflated to flatten this atheroma against the wall and widen the vessel. This method is suitable for patients who are poor operative risks and who have short segments of disease. The longterm results are less good than those of grafting operations.

5. *Sympathectomy*

When the arterial involvement is diffuse and severe it may be impossible to reconstruct the arterial tree. In these cases, treatment is only offered for limb salvage. Reduction of sympathetic tone may divert blood from the muscles to the superficial tissues which are threatened with gangrene. This can be effected in the case of the lower limb by division of the sympathetic chain in the lumbar region. Traditionally, this was carried out as a formal operative procedure. Now, it is more common to destroy the sympathetic chain by the injection of phenol percutaneously.

Upper limb sympathectomy can be achieved by surgical excision of the stellate ganglion or by injection of the ganglion with phenol. This procedure is less common than lumbar sympathectomy and the usual indication is Raynaud's disease. Recurrence is, however, common and the operation is less frequently carried out than in the past.

6. *Amputation*

When limb salvage fails or is impossible the only alternative is amputation. The amputation must be at a level at which healing can be expected. In most vascular cases a below-knee amputation is the minimum amputation acceptable. This operation preserves the knee joint with its sensitive pressure and position receptors and the patients usually are able to learn to walk with a prosthesis. Sometimes the blood supply below the knee is so poor that healing is unlikely. In these patients an above-knee amputation is necessary. While healing is more certain, walking afterwards is much more difficult and many elderly patients cannot learn to walk after this operation. When the patient is confined to bed this does not, of course, matter and the

◄ Amputation may eventually be necessary if sufficient blood supply cannot be achieved

better healing would lead one to an above-knee amputation as a matter of choice.

In diabetic patients with normal distal pulses where gangrene is due to small vessel disease it is necessary only to remove the diseased tissue. In such patients very limited amputations are undertaken.

After any amputation intensive rehabilitation is essential to ensure that the patient returns to the maximum possible mobility as soon as possible. In the early stages after operation the patient learns to walk with a frame. Once confident with the frame he progresses to crutches and learns to negotiate steps and stairs. By this stage his stump is sufficiently healed to allow the fitting of a temporary prosthesis and the patient can start to re-learn 'normal' walking. In due course a made-to-measure prosthesis is fitted and the patient should be able, with a below-knee amputation, to walk without the aid of a stick.

Outcome of peripheral vascular disease

Although the short term results of surgery are good, patients with peripheral vascular disease have a poor longterm prognosis because of associated atheroma in the cerebral and cardiac circulation. The 5-year survival for a patient who has undergone bypass grafting is a figure comparable to many cancers.

Respiratory diseases 5

The cardiovascular and respiratory systems share the major function of provision of adequate amounts of arterialized blood to all tissues of the body according to their need. The important process in this complex series of events that is the primary function of the lung is the loading of blood in the lungs with enough oxygen at high enough pressure and the unloading of carbon dioxide. Transport of blood to and from the lungs and the exchange of O_2 and CO_2 between blood in capillaries and tissue cells are functions of the cardiovascular system.

The arterialization of venous blood returning to the lung involves three stages: ventilation, which includes the volume and distribution of air ventilating the alveoli; diffusion, by which O_2 and CO_2 pass across the membranes between air and blood; and pulmonary capillary blood flow, which must be distributed evenly to all alveoli according to their ventilation.

Table 5.1.   Simple tests of pulmonary function

Forced Expiratory Volume (FEV_1)
    1·7–3·8 litres
    (varies with age, sex and height)
Forced Vital Capacity (FVC)
    1·9–5·3 litres
    (varies with age, sex and height)
FEV_1/FVC greater than 75%
    reduced in diseases causing airways obstruction. Not in restrictive lung disease
Peak Expiratory Flow Rate (PEFR) (litres per minute)
    400–650 litres/min.
FEV_1, FVC, PEFR reduced in all forms of lung disease but FEV_1/FVC reduced in airways
    obstruction (bronchitis, emphysema, asthma) and normal in fibrosing pulmonary
    diseases

Inspired air passes through the conducting airways (the bronchi and bronchioles) to reach the alveoli where gas exchange occurs. The volume of inspired air reaching each alveolus is not uniform, so that not all of this ventilation is useful in arterializing venous blood; some is wasted or ineffective, the proportion being small in health but much larger in disease where there is damage to the conducting airways, such as bronchitis and asthma.

◄ A small amount of ventilation is ineffective ('wasted') in arterializing blood in normal individuals, this is greatly increased when there is airways disease

The exchange of gases between alveolar air and pulmonary capillary blood occurs by a passive physical process of diffusion. The process is limited by the distance that gas must travel, being reduced when the alveolar and/or capillary membrane is thickened by abnormal tissue or by exudate, as in left heart failure. A second limitation to the process of diffusion is the surface area of contact between ventilated alveoli and functioning pulmonary capillaries, which can be altered by both disorders of ventilation and of the pulmonary circulation.

The functional parts of the pulmonary circulation are the lung capillaries. Normally, resistance to blood flow through the pulmonary arteries and capillaries is low, so that mixed venous blood returning to the right side of the heart is distributed uniformly to the alveoli. In disease, both pulmonary and cardiac, resistance to blood flow is increased with disturbance of this even distribution so that blood entering the lungs may not come into contact with alveolar gas, resulting in hypoxaemia, a process referred to as 'arterio-venous shunting'.

◄ Changes in the pulmonary circulation affect gas exchange and occur in cardiac as well as lung disease

Symptoms of respiratory disease

The most common and disabling system of respiratory disease is difficulty in breathing, *dyspnoea*. Dyspnoea is a symptom, an uncomfortable experience that can only be judged by the patient and should not be confused with overbreathing (hyperventilation), such as occurs in the anxious individual, or rapid breathing (tachypnoea), such as may be noted in cardiac and pulmonary disorders. The dyspnoea of respiratory disease may be difficult to distinguish from that associated with left

◄ Dyspnoea is a symptom and should not be confused with altered patterns of breathing

heart failure, orthopnoea occurring in both although some patients with respiratory illness find that lying on one side may provoke discomfort. Some patients with respiratory disorder complain of difficulty with inspiration, that the lungs 'cannot be filled', a symptom associated with overinflation of the lungs with airways obstruction, such as bronchial asthma.

There are probably many factors that cause dyspnoea (*see Table* 5.2), although tests of lung function show little correlation with the patient's discomfort: one patient having hypoxaemia but no symptoms, even on severe testing with exercise on a treadmill; another complaining of severe breathlessness, but pulmonary function tests being normal. The evaluation of dyspnoea depends on the patient's description of the sensation and provocative factors, such as exercise, position, and environmental factors.

Noises associated with breathing may be either high-pitched (wheezing) or low-pitched (snoring sounds, or stridor) and are caused by narrowing of airways; wheezing is associated with narrowing of small airways, as in asthma, and stridor with narrowing of major bronchi or the larynx, as with mediastinal mass. Noisy breathing is not always associated with breathlessness nor — in asthma or other diseases, such as bronchitis, causing small airways obstruction — is there relationship between dyspnoea and wheezing; in severe asthma, for example, wheezing may be almost inaudible even with a stethoscope.

Stridor, which indicates major airways obstruction, has importance in assessment of the patient being

◀ Noisy breathing indicates airways obstruction, the higher the pitch the smaller the airways. But severe airways obstruction does not always cause noises

Table 5.2.   Dyspnoea

Respiratory
    airways obstruction — larynx (stridor)
                               — bronchi (wheezing)
    pulmonary collapse — pneumothorax, pleural effusion
    loss of elasticity — emphysema
Cardiac — L. heart failure
Severe anaemia — reduced supply of haemoglobin to pulmonary capillaries for oxygen
                     transport
Metabolic — acidosis (diabetic, chronic renal failure)
Voluntary hyperventilation — anxiety, hysteria

considered for general anaesthesia for dental treatment; airways obstruction may increase when the patient is unconscious or when respiration is depressed, particularly when caused by mediastinal masses such as malignant lymph nodes or goitre. Severe obstruction in the upper mediastinum is also associated with the sensation of facial fullness, made worse by coughing or straining, as well as stridor.

Most patients with pulmonary disease complain of *cough*, with or without expectoration of sputum. Coughing results from stimulation of vagus nerve endings in the pharynx, larynx, trachea or bronchi by stimuli such as mucosal inflammation, inhaled gases or foreign bodies, chemical inhalation including anaesthetic gases and even very hot or cold air. The cough reflex plays an important role in clearing the airways of foreign material, along with the ciliary activity of the epithelium in the upper air passages, bronchial mucosal cell secretions and respiratory movements.

Although cough is usually a symptom of pulmonary disorder, left heart failure with pulmonary oedema may begin with paroxysmal coughing, associated with wheezing but rarely sputum, except in the most florid cases when frothy, blood-stained secretions may be expectorated. Tumours in the mediastinum, not originating from the lungs (retrosternal goitre), may also cause cough.

◄ Distressing unproductive cough may be an early symptom of left heart failure and bronchial asthma

Cough may occur only in the morning on rising, a feature of chronic bronchitis; or mainly at night, as may occur in asthma or left heart failure; or throughout the day, for example with carcinoma of bronchus and bronchiectasis. Sputum may be expectorated in most pulmonary diseases, especially chronic bronchitis,

Table 5.3.   Haemoptysis

Chronic simple bronchitis
Bronchiectasis
Pulmonary tuberculosis — active
Carcinoma of bronchus
Pulmonary embolism with infarction, vascular abnormalities (arteriovenous shunts)
Pneumonia
Haemorrhagic disorders — coagulation defects, anticoagulant therapy
L. heart failure

where the sputum is usually mucoid, tenacious and difficult for the patient to bring up; and with bronchiectasis, in which the volume is much greater, the colour usually yellow or green, being easy to expectorate.

Haemoptysis, the presence of blood in the sputum, is an important feature of other disorders including left heart failure (*see Table* 5.3). Patients may find difficulty in deciding where the blood has come from, often thinking that bleeding has occurred from the mouth and consult their dentist, without realizing that the blood is from the lungs. Similar confusion may occur with the vomiting of small amounts of blood.

◀ The patient may think that blood in the sputum is from the oral cavity

Some patients with respiratory disease complain of pleuritic *chest pain*, usually lateral but at times central, of a sharp character and made worse by coughing, deep breathing, and other movements of the thorax. Pleurisy can be differentiated from cardiac pain but can be difficult to distinguish from that due to pericarditis. Central chest pain may occur with tracheobronchial diseases or with foreign bodies lodged in the upper airways; it is usually felt beneath the sternum and made worse by coughing.

Signs of respiratory disease

Central cyanosis is an important sign of respiratory disease indicating that the normal gas exchange between alveoli and pulmonary capillary blood is disturbed. Central cyanosis is also a feature of congenital heart disease with right-to-left shunting of mixed venous blood; in effect what happens to pulmonary capillary blood that does not come into contact with alveolar gas in its passage through the lungs. Pulmonary cyanosis disappears with inhalation of oxygen within a few minutes, whereas in congenital heart disease this change may take much longer (*see* Chapter 3).

◀ Central cyanosis is a feature of severe pulmonary disease or congenital heart disease with right-to-left shunt

Noises with respiration indicate airways obstruction. Stridor is usually best heard with mouth-breathing and may be both inspiratory and/or expiratory; it is usually a snoring sound and is caused by narrowing of larynx, trachea or either main bronchus by tumour, foreign body or external pressure on the air passages by enlarged lymph nodes or by goitre, particularly retrosternal. Wheezing is a higher pitched sound, more often expiratory but occasionally inspiratory as well; it is caused by narrowing of small airways, as in asthma, but its intensity does not indicate the severity of obstruction. Severe asthma may be associated with quiet, albeit rapid breathing.

A fast respiratory rate may be a sign of respiratory disorder and is usually accompanied by the symptom of breathlessness, although it may also be noted in the anxious patient and in patients with intra-abdominal lesions, where breathing causes pain or where movement of the diaphragm is prevented by fluid collection in the peritoneum (ascites). The normal respiratory rate is 12–14 per minute, but may increase in respiratory disease to 30 or more cycles. Rapid respiration occurs most commonly with diseases that cause stiffening of the lung (pulmonary fibrosis) or loss of elasticity of the lung (emphysema). In these examples the amount of air moved in and out of the chest (tidal volume) is normal or slightly reduced. In patients with acidosis, diabetics with ketosis and patients with renal failure, the respiratory centres are stimulated, and the tidal volume is increased (hyperpnoea or Kussmaul's respiration). Tidal volume in voluntary hyperventilation may be shallow or deep, and associated with a tingling sensation in the hands, feet and around the mouth, sometimes with cramps, due to reduction in arterial carbon dioxide tension and alkalosis caused by overbreathing.

Clubbing of the fingers (*see Table* 5.4 and *Fig.* 1.7) is associated with some respiratory diseases but not with

◀ Tachypnoea and hyperventilation should not be confused with the symptom of breathlessness

Table 5.4.   Digital clubbing

Carcinoma of bronchus
Bronchiectasis
Fibrosing alveolitis (idiopathic or extrinsic: e.g. pigeon fancier's disease)
Malabsorption (coeliac disease)
Hepatic cirrhosis
Inflammatory bowel disease (Crohn's disease and ulcerative colitis)
Idiopathic

---

others; it occurs with carcinoma of bronchus, bronchiectasis and pulmonary fibrosis, but not with chronic bronchitis, asthma or emphysema. Recognition of finger clubbing should alert the dentist to the possibility that the patient may have respiratory disorder, although the other causes of this physical sign must be considered (*see Table* 5.4).

Chronic bronchitis

The most common respiratory disorder and one of the most important causes for time lost from work in the U.K. is chronic bronchitis. The earliest symptoms of the disease are cough productive of mucoid sputum, usually in the morning on rising. The sputum is difficult to expectorate because it is tenacious and viscid, although the volumes produced are small. These symptoms, occurring at least three months during the year, usually in winter, for two consecutive years, are those of chronic simple bronchitis. Distinction is made from chronic obstructive bronchitis in which the patient complains, in addition, of breathlessness on exertion, usually associated with wheezing, and is a later stage of the disease process.

Although 'bronchitis' suggests that the disease is one of chronic inflammation, there is little evidence for the role of infection in the aetiology of the disorder other than the acute exacerbations that occur during the course of the disease. The sputum between these exacerbations is sterile on culture and the most important abnormality is that the secretions are viscous and difficult to expectorate. Sputum is produced in larger volumes than normal and is associated with histological changes in goblet cells of the bronchial mucosa. Apart from the physical abnormalities of sputum an additional factor in the difficulty with expectoration is impaired ciliary function, with slowed clearance of small particles from the upper airways. Impaired clearance of particles from the airways and lungs carries the risk of infection or collapse of part of the lung, particularly if inhalation of a foreign body, such as part of a tooth or bits of amalgam, occurs during dental procedures, usually under general anaesthesia.

◄ Broncho-pulmonary clearance of secretions and foreign bodies is impaired in chronic bronchitis because of the physical properties of the sputum and impaired ciliary function

Impaired clearance of viscid sputum also results in narrowing of the airways, some being plugged with mucus. An additional factor in airways obstruction is structural changes in the bronchiolar wall which collapses during expiration.

The aetiology of the disease is unknown but environmental factors play an important part, the disease showing a geographical distribution not only within the U.K. but in the world. Air pollution with dust, fumes and chemical irritants in certain industries play some role in causation as well as smoking. Whether repeated acute infections play a role in causing chronic bronchitis, or whether they are a reflection of the natural history of the disorder is not known. The cause is probably multifactorial, including genetic factors as well as those already mentioned.

Patients with chronic simple bronchitis are a frequent problem in dental as well as in medical practice, principally because of the risk of inhalation during oral procedures under general anaesthesia or when intravenous sedatives, such as diazepam, are given. Local anaesthesia is to be preferred in these patients, and if general anaesthesia is necessary care must be taken to avoid inhalation, including packing of the pharynx.

◀ The patient with chronic bronchitis is at risk of aspiration pneumonia during dental treatment, particularly with general anaesthesia

Inhalation is a more serious complication in the patient with obstructive bronchitis, often producing an acute worsening of airways narrowing. Aspiration pneumonia is also a more serious complication in these patients. The preference for local anaesthesia is therefore stronger in those with obstructive symptoms.

Airways narrowing in chronic bronchitis is usually associated with mismatching of ventilation and blood flow in parts of the lung and consequent impairment of gas exchange, *respiratory failure (see Table* 5.5). Recognition of respiratory failure depends on the detection of central cyanosis. However, minor degrees of hypoxaemia cannot be recognized from the colour of the mucosa. Severe hypoxia is usually associated with impaired pulmonary exchange and increase in blood content of carbon dioxide — hypercarbia. The clinical features of hypercarbia are warm hands associated with a full and bounding pulse. There may be fluid retention. The patient's movements may be clumsy, due to a coarse flapping tremor of the hands, and he may drop objects or spill the contents of cups, and so on (*see* Chapter 11).

Patients with chronic bronchitis and respiratory failure (hypoxaemia and hypercarbia) frequently develop fluid retention with signs of congestive heart failure, raised venous pressure and dependent oedema; this combination of cyanosis with fluid retention being termed euphemistically the 'blue bloater' syndrome. The mechanism of fluid retention in these patients is not known but the term 'cor pulmonale' is misleading since there are many factors that play a role in oedema formation in such patients other than the effects of the lung disease on right heart function. The appearance of oedema is usually late in the natural history of the disease, by which time the degree of breathlessness is very severe and the patient is unable to do any work that involves physical effort.

The management of the patient with chronic bronchitis combines the use of antibiotics for exacerbations of infection, with bronchodilators and diuretics, for fluid retention. In some selected patients long-term domiciliary oxygen therapy may be helpful, particularly when hypoxaemia is severe and there are secondary complications such as polycythaemia and pulmonary arterial hypertension. Prophylactic antibiotics have not been shown to have value in the long-term management of these patients because the organisms that are associated with acute exacerbations, commonly *Haemophilus influenzae* and *Streptococcus pneumoniae*, occasionally *Escherichia coli* and *Klebsiella aerogenes*, develop resistant strains. If there is risk of inhalation during oral treatment an oral penicillin, tetracycline or co-trimoxazole should be used to prevent aspiration pneumonia.

Table 5.5.   Respiratory (ventilatory) failure

Type 1	Hypoxaemia, normal or reduced arterial P_{CO_2} Examples — pneumonia, pulmonary fibrosis Clinical features — usually obvious tachypnoea; central cyanosis
Type 2	Hypoxaemia and hypercapnia Examples — end stages of chronic bronchitis Clinical features — full bounding pulse, warm peripheries, tremor of hands, episodes of fluid retention, cyanosis

Some patients respond to bronchodilators, either by inhalation or by mouth, and this can be predicted by measurement of forced expiratory volume (FEV) (*see Table* 5.1) before and after a beta-2-adrenergic stimulant, such as salbutamol. In those patients with severe airways obstruction, greatly disabled by breathlessness and wheezing, oral and inhaled steroid therapy may be used, although there is risk of hypoadrenalism at the time of stress, such as infection or surgical procedure, and with oral treatment.

Diuretic therapy is given to patients with chronic bronchitis when oedema develops. Abnormalities of cardiac rhythm are uncommon in these patients and digoxin is rarely used.

◄ Fluid retention may complicate chronic obstructive bronchitis

Oxygen therapy has to be given with caution to any patient who has chronic obstructive bronchitis. In some patients therapy may cause depression of ventilation, somnolence and coma. Chronic hypoxaemia and hypercarbia are associated with important changes in chemoreceptor respiratory reflexes, such that the sensitivity of the medullary centres to hypercarbia is diminished and respiratory drive depends on stimulation of the carotid receptors by reduced arterial oxygen tension. Oxygen therapy in patients with chronic pulmonary disability produces an increase in oxygen content of arterial blood but reduced stimulation of chemoreceptors, with slowing and reduction of the volume of ventilation. Oxygen therapy can, however, be beneficial in these patients provided that it is given in carefully controlled concentrations of 24–28%. Ordinary oxygen face masks provide much higher concentrations (36% upwards) but some, operating on a Venturi principle, mix oxygen with air and the concentration can be fairly accurately controlled. Oxygen should not be administered to a patient with chronic respiratory problems other than with a Venturi mask.

◄ Oxygen therapy can be harmful in chronic obstructive bronchitis and should be administered in concentrations of 24–28%

Emphysema

By definition emphysema is a condition of the lung characterized by increase, beyond the normal, in the size of air spaces distal to the terminal bronchiole, either from dilatation or from destruction of their walls.

Pathologists classify emphysema according to its anatomical distribution, based on studies of the lung by inflation/fixation techniques, into that associated with destruction of walls of air spaces (centrilobular emphysema) and that with generalized dilatation of air spaces (pan-acinar) emphysema. The centrilobular form is associated with chronic bronchitis. The pan-acinar form is of unknown cause in most instances, although there are some younger subjects who develop the disease in early years (35–50) associated with absence of an enzyme in the blood (alpha-1-antitrypsin deficiency).

The diagnosis of emphysema during life is difficult, even using sophisticated tests of lung function and X-rays, the classification described being based on post-mortem studies. The pan-acinar form is associated at the advanced stage with distension of the thorax, the barrel-shaped chest, and with a rapid respiratory rate, the patient breathing noisily through pursed lips. These clinical features, sometimes referred to as the 'pink puffer' syndrome, do not always relate to the pathological changes. Cough is unusual in emphysema, except when complicated by infection. The predominant symptom is increasing breathlessness.

There is airways narrowing in emphysema, due to collapse of the smaller airways during expiration, and it is not reversible by bronchodilator drugs. Hypoxaemia is uncommon, except in the late stages of the disease, despite severe disability, and hypercarbia does not occur, arterial CO_2 content being low because of the rapid respiratory rate. Oxygen therapy is, therefore, safe in these patients but produces little lasting relief of symptoms. The principal disturbance of pulmonary function is loss of elasticity of the lung due to over-expansion of the air spaces, with loss of diffusing capacity and disordered distribution of ventilation.

There is no specific treatment for emphysema, bronchodilators and oxygen therapy having little benefit. The prevention of inhalation of foreign material during oral treatment is important since respiratory infections may be life-threatening. Coughing is weak and ineffective in clearing the bronchial tree after inhalation because of diminished elastic recoil. These mechanical problems present difficulties during general anaesthesia, since active

◄ The clinical features of pan-acinar emphysema are breathlessness and noisy breathing but no cough or sputum

expiration due to contraction of muscles is diminished, and, together with poor elastic recoil, results in impaired ventilation and trapping of gas in the lungs due to airways collapse.

Bronchial asthma

By definition bronchial asthma is a condition of narrowing of the smaller airways, with breathlessness and wheezing, that is reversible either with the passage of time or in response to bronchodilator therapy. In some patients the stimulus to airways narrowing can be identified and is usually bronchial smooth muscle contraction induced by an inhaled or ingested substance, pollen or some shell fish for instance; this form of asthma is termed 'extrinsic'. In other patients, usually with late-onset (aged 25 onwards) symptoms, there are no detectable extrinsic factors; this is called 'intrinsic' asthma.

Extrinsic asthma usually starts early in life, almost invariably before the age of 20 and may be associated with eczema, hay fever or urticaria in the affected person, or in other members of the family. This history of so-called 'atopy' is the clue to the diagnosis of extrinsic asthma, otherwise called 'allergic airways disease', and confirmation may be obtained by tests with intradermal injections of allergens or by challenge with the known provocative agent, which produces breathlessness and wheezing. The symptoms of extrinsic asthma are usually closely related to contact with the allergen, although some patients with hypersensitivity may have delayed (12–18 hours) symptoms.

Extrinsic asthma is very often seasonal and may be preceded by symptoms of allergic rhinitis (hay fever) — nasal stuffiness, sneezing and a copious, clear discharge from the nose. The symptoms are usually of sudden onset, lasting a few days or weeks, and may occur at any time of day, but particularly at night. Symptoms are usually mild and become less frequent and troublesome with age, even though the problem of allergic rhinitis persists.

There are no such provocative factors in patients with intrinsic asthma, symptoms of which usually begin in the third or fourth decade. Breathlessness, wheezing

◀ Extrinsic asthma is of early onset and associated with a personal or family history of hay fever, eczema, hives or other allergy

◀ Intrinsic asthma is of late onset and, when persistent, may be difficult to distinguish from chronic obstructive bronchitis

and an unproductive cough are the symptoms of this as well as the extrinsic form, but attacks are both more severe and persistent, in some patients lasting for many months, making it difficult to distinguish from chronic obstructive bronchitis. Intrinsic asthma, in contrast to the extrinsic form, shows no family tendency, no seasonal variation or increase in symptoms at certain times of the day. This form is more disabling and most deaths due to asthma occur in this group.

Attacks of asthma can be difficult to differentiate from left heart failure (LHF) on clinical grounds, even with the additional information provided by chest X-ray, lung function tests and electrocardiograph (*see Table* 5.6). Both occur at night or with exertion, and are often preceded by an unproductive cough. Wheezing may occur in LHF although it is more typical of bronchial asthma. The patient with a severe attack of bronchial asthma uses the accessory muscles of respiration, sternomastoid and pectoralis major, often fixing the shoulder girdle by grasping objects to enhance the effect of these muscles. Patients with LHF sit up because breathlessness is eased (orthopnoea), although patients with bronchial asthma are also more comfortable when upright, which might be predicted from the change in lung function from supine to erect positions.

Patients with LHF and bronchial asthma are not usually cyanosed except in extremis. The venous pressure may be increased in LHF whereas in patients with bronchial asthma the level fluctuates widely, increasing during expiration, falling during inspiration.

◄ Patients with severe asthma may not appear cyanosed even though there is significant hypoxaemia

Table 5.6. Comparison of bronchial asthma and L.H. failure

	Asthma	*L.H. failure*
Onset	Usually sudden	Sudden — related to posture
Cough	May be early feature	Yes
Appearance	Cyanosis rare	Often cyanosed
Respiratory noises	Wheezing	Rarely wheezing
Pulse	Regular	Often irregular
Venous pressure	Wide variation	Usually increased
Medical history	Previous paroxysms	Heart disease. Progressive breathlessness on effort

Patients with LHF may have abnormalities of the pulse rate and rhythm, frequently atrial fibrillation or multiple ectopic beats. The pulse in the patient with bronchial asthma is usually regular but often rapid, especially when sympathomimetic drugs are being used, and there may be variation in volume with respiration becoming weak during inspiration, termed 'pulsus paradoxus'.

The medical history is probably most helpful in making the distinction, and any questionnaire that the patient answers should enquire whether there is a history of heart disease and cardiovascular disorders, allergy, asthma or hay fever, hives or eczema. Awareness of the possibility that breathlessness may be provoked by lying the patient flat, by emotion or by drugs, such as adrenaline, should have important influences on dental management.

Attacks of asthma are usually treated with beta-2-adrenergic agonists, such as salbutamol, either by mouth or by inhalation as an aerosol, which produces rapid relief of symptoms. Although salbutamol and other drugs in the same class are predominantly stimulants of the beta-2 receptors, found in bronchi, bladder, bowel and pancreas, in large doses they have cardiac effects, notably tachycardia. The excessive use of salbutamol by the patient may cause tachycardia in excess of 160/minute and patients are advised that they should not use aerosols more than 8 times/day.

◄ Repeated use of beta-2-adrenergic stimulants in patients with bronchial asthma may cause tachycardia and be associated with loss of bronchodilator response

Anticholinergic drugs may also be used to relieve airways obstruction and are most effective as an aerosol. Oral therapy with theophylline derivatives is also effective in controlling asthma but does not provide the same rapid relief as aerosols.

Acute attacks of asthma may be relieved by intravenous injections of aminophylline and subcutaneous administration of adrenaline, the latter being popular before the use of aerosols which have fewer cardiac effects. Addiction to salbutamol does not occur, but can be a problem with adrenaline.

Prolonged, severe attacks of asthma that do not respond to aerosol or oral therapy with bronchodilators are termed 'status asthmaticus'. If the attack persists for some days the patient may find that eating and eventually drinking become difficult because of severe breathlessness. Most of the sudden deaths from asthma occur in this group, in whom there is resistance to bronchodilators.

Patients with status asthmaticus and those with symptoms resistant to treatment with simple bronchodilators are treated with steroid therapy. In status, steroids are administered intravenously, oral therapy being given later when absorption from the gut is reliable and when dehydration has been corrected. The initial doses are often large, 500–600 mg hydrocortisone or 60 mg prednisolone daily, although the object of treatment is to reduce the amount to as small a quantity as possible to avoid the side-effects of such therapy. A reduction in the dose of oral steroid needed can sometimes be achieved, in the long term, by use of inhaled steroids, usually beclomethasone, which is frequently tried in patients with symptoms resistant to other treatment before giving oral prednisolone. Some patients seem to respond better to ACTH, which has the advantage that it stimulates adrenal cortical production of steroids, unlike oral corticosteroids, which cause adrenal atrophy after prolonged use. ACTH has, however, to be given by intramuscular injection and may be less effective than expected in status asthmaticus because of impaired adrenal response to stimulation.

Patients with asthma present several problems to the dentist, not the least being that paroxysms may be provoked by anxiety about dental treatment. Such attacks usually respond rapidly to inhaled sympathomimetic drugs. The complications of steroid therapy are described elsewhere (*see* Chapter 9). Extensive thrush with oral ulceration that may involve the palate can sometimes necessitate the withdrawal of inhaled beclomethasone. However, the advantage of this route for steroid therapy is that, with the exception of candidiasis, there are few side-effects and, in particular, no evidence of suppression of adrenal function.

◀ Patients with asthma may be treated with short- or long-term steroids

Aspiration pneumonia (*Table* 5.7)

Reference has been made to inhalation of foreign bodies and infected material from the mouth and upper respiratory tract and the added risk that this may occur during general anaesthesia and in patients with chronic respiratory disorder, such as emphysema and bronchitis. Unless the foreign body is removed within a few hours suppuration occurs in the lungs which, initially, shows the macroscopical appearance of bronchopneumonia but later cavitates, with surrounding fibrous tissue (lung abscess). The usual infecting agents are staphylococci, streptococci, *E. coli* and *Klebsiella aerogenes*.

Aspiration pneumonia is more common in the right lung, the main bronchus on that side being shorter, wider and anatomically more in direct line with the trachea. The segment of the lung in which the pneumonia occurs is determined by the position of the patient at the time of inhalation. If, as is usually the case in dental practice, the patient is lying supine the infected material enters the most dependent segments of the lung in that position, the posterior of the upper lobe and the apical of the lower lobe.

The symptoms that suggest pneumonia are fever and cough, initially unproductive but later with purulent, often offensive and blood-stained sputum. Pleurisy is a late symptom and breathlessness is also unusual.

◄ Swinging fever, cough with purulent sputum and pleurisy are the features of aspiration pneumonia

Initially there are few signs, and examination of the chest is normal. Finger clubbing may develop much later and this reverses with resolution. Diagnosis depends on the awareness that aspiration of teeth, amalgam and other infected material may have occurred and also on appearances of the chest radiograph.

Table 5.7. Aspiration of foreign material into the airways

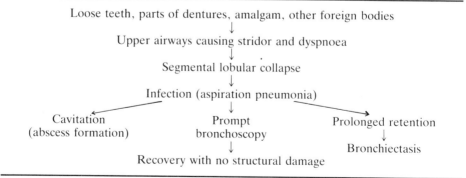

Loose teeth, parts of dentures, amalgam, other foreign bodies
↓
Upper airways causing stridor and dyspnoea
↓
Segmental lobular collapse
↓
Infection (aspiration pneumonia)
↓
Cavitation (abscess formation) · Prompt bronchoscopy · Prolonged retention
↓
Recovery with no structural damage · Bronchiectasis

Treatment consists of a broad spectrum antibiotic, one of the penicillins or, in the patient with hypersensitivity, cotrimoxazole, and attempts to remove the foreign body with a bronchoscope. If there is failure of radiographic resolution with prolonged (1 month and more) antibiotic treatment, this will require thoracotomy and resection.

Prevention of inhalation is the most important feature of management in the patient at risk, particularly those with chronic respiratory disorder or neuromuscular disease affecting the oropharynx, who show impaired cough reflex. Inhalation may occur in the normal patient, without any preceding history of respiratory illness, during general anaesthesia, if inadequate measures are taken to prevent amalgam or teeth falling into the upper airways. Inhalation of foreign bodies may occur without initial symptoms or signs, although in most patients persistent cough, with wheezing, suggests that there is obstruction of the airways.

◄ Aspiration pneumonia can be prevented by identifying those patients at risk and avoiding inhalation of amalgam or teeth during GA in normal subjects

If inhalation occurs early bronchoscopy is of greatest importance, usually with a rigid rather than a fibreoptic, flexible instrument, in most instances the foreign body being within the view of the instrument and removable with forceps. Chest X-ray is of little help in locating amalgam or teeth in the lungs until collapse of a lobule has occurred, which may take some days to develop. Having removed the foreign body prophylactic antibiotics should be given for approximately 5 days, or longer if follow-up X-ray or symptoms and signs suggest that pneumonia has developed.

◄ Rigid bronchoscopy is of greater value in the management of suspected or known inhalation than chest radiography

Bronchiectasis (*see Fig.* 5.1)

If an inhaled foreign body is not removed within a few hours collapse of part of the lung occurs due to obstruction of a bronchus and resorption of air in the lobule being supplied. Secretions and pus accumulate within the bronchus and infection extends into the lung parenchyma, a sequence of events that occurs in aspiration pneumonia. In some patients, when the foreign body has not been removed at an early stage,

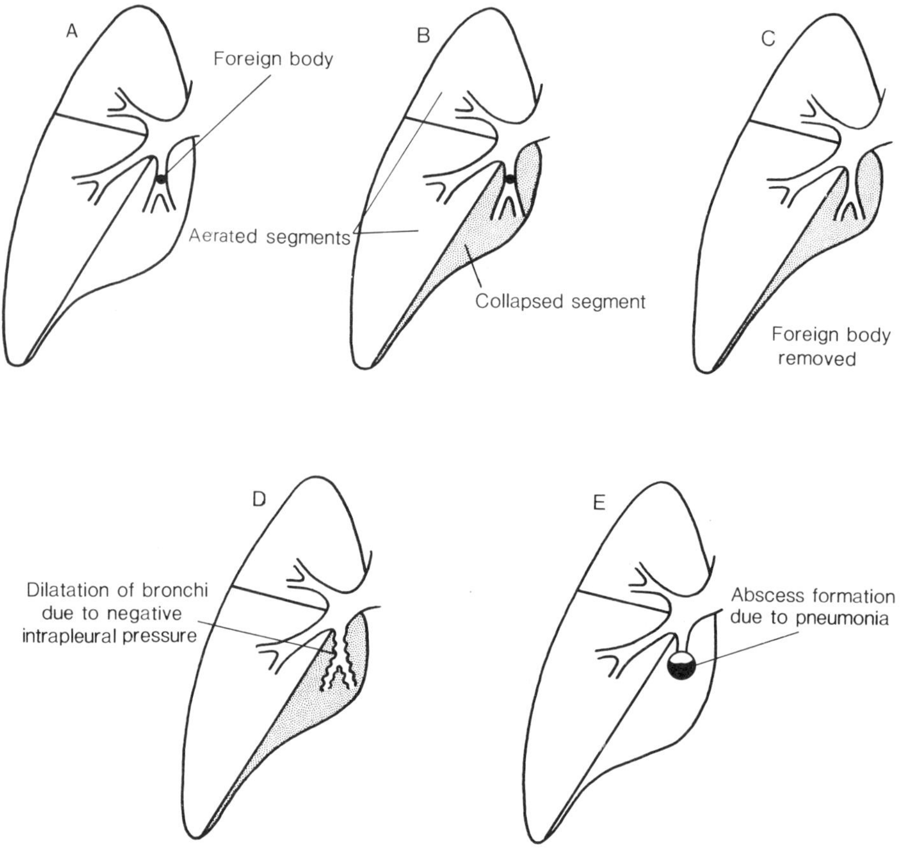

Fig. 5.1. Inhalation of foreign body (A) leads to collapse (B) which persists if obstruction is removed some weeks later (C). Bronchi in the collapsed segment dilate due to negative intrapleural pressure (D); or abscess develops due to pneumonia in collapsed lung (E).

the bronchial wall is damaged. Dilatation of the weakened bronchus occurs as the result of negative intrapleural pressure transmitted through the collapsed lung tissue. Dilated bronchi are further distended by retained excessive secretions which are persistently infected. This dilatation of bronchi with persistent pus formation is called 'bronchiectasis'.

Bronchiectasis occurs most frequently in the lower lobes, lingula and middle lobe. The symptoms vary from unproductive cough to severe respiratory disability associated with large volumes of offensive purulent sputum, and brisk haemoptysis. There is a risk of lung abscess, frequent episodes of pneumonia and pleurisy, and pus accumulation in the pleural space, empyema. Most patients produce 50 ml of sputum per day (a cupful) over several hours, these symptoms developing within 3–6 months of an episode of inhalation.

The signs that suggest bronchiectasis are the appearance and volume of sputum, the development of finger clubbing, although this does not appear in all cases, and signs on examination of the chest that suggest collapse and fibrosis. Diagnosis is confirmed by a straight chest radiograph and by the injection of radio-opaque oily solutions into the upper airways, which outlines the lower bronchial dilatation and irregularity.

◀ Large volumes of consistently purulent sputum and finger clubbing should suggest bronchiectasis

The treatment of bronchiectasis involves the intermittent use of antibiotics. Long term therapy is of no value since large sputum volumes persist, even after acute exacerbations have been treated. Local areas of bronchiectasis with frequent and troublesome exacerbations of symptoms are usually treated by surgical resection, but extensive disease involving lobes in both lungs may be unsuitable for surgery.

Bronchiectasis may be complicated by progressive respiratory disability culminating in heart failure, and local effects of exacerbations such as empyema, and by metastatic brain abscess.

Carcinoma of bronchus (*Table* 5.8)

There has been a great increase in the incidence of bronchial carcinoma over the past three decades

Table 5.8.   Lung tumours

Benign — rare, adenoma, presentation with same
respiratory symptoms as carcinoma
Malignant
    carcinoma   squamous 60%
            oat-cell 30%
            adenocarcinoma 10%
    metastases to brain, bone, liver

although there is now some evidence that the rise has been halted and that there may be a fall in some social classes. It is the most common cause of cancer deaths in U.K. (approximately a quarter) and is the cause of 1 in 20 deaths. There has been a predominant incidence of the disease in males but this is diminishing and there is now an increase in females.

Several aetiological factors have been suggested including smoking, atmospheric pollution, occupational hazards, X-irradiation and, more contentiously, genetic influences. There are several histological types, squamous cell, adenocarcinoma and undifferentiated carcinoma with varying prognosis and incidence of distant metastases.

Most patients (60–70%) present with respiratory symptoms. Cough, with or without sputum, is the most frequent complaint. The character of the cough often has a high pitch due to abnormal movement of the vocal cords. Paralysis of the vocal cords occurs when there is damage to the recurrent laryngeal nerves, usually on the left because of its intrathoracic course, and the altered size of the larynx during forced expiration changes the noise of the cough and reduces its effectiveness in expectorating sputum. Although the patient may have had a cough, due to chronic simple bronchitis, for some years it is the change in character which alerts him, either because of alteration in noise, such as the 'bovine' cough described, or change in the volume of sputum.

◄ The most common complaint of patients with carcinoma of bronchus is cough

Nearly 15% of patients with carcinoma of bronchus have distant metastases when diagnosed, either bloodborne to the brain, liver and adrenals or lymphatic spread to cervical and mediastinal nodes causing compression of the superior vena cava and trachea. Metastasis to the base of the skull may cause non-dental facial pain; mainly in the maxillary area, associated with lacrimation and dilatation of the pupil on the same side, Reader's neuralgia (*see* Chapter 11).

◄ 15% of patients with carcinoma of bronchus present with non-pulmonary non-metastatic features and 15% with distant metastases, often intracranial

Approximately 15% of patients present with non-metastatic complications such as peripheral neuropathy, which usually involves the limbs but may affect the cranial nerves. Undifferentiated carcinoma of bronchus may produce hormones or hormone-like substances that cause endocrine disorders — most frequently Cushing's syndrome due to excessive blood levels of ACTH, produced ectopically by the tumour (*see* Chapter 9). Other hormones, such as antidiuretic hormone and possibly thyroid-stimulating hormone, may be produced ectopically by oat-celled carcinoma.

Approximately 5% of patients with carcinoma of bronchus have no symptoms and are discovered by routine chest X-rays, by mass miniature radiography or because the patient is noted to have finger clubbing. Unfortunately, many of these patients have distant, asymptomatic metastases and this form of screening has been less successful than for other carcinomas, such as those of breast and cervix.

Carcinoma of bronchus may be treated surgically, with the best results, by X-irradiation, and with cytotoxic drugs. Surgical procedures consist of lobectomy, for an early or localized tumour, and pneumonectomy when the tumour is more extensive and near to the mediastinum. There is remarkably little effect of either operation on lung function and some patients are improved symptomatically, particularly if they had been breathless. Inhalation of foreign material into the remaining lung or lobes is obviously more serious, and greater care needs to be taken in such patients to avoid this.

X-irradiation for carcinoma of bronchus is often dramatically effective in relieving symptoms, especially in patients with superior mediastinal obstruction and in those with severe pain due to bone metastases. Altered immunity is a rare complication of modern radiotherapy, which minimizes total body radiation. Extensive oral ulceration during or after treatment may occur, however, as well as candidiasis, usually associated with leucopenia, impaired immunity and, in some instances, secondary to irradiation damage to the oesophagus, which causes painful dysphagia even for fluids. Late effects of irradiation, such as fibrosis, are unusual in such patients since they die of metastatic disease before this reaction is fully developed.

Attempts to treat carcinoma of the bronchus by immunotherapy — a combination of steroids, cytotoxic drugs and large doses of the anti-tuberculosis vaccine BCG — have proved unsuccessful. Extensive oral ulceration, systemic candidiasis and other opportunistic infection may occur during such treatment as well as a bleeding tendency, due to thrombocytopenia.

◄ Cytotoxic drugs used in the treatment of inoperable carcinoma of bronchus may cause oral ulceration and opportunistic infection

Pulmonary tuberculosis (*Table* 5.9)

The lungs are by far the most common site of tuberculosis. Although the death rate for pulmonary tuberculosis in countries such as England and Wales has fallen dramatically since 1945, the disease still occurs, however, and remains important to the dentist because of the risk of spread of infection to others. Many, but not all, new cases notified are amongst immigrants from the Indian sub-continent.

The organism *Mycobacterium tuberculosis* is inhaled in the form of droplets or in dust particles. Among factors that predispose to the infection are close contact with patients who are producing sputum that contains the organism (the open case), racial factors, malnourishment and systemic diseases such as diabetes mellitus.

Two forms of tuberculosis infection, primary and secondary, occur whether the site of entry is the respiratory tract, the mouth or the small bowel. Primary infection usually occurs in the young or in adult life and consists of a small focus in the lung parenchyma, the tonsil, or the bowel. Associated with the focus are enlarged regional lymph nodes which may break down (caseate) and, when in the neck, are associated with overlying skin changes, including discharging sinuses. Except in the cervical region the

◀ Primary tuberculous infection usually occurs in the lungs or pharynx

Table 5.9.   Pulmonary tuberculosis

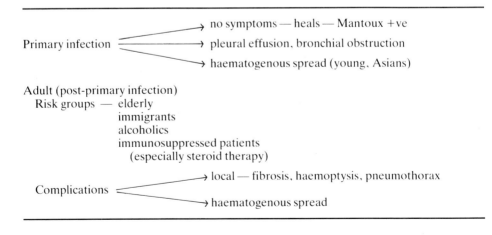

primary infection is invariably subclinical and passes unnoticed. Evidence of past primary infection is discovered by the chance finding of a calcified focus on a routine chest X-ray or a positive Mantoux test, during screening at a school or before entry to a college. The latter indicates hypersensitivity to a protein derivative of the organism, tuberculin.

The primary pulmonary infection rarely produces signs or symptoms at the time. In a few patients an unproductive cough with breathlessness may appear due to pleural effusion and in some there may be red, raised, painful and tender skin lesions on the shins which fade slowly through the colour changes of a bruise. This skin lesion (erythema nodosum) is not specific for primary tuberculosis and may occur with streptococcal infections, or sarcoidosis.

The primary infection may also cause progressive destruction of lung tissue and thus spread via the bronchial tree to produce tuberculous bronchopneumonia or, via the blood, producing tuberculous lesions throughout many organs of the body (miliary spread), particularly the brain and meninges, or to a single organ such as a joint, bone or one kidney.

Secondary tuberculosis occurs in an older population and may be due to reinfection following inhalation or reactivation of organisms in an old primary complex. Unlike the primary lesion, secondary disease almost always causes symptoms, although a few patients are discovered by chance when a routine X-ray is done or during a mass miniature radiography campaign. The usual symptoms are cough with sputum, which is often blood-stained; breathlessness; weight loss and anorexia; fever and sweating, which occurs classically, but not always, at night.

The patients are more often male, smokers, over the age of 45 and frequently Asian. Diagnosis depends upon an awareness of the possibility of the disease in this population, who are often socially deprived. X-ray may show fibrosis only, but in the very active disease there is cavitation. Activity is confirmed by the finding of the mycobacterium in the sputum on direct examination, with Ziehl–Neelsen staining, or on culture, which may take up to 6 weeks.

Treatment of tuberculosis is largely by drugs. Surgical resection is rarely needed, and attempts to

◀ Secondary tuberculosis is most common in middle-aged men, smokers and Asians and presents with fever, haemoptysis, weight loss and anorexia

collapse the lung, or the part affected, by procedures such as artificial pneumothorax and thoracoplasty are never used, although they were widespread before chemotherapy became available and some patients survive thirty or more years after such treatment. Drug therapy usually consists of two or three of the orally effective agents (isoniazid, ethambutol and rifampicin) which are given for periods of 9 months or longer according to the sensitivities, *in vitro*, of the cultured bacillus. Occasionally, because of lack of sensitivity of the organism to these three drugs, second-line agents such as streptomycin and ethionamide have to be used, with an increased risk of important side-effects.

If the patient's sputum is positive for tubercle bacilli on smear examination he/she is admitted to hospital for isolation and chemotherapy. Contact tracing, plus investigation of the source of infection, begins without delay. Before treating a patient who is known to have pulmonary tuberculosis, for which he receives drug therapy, the dentist should enquire of the chest physician treating the disease what is the risk to his staff, to other patients and to himself, so that they can be prevented from contracting the disease. General anaesthetic using inhalation techniques should be avoided since the bacillus may remain active for some weeks in saliva and sputum that can contaminate the apparatus.

◀ New cases of tuberculosis are reported to the Medical Officer for Environmental Health so that contact tracing and the source of infection can be found as soon as possible

The dentist should ensure that Mantoux testing is done and, if necessary, BCG is given to his staff, particularly if there has been contact in the surgery. He should always be aware of the possibility of active disease in the middle-aged male, a smoker, who complains of weight loss and attributes this to his poor dental health, since pulmonary tuberculosis may well be the cause of general health problems.

Pulmonary collapse

Absorption of air from the whole or part of a lung (collapse) may occur because of blockage of the supplying bronchus (by foreign body, a tooth, mucus, tumour or inhaled vomitus) or pressure on the lung from air or fluid in the pleural space. The physiological effects of pulmonary collapse are to reduce the amount of functioning lung available for gas exchange, and mismatching of ventilation and pulmonary blood flow, causing hypoxaemia. Whatever the cause the clinical features of collapse are cyanosis of varying degree and breathlessness.

Additional features of bronchial obstruction are cough, with or without sputum, and fever, when infection has developed distal to the foreign body etc. Pleurisy may develop once infection is established and, if the obstruction is not removed, lung abscess may occur. Treatment depends on the cause of obstruction, which is removed by bronchoscopy where possible. When the obstruction is by tumour (adenoma of bronchus or carcinoma) resection of the collapsed part is necessary.

Air in the pleural space causes contraction of the elastic tissue in the lung, which collapses to a smaller size, the degree of collapse depending on the volume of air in the cavity.

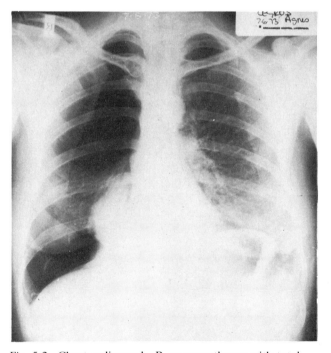

Fig. 5.2. Chest radiograph. R. pneumothorax with total collapse of lung.

Pneumothorax may occur spontaneously (due to rupture of a small vesicle on the lung surface; often associated with emphysema and occurring in the tall, thin young man) or may be due to trauma (rib fracture). Pneumothorax may occur secondarily to lung abscess, pulmonary tuberculosis and with bronchial carcinoma which acts as a ball valve, allowing air into but not out of a pulmonary segment.

Pneumothorax is usually of sudden onset with pleuritic pain followed by breathlessness. Increasing dyspnoea and cyanosis suggest that the pressure of air in the cavity is increasing, causing displacement of the mediastinum towards the unaffected side and impaired ventilation of the normal lung (tension pneumothorax). Small amounts of air in the pleural space may absorb without treatment but, if large, a drainage tube is inserted into the chest and the air allowed to escape through an underwater seal. Repeated episodes of pneumothorax may require attempts to obliterate the cavity, and any secondary cause is treated appropriately, once the urgent situation has been dealt with.

Fluid in the pleural cavity (*pleural effusion*) also causes pulmonary collapse due to contraction of elastic tissue in the lung with features of breathlessness, with or without cyanosis and sometimes preceded by pleurisy. Small volumes of fluid do not cause symptoms and may only be discovered on chest X-ray.

Pleural effusion may occur in heart failure and with diseases that are complicated by fluid retention (cirrhosis of the liver; nephrotic syndrome). Inflammation of the pleura due to underlying pneumonia and tuberculosis; trauma and infiltration by tumour, bronchial carcinoma or pleural neoplasm (mesothelioma), may also cause effusion.

The cause of pleural effusion can usually be determined from examination of the fluid. Treatment is to remove the fluid and allow the affected lung to re-expand, in addition to treatment of the underlying cause. The effusion due to cardiac, hepatic and renal disease usually disappears with diuretic therapy.

Pulmonary infarction

Infarction of the lung is associated with haemorrhage into the necrotic tissue because of the two separate blood supplies. The usual cause is embolism arising from thrombus in other parts of the circulation, most frequently the veins in the leg, which may complicate periods of inactivity when patients are confined to bed after operation or serious illness. Embolism may also arise from the right atrium in patients with atrial fibrillation.

The clinical features depend on the size of the embolism, massive emboli causing dramatic 'collapse' and sudden death. Smaller emboli cause pulmonary infarction with clinical features of dyspnoea, haemoptysis and pleurisy. Treatment with anticoagulants prevents further embolization. Small amounts of heparin are given subcutaneously in the perioperative period in patients at risk, particularly those having orthopaedic operations on the legs.

Pulmonary fibrosis

Localized pulmonary fibrosis may follow tuberculosis, pneumonia or infarction but generalized lung disease occurs with inhaled industrial chemicals (silicosis, coal-workers' pneumoconiosis, and asbestosis) and hypersensitivity to certain allergens (farmer's lung, bird-fancier's lung). Generalized fibrosis may occur with systemic disorders such as sarcoidosis, rheumatoid disease and following radiation damage. In some patients no cause is found.

The clinical features of generalized pulmonary fibrosis are dyspnoea with effort, a rapid respiratory rate at rest, cyanosis and finger clubbing. The treatment depends on the cause. Oxygen therapy is helpful in some patients who may carry a portable cylinder. Corticosteroids are given to many patients with little benefit, although they may have dramatic effect in sarcoidosis and systemic lupus erythematosus.

Sarcoidosis

Sarcoidosis is a granulomatous inflammation due to a cell-mediated immune response to an unknown antigen. It affects many tissues in the body but predominantly the lungs and skin. The histological appearance of tissue damaged by the disease, which is the way in which the diagnosis is made, is similar to tuberculosis, except that there are no bacilli seen nor does caseation occur. Patients with sarcoidosis usually have negative Mantoux tests but show reaction to extracts of tissues damaged by the disease, when injected intradermally (Kveim test).

Sarcoidosis may occur in an acute form presenting as fever, enlarged lymph nodes (usually intrathoracic), joint pains and erythema nodosum. Few patients with acute sarcoidosis progress to the chronic form, the clinical features of which are those of pulmonary fibrosis, enlarged lymph nodes, skin lesions, cardiac failure and disturbances of rhythm, as well as a variety of neurological presentations, including cranial nerve lesions.

The acute form of the disease does not often require treatment but chronic pulmonary, cardiac and CNS involvement may threaten life and are treated with corticosteroids.

Problems of respiratory diseases for the dentist

The principal problem that the dentist faces in patients with chronic pulmonary disorders is the recognition of severity of disability on the basis of the symptoms and simple tests of lung function, which will decide whether the patient is fit for general anaesthesia. The risks of inhalation of foreign material from the oral cavity into the respiratory tree are greater in the patient with impaired broncho-pulmonary clearance, such as chronic bronchitis and asthma. Inhalation may occur in the patient with a normal respiratory tree, however, and due care to avoid this complication of oral surgery must be taken.

By recognizing clubbing of the fingers the dentist may be the first health care person to realize that the patient may be seriously ill. Similarly, the dentist may have to recognize the differences between breathlessness of cardiac and respiratory origin, since both may occur in the dental clinic, particularly when the patient lies flat.

Finally, the dentist must appreciate the risks of pulmonary tuberculosis for his staff, patients and himself and take care to enquire about the safety of dental treatment in a patient undergoing chemotherapy for the disease, and ensure that his staff have received BCG, if necessary.

Gastrointestinal diseases

6

Symptoms of gastrointestinal disorder are common in the general population and some, such as indigestion and difficulty in swallowing, can be related by patients to poor dental health. A precise history of the patient's complaints will usually determine the exact relevance of symptoms and abnormal findings.

Dysphagia is the term used for pain and/or difficulty in swallowing. True dysphagia begins within seconds of the initiation of swallowing; it may be painful but is usually described as the sensation that food has 'stuck'. Some patients complain of pain and discomfort several minutes after swallowing (pseudodysphagia). It is important to distinguish between true and false dysphagia; the former is invariably due to organic disease in the pharynx and oesophagus, the latter to gastric or functional disorders. Patients often localize the site at which the food bolus is held up but this does not always correspond, anatomically, with the lesion. The usual sites to which the patient refers are the cricoid cartilage, mid-sternum and epigastrium.

◀ True dysphagia is the sensation, sometimes painful, of the food bolus having stuck in the throat or chest within 1–3 seconds of swallowing

Table 6.1.   Patients' interpretation of the term 'indigestion' (dyspepsia)

Nausea
Bad taste in the mouth
Post-prandial abdominal fullness
Epigastric burning
Heartburn
Abdominal pain
Wind — flatus usually upwards
Constipation

Table 6.2.   Causes of chronic or repeated episodes of nausea

Local causes
    alcohol
    drugs (phenylbutazone)
    tumour/ulcer
Neurological
    raised intracranial pressure
    vestibular dysfunction (vertigo)
    migraine
Biochemical
    chronic renal failure
    hypercalcaemia (hyperparathyroidism)
Pregnancy
Autonomic response to pain
Endocrine
    Addison's disease or hypoadrenalism
      (patients with stress on steroids)

Indigestion is a vague term used by patients to imply nausea, a bad taste in the mouth, fullness in the abdomen after meals, epigastric burning, heartburn, abdominal pain, wind (burping or flatus) or a change in bowel habit. Food-related pain or discomfort occurs with many abdominal disorders including peptic ulcer, gastric carcinoma, gallbladder and pancreatic disease and non-organic problems. Nearly 1 apparently healthy person in 5 has several attacks of abdominal discomfort each year, called 'indigestion', which are sometimes attributed to dental problems preventing proper mastication of food.

Chronic or recurrent nausea and vomiting occur not only with gastrointestinal disease but also with neurological disorders, renal failure, hypercalcaemia and pregnancy. Duodenal ulcer may cause pain and nausea, the former being relieved by vomiting unlike the pain of gastric cancer which can be similar. Obstruction of the stomach outlet by ulcer, scarring or carcinoma (pyloric stenosis) presents as vomiting of large amounts of food, often several hours after a meal, preceded by acute spasms of upper abdominal pain. Raised intracranial pressure, disturbance of vestibular function, migraine and neuropathy due to diabetes can all cause painless nausea and vomiting (*see* Chapter 11).

Recurrent vomiting results in dehydration with electrolyte disturbance, and the risk in a sedated or unconscious patient of inhalation.

To a patient the term *wind* may mean excessive belching, the passage of large amounts of flatus, abdominal discomfort and, sometimes, audible bowel sounds. Belched wind is air that has been swallowed; gas is produced in the stomach only with severe pyloric stenosis. Dryness of the mouth, profuse salivation and bolting of food can cause excessive air swallowing with abdominal discomfort and belching. The amount of flatus passed per rectum is determined by the gut flora and food eaten, particularly large amounts of carbohydrate.

Constipation is usually harmless and is often due to a diet lacking adequate amounts of roughage. Constipation of recent origin can be serious, especially if associated with weight loss, and may be due to malignant disease, diverticular disease, endocrine disorder (e.g. hypothyroidism) or, simply, a painful anal lesion.

Diarrhoea — the frequent passage of loose or watery stools, sometimes with pus and blood — may be an acute condition due to infection (*Salmonella* or *Yersinia*) or toxic effects of staphylococci in food. Chronic diarrhoea (lasting longer than one month) can be due to a large variety of causes including infections (amoebiasis and giardiasis), inflammatory disorders of bowel (Crohn's disease and ulcerative colitis); large bowel cancer; small bowel disorders (malabsorption and surgical resections); metabolic problems (hyperthyroidism); neuropathic complications of diabetes; functional disorders (irritable bowel syndrome); and drugs (antibiotics and the anti-rheumatic indomethacine). Alternating constipation and diarrhoea are typical features of irritable bowel syndrome — the commonest cause of chronic diarrhoea in the U.K.; associated with pain anywhere in the abdomen, chest, back and thighs.

Oral manifestations of general medical diseases

Being an exposed site the oral cavity is subject to local and environmental irritants, so that many of the abnormalities seen in the mouth are due to local disease. However, genetic, nutritional, hormonal, haematological and bowel disorders can cause changes in the oral cavity as the first manifestations of general medical disease.

Pallor of the mucous membranes, bleeding gums, gingival ulceration, petechiae, infection, uncontrolled bleeding, cheilitis and tongue abnormalities are common presenting features of *blood disorders*. The early involvement of the mouth is probably due, in some instances, to the constant trauma to the gums and buccal mucosa by food, teeth or dentures. Oral mucosal cells are normally shed and replaced from the deeper layers at a fast rate; in vitamin B_{12} deficiency, however, replacement is slow, the mucosa becoming atrophic and more susceptible to trauma (*see* Chapter 8).

Iron deficiency anaemia may result in a burning sensation in the tongue, provoked by eating 'sharp' or acid foods, with mucosal atrophy and depapillation of the dorsum of the tongue, frequent *Candida* infections and angular cheilitis. A furry red glossitis of the tongue, involving the lateral margins and tip, with papillary atrophy occurs in pernicious anaemia. The patient complains of a sore tongue and difficulty in wearing dentures. Jaundice of the oral mucosa may be noted in patients with pernicious anaemia and haemolytic disorders, such as sickle cell disease (*see* Chapter 8).

◀ Mucosal jaundice is most readily seen on the palate and in the sublingual area

The purpuras, both thrombocytopenic and non-thrombocytopenic, can present with petechiae, gingival haemorrhage, bleeding from any part of the oral mucosa and after dental extraction. Coagulation disorders may also present as heavy bleeding (*see* Chapter 8).

◀ Spontaneous or post-extraction gingival haemorrhage may be the first symptom of thrombocytopenia

Agranulocytosis and leucopenia, whether idiopathic or drug-induced, should be suspected when necrotizing ulceration is seen in the mouth. Gingival swelling and bleeding also occur. Ulcerative and gangrenous lesions affect the gums, cheeks or palate but are not usually painful and do not show marked inflammatory changes, have a dirty yellowish-green base and cause halitosis (*see* Chapter 8).

◀ Painless ulcers showing little inflammatory change, without pus formation but malodorous breath are typical features of agranulocytosis

Oral lesions occur frequently in both acute and chronic leukaemias. Gingival hyperplasia is particularly common in monocytic leukaemia, but gum hypertrophy, petechiae, ulceration, bleeding, loosening of teeth and alveolar bone loss, seen in radiographs, may be presenting signs in all varieties. Many drugs used to treat leukaemia predispose to oral ulceration and contribute to the frequent orofacial infections with herpes virus and *Candida* in these patients (*see* Chapter 8).

Enterovirus and other infections can involve the oral cavity as well as the skin and other organs. Hand, foot and mouth disease is one of the most common, caused by coxsackie A virus, occurring in outbreaks in schools and nurseries (*see* Chapter 15).

Syphilis is the sexually transmitted disease most likely to present with oral lesions. The primary chancre can occur on the lips, and appears as a painless papule, which ulcerates and exudes serum rather than blood. It is associated with enlarged submandibular lymph nodes and heals in 3–8 weeks. The *secondary stage* of acquired syphilis occurs 6–8 weeks after the primary chancre and a third of patients have oral mucosal ulceration and a maculopapular rash that can affect the palms. The mucosal lesions have a greyish-white base and may coalesce to produce a serpiginous lesion — the 'snail-track' ulcer.

Tertiary syphilis, developing 3–10 years after the untreated primary stage, is rarely seen. The characteristic lesion is the gumma, histologically a granuloma, sometimes occurring in the mouth and throat. The submucous tissues are initially involved, followed by ulceration, with a characteristic punched-out appearance, and a 'wash leather' slough at the base. Diffuse gummatous infiltration may occur in the tongue — 'chronic superficial glossitis'. Destruction of deep tissues occurs and perforation of the palate and nasal septum are also features of the tertiary stage.

Several inherited disorders produce fairly characteristic oral manifestations. *Peutz–Jeghers' syndrome* is the association of intestinal polyposis with oral melanin pigmentation, particularly on the lips. It may be difficult to distinguish from pigmentation due to chronic adrenal insufficiency (*see* Chapters 2 and 9).

Tuberous sclerosis may present with gingival fibromas and angiofibromas around the mouth, red to pink nodules with a smooth surface on the cheeks, chin, and also under the nails. Other features of the disease are epilepsy, mental retardation and benign tumours in brain, heart and kidneys.

Hereditary haemorrhagic telangiectasia affects the mucous membranes of the conjunctiva and lips, tongue and mouth in almost all patients. Nose bleeding is the most common presentation, but bleeding may occur from the mouth and gums after dental extraction. The disease is inherited by a non sex-linked dominant gene and tends to worsen with age (*see* Chapter 8).

◄ Epistaxis is the most common complication of hereditary telangectasia but bleeding may also occur from the lips and gums

Blistering diseases of the skin may be accompanied by mouth changes. Both pemphigus vulgaris and pemphigoid produce haemorrhagic blebs on the lips, tongue, buccal and palatal mucosa (*see* Chapter 15). Other mucosal surfaces may be involved including the conjunctiva, vagina and rectum.

◄ In more than half the patients with pemphigus vulgaris the oral lesions precede the skin blisters

Erythema multiforme is another lesion with subepidermal blisters, severe forms of which are accompanied by bullous mucosal lesions of the mouth, eyes and genitalia, that rupture easily, the lips and buccal mucosa becoming encrusted with blood, making eating and drinking difficult (*see* Chapter 15).

◄ The lips and oral mucosa become encrusted with blood and eating becomes difficult in Stevens–Johnson syndrome

Collagen vascular diseases such as scleroderma and systemic lupus erythematosus present with oral lesions in some patients (*see* Chapter 12).

Table 6.3. Comparison of major and minor aphthous ulceration

	Major	*Minor*
Size	Larger than 1 cm	Smaller than 1 cm
Numbers	Up to 10	1 to 5
Scarring	Yes	No
Associated disorder	Yes (Behçet's)	No
Duration	Up to 30 days	Heal within 10 days
Palatal and pharyngeal	Yes	No

Aphthous ulceration in the mouth is not commonly associated with systemic disorder except when the ulcers are large, occur in numbers of five or more, persist for up to two weeks, and heal by scarring, when Behçet's syndrome should be suspected. Ulceration may occur in other areas, particularly the genitalia, and there can be ocular inflammation. The mouth ulcers are characteristically painful, recurrent, shallow or deep ulcers with a yellowish necrotic base, and can occur on the tonsils. The disease has systemic features including joint, CNS and vascular (usually thrombophlebitis) involvement with skin pustules (*see* Chapter 12).

Mouth lesions occur with both ulcerative colitis and Crohn's disease. Major or minor aphthous ulceration can be a feature of either but characteristic oral mucosal changes are found in Crohn's disease including cobblestone nodularity, hyperplastic ridges and a granulomatous cheilitis, suggesting a direct relationship between mouth and bowel changes. The vestibule is a frequent site for these changes which may, occasionally, precede bowel symptoms.

◀ The mouth lesions of Crohn's disease consist of ulcers, with 'cobblestone' nodularity, hyperplastic mucosal ridges and cheilitis which may precede the bowel symptoms

Diseases of the oesophagus and pharynx

Functionally the pharynx and oesophagus act as a single unit that conveys food by peristalsis from the mouth to the stomach. The symptoms of disorders of both are true dysphagia and oesophageal pain.

The pharyngeal muscles may be affected by neurological lesions that cause bulbar and pseudobulbar palsy with the risk of inhalation of food and secretions from the mouth, and nasal regurgitation of liquids when the patient attempts to swallow. *Pharyngeal diverticulum (pouch)* is a bulging of mucosa through a weakened portion of the posterior muscle at the junction of pharynx and oesophagus, causing varying degrees of dysphagia over several years associated with a variable mass in the left side of the neck. The contents of the pouch, stale undigested food, may be regurgitated several hours after eating or may be inhaled, particularly in the elderly, at night. Surgical excision and repair of the muscle defect is the ideal treatment provided that the patient's general condition is good. The condition is probably due to a defect of upper oesophageal sphincter relaxation.

Tumours of the oesophagus are usually malignant and squamous carcinoma is the most common (90%). There are marked geographical variations of incidence: it is the most common malignancy in Asia. The most

◀ Progressive dys-
phagia, to the point of
difficulty in swallowing
liquids and saliva, is the
feature of carcinoma of
oesophagus

frequent sites are in the mid and lower oesophagus although postcricoid lesions do occur. Progressive dysphagia is the usual presenting symptom, becoming so severe that eventually liquids and saliva cannot be swallowed. There is rapid weight loss and pulmonary complications can occur, either due to overspill or development of a fistula between the trachea and oesophagus.

Surgical resection of the tumour offers the only chance of cure but the procedures required are major (mortality approximately 20%), mobilization of the stomach being necessary to maintain the continuity of the gut if the lesion is at the lower end of the oesophagus. Mid-oesophagus and the postcricoid lesions may require mobilization of part of the colon through the thorax to maintain continuity. Correction of malnutrition before surgery is essential, particularly as postoperative wound and pulmonary complications are very common.

Radiotherapy may be an alternative form of treatment if surgery is considered impossible. Palliative operations, to relieve dysphagia, involve passage of tubes through the tumour from above, during endoscopy, or from below via the stomach, using a small laparotomy.

Achalasia of the cardia is a condition in which the body of the oesophagus becomes dilated due to narrowing, caused by muscular hypertrophy and spasm of its lower sphincter. Intermittent dysphagia, which may be painful, and inhalation are the earliest symptoms of the disease. Differential diagnosis may be difficult, particularly exclusion of a small carcinoma with spasm. There is an excess incidence of carcinoma of oesophagus in patients with long-standing achalasia.

Treatment of achalasia is usually to incise the hypertrophied muscle at the lower end of the oesophagus (Heller's operation), but some patients learn to swallow oesophageal dilators, a treatment used more often for benign oesophageal stricture.

Hiatus hernia is the term used to describe herniation of part of the stomach through the oesophageal hiatus of diaphragm. In some the cardia (the junction between the stomach and oesophagus) lies above the diaphragm (sliding variety), in others only a pouch of stomach passes through the hiatus, the cardia remaining in its normal site (rolling type). Many patients are asymptomatic, others complain of pain in the abdomen or lower chest, radiating upwards to the throat, related to food. Regurgitation of acid on lying flat and bending, intermittent dysphagia and vomiting can occur. Chronic anaemia due to blood loss may be the presenting feature of the para-oesophageal (rolling) hernia.

Treatment of hiatus hernia includes antacids and histamine-2 receptor antagonists to reduce acid secretion by the stomach, or surgical attempts to reduce the hernia. Simple measures such as weight reduction are also helpful, the hernia being symptomatically more troublesome in obese subjects, and during pregnancy.

Benign stricture of the oesophagus usually occurs as a complication of acid reflux due to an abnormal lower sphincter or following peptic ulcer, which has healed. Stricture causes varying degrees of dysphagia, pain and heartburn. The usual treatment is progressive dilatation until the patient is able to swallow mercury-filled bougies at regular intervals, so as to maintain food passage plus measures to reduce reflux and gastric acidity.

Peptic ulcer

A peptic ulcer occurs in any part of the gastrointestinal tract exposed to acid-pepsin secretion, chiefly the stomach and duodenum but also the oesophagus and the small bowel, at the anastomosis of a gastroenterostomy. The cause of peptic ulcer is not known but a highly acid gastric juice is not sufficient in itself to account for all cases, particularly gastric ulcer in which acid production may be low, and an additional factor of mucosal resistance has to be proposed. Hormones may be involved in the cause of peptic ulcer including gastrin, a hormone produced by the antrum of the stomach which stimulates acid and pepsin secretion, and can be produced ectopically by certain tumours of the islet cells in the pancreas — the Zollinger–Ellison syndrome of duodenal and jejunal ulceration often accompanied by malabsorption and diarrhoea. Other influences on the incidence of peptic ulcer include smoking, other hormones (parathormone and cortisol), and the ABO blood group of the patient, blood group O being associated with twice the usual liability to develop duodenal ulcer than groups A, B or AB.

The characteristic symptom of peptic ulcer is pain, usually in the upper abdomen but sometimes in the lumbar region and thorax, related to food, and relieved by eating. The pain is usually burning in character, sometimes called 'hunger pain', and relieved by alkali and vomiting. Symptoms are usually periodic, lasting for a few days to several weeks, with trouble-free intervals of some months. The sudden filling of the mouth with tasteless fluid (waterbrash) occurs with both duodenal and other peptic ulcers.

◀ Food-provoked abdominal or lower thoracic pain, relieved by vomiting and by alkali, is the characteristic symptom of peptic ulcer

Diagnosis of peptic ulcer is made on the history, visualization by barium meal series or gastroduodenoscopy and biopsy, particularly of gastric ulcers which may be malignant. Repeated gastroduodenoscopy at intervals helps to assess healing.

◀ Gastroduodenoscopy is probably indicated in patients with 'indigestion' if a barium meal X-ray is normal or shows only minor abnormalities

Medical treatment of peptic ulcer consists of attempts to neutralize or reduce acid secretion and increase resistance to ulceration. Large volumes of antacids, H_2-receptor antagonists, bismuth suspension and liquorice derivatives are all used and there is, possibly, little difference between their efficacy. Cimetidine, one of the H_2-receptor antagonists used, is an hepatic enzyme inhibitor and may potentiate the effects of diazepam (*see* Chapter 16).

Many surgical procedures have been suggested for the treatment of duodenal ulcer. Surgical treatment is indicated when symptoms are not controlled by medical measures, when uncontrollable bleeding occurs, following perforation and if there is pyloric stenosis. The procedures are either attempts to drain the stomach contents, by enlarging the pylorus or via a gastroenterostomy; or denervation of the stomach by division of the vagus, to reduce acid secretion. Both procedures are commonly performed together (e.g. vagotomy and pyloroplasty, one of the most popular operations for duodenal ulcer).

Gastric ulcer that does not respond to medical treatment or which is suspected as malignant is treated by partial gastrectomy and gastroenterostomy. Complications can follow this operation, including malabsorption, anaemia and sudden, rapid emptying of

Table 6.4. Complications of peptic ulcer

Haemorrhage
   haematemesis — frank or coffee-ground appearance
   melaena (black stools due to altered blood)
   slow — iron deficiency anaemia
Perforation
Penetration of other organs
   pancreas
Narrowing of the outlet of the stomach (pyloric stenosis)

---

the stomach (dumping syndrome) causing faintness and palpitations in some and symptoms of hypoglycaemia in others.

The complications of peptic ulcer include haemorrhage, which may be brisk (haematemesis) or slow causing chronic iron deficiency anaemia; perforation; penetration of other organs, particularly the pancreas; and pyloric stenosis. Malignant transformation does not occur in duodenal ulcer, and it is questionable whether it occurs in gastric ulcer.

Tumours of the stomach

Carcinoma is the most common gastric tumour. Inflammatory and adenomatous benign polyps also occur as do submucosal tumours, including smooth muscle neoplasms (leiomyoma), and non-Hodgkin's lymphomas (*see* Chapter 8).

Although polyps are frequently asymptomatic and discovered by chance, most tumours cause 'indigestion'. Dysphagia may occur when the lesion is in the cardiac region of the stomach; pseudodysphagia can also occur. Haematemesis may be the presenting feature of any gastric tumour and, although not usually as profuse as with peptic ulcer, may require emergency treatment. Carcinoma usually presents with anorexia, nausea, vomiting with weight loss and increasing weakness.

Diagnosis depends on radiology, gastroscopy and biopsy. Some areas of the stomach (the fundus) are difficult to visualize, requiring special manoeuvres with the flexible gastroscope. Endoscopy may be used to remove polyps, which are regarded as pre-malignant until proved otherwise.

The results of gastric surgery for carcinoma are poor, the majority of patients having inoperable disease by the time diagnosis is made (5-year survival 8%). Palliative surgery may be performed to relieve recurrent vomiting due to pyloric obstruction, but the treatment of choice, attempting to cure, is subtotal or total gastrectomy.

Small bowel diseases

The primary functions of the small intestine are digestion and absorption. Failure of digestion can also result from pancreatic and stomach disease.

Failure of digestion due to pancreatic enzyme deficiency can occur with chronic pancreatitis, an inflammatory disease related to heavy alcohol consumption (see Chapter 7), or fibrocystic disease, an inherited condition associated with abnormally viscid secretions produced by all mucus glands, in the respiratory as well as digestive tract. Failure of digestion also occurs when the small bowel fails to produce specific enzymes, usually those which split sugars such as lactose (alactasia).

Bile salts are necessary for the solubilization of the products of digestion prior to absorption. Obstructive jaundice and fistula between gallbladder and colon are associated with malabsorption, particularly of fats and fat-soluble substances (e.g. vitamin K). Bile salts are absorbed in the terminal ileum and re-secreted in bile. When this enterohepatic circulation is interrupted as, for example, by small bowel disease (Crohn's disease) or surgical resection, malabsorption occurs.

Failure of absorption also occurs with generalized disease of the small bowel, either by reduction in size of the absorptive area following mucosal damage or by formation of fistulae and short circuiting between proximal and distal parts of the gut. Coeliac disease (gluten-induced enteropathy) is an example of the former and Crohn's disease of the latter. In these disorders there is a generalized failure of absorption although, for reasons unknown, in some instances the presenting feature may be malabsorption of a specific substance, such as vitamin D, causing bone pain due to osteomalacia. Failure to absorb substances, such as vitamin B_{12} in pernicious anaemia and with terminal ileum disease or resection can also be classified as malabsorption syndromes. Some drugs may cause malabsorption when given by mouth (e.g. antibiotics), and although the mechanism is not always understood it can be specific for some substances (e.g. malabsorption of folate due to phenytoin).

Although the underlying cause for malabsorption may cause some typical features, such as the skin changes of scleroderma, the clinical manifestations of malabsorption are similar. Some patients remain asymptomatic for many years, particularly those with coeliac disease, and in most the onset is insidious. Symptoms can fluctuate in severity with long remissions punctuated by acute exacerbations, comprising profuse diarrhoea, weight loss and abdominal distension.

Diarrhoea is not a constant feature of malabsorption, some patients complaining of episodes of constipation. Characteristically the complaints are of the passage of frequent, loose, bulky, pale, foul-smelling motions which float on water and may obviously contain fat. The diarrhoea is painless, and the motion does not contain blood or mucus. Weight loss can be marked or, in the child, there may be failure to thrive or delay in growth and the onset of puberty. The abdominal distension, due to gaseous dilatation of the small intestine, is in striking contrast to wasting of muscles in the limbs.

◀ Diarrhoea is not essential for the diagnosis of malabsorption syndrome

Other manifestations of malabsorption are the signs and symptoms of specific deficiencies, most often a microcytic hypochromic anaemia due to failure of iron absorption. Megaloblastic anaemia is a less frequent presenting feature, usually due to folic acid deficiency. A rare haematological complication is excessive bleeding and bruising due to hypoprothrombinaemia secondary to vitamin K deficiency (see Chapter 8).

◀ The commonest abnormal investigation in malabsorption syndrome is hypochromic microcytic anaemia, due to iron deficiency

Failure of absorption of vitamin D results in osteomalacia in adults and rickets in children, presenting as bone pain, deformity, increased fragility and, in some patients, proximal muscle weakness (see Chapter 12). In severe malabsorption negative protein balance develops with hypoalbuminaemia and fluid retention, plus impaired synthesis of immunoglobulins and increased risk of infections. Absorption of drugs given orally may also be affected. Every patient with an unexplained nutritional deficiency should be investigated for malabsorption.

Table 6.5.   Signs and symptoms of coeliac disease

Patient may be asymptomatic for long intervals
Lassitude and weight loss
Diarrhoea
Abdominal pain (non-specific)
Nausea and vomiting
Symptoms of specific deficiencies
    purpura (vitamin K)
    tetany (vitamin D)
    bone pain and muscle weakness
      (vitamin D)
    paraesthesiae of limbs (vitamin B_{12})
Signs
    anaemia
    glossitis
    finger clubbing
    pigmentation (hands and occasionally oral mucosa)

Coeliac disease is a disorder of the small bowel due to hypersensitivity to the wheat protein gluten that occurs in 1/1000–2000 of the population in U.K. The effects of gluten sensitivity are on the small bowel surface cell, the enterocyte, which is destroyed at a rapid rate, leading to broadening and shortening of villi, reducing the absorptive surface of the intestine. The changes revert towards normal after a few months when the patient is on a strict gluten-free diet.

Coeliac disease may be diagnosed at any age although there are peaks in infancy; during puberty, especially in the female; during childbearing years in women; and in the fifth and sixth decades in both sexes. The diagnosis may even be made for the first time in patients more than 70 years of age. The symptoms vary from non-specific features of general ill health (lassitude and loss of weight) and abdominal complaints (diarrhoea, flatulence, abdominal pain, nausea and vomiting) to those of nutritional deficiencies. Digital clubbing occurs in some patients and glossitis is common, the whole buccal mucosa being red and sore, with frequent aphthae, which may be the sole presenting feature. There may be increased melanin pigmentation on exposed areas and, occasionally, the buccal mucosa in some patients. Most patients are clinically anaemic.

The diagnosis of gluten-sensitive enteropathy is made by peroral small bowel biopsy, and subsequent improvement with diet. Some patients excrete large amounts of fat in the stool, hence the alternative term 'idiopathic steatorrhoea', but this is not essential for diagnosis.

A gluten-free diet is one essential feature of treatment of coeliac disease; although some patients may be indiscreet without suffering ill-effects, others have serious relapse after eating a small amount of gluten in bread or pastries. Correction of specific deficiencies is the other basic treatment.

Inflammatory bowel disease

Both ulcerative colitis and Crohn's disease present with the symptoms of large bowel disorder — diarrhoea with rectal bleeding and the discomfort in the rectum of incomplete evacuation (tenesmus). The symptoms vary in severity according to the site and extent of involvement; in some patients only the rectum is affected. Generalized abdominal pain, relieved by opening of the bowels, occurs in most patients as does weight-loss.

The disease is usually of long standing but can occur in an acute form, and some patients have only one episode with complete recovery. Relapses may cause heavy blood loss and severe constitutional disturbance, fever and dehydration. Other patients have milder but persistent symptoms. Perianal lesions, such as fistula and abscess formation, are more common in Crohn's disease.

Although ulcerative colitis is confined to the large bowel, Crohn's disease may affect any part of the gastrointestinal tract, especially the ileum. The disease can be differentiated from colitis by the involvement of

◀ The symptoms of ulcerative colitis and colonic involvement in Crohn's disease are usually indistinguishable

Table 6.6.　Non-enteropathic features of inflammatory bowel disease

---

Skin lesions
  pyoderma gangrenosum (10%)
  erythema nodosum (5%)
Joint disease
  sacroiliac disease (20%)
  monoarthritis (acute 10%)
Eye complications
  iritis and conjunctivitis (5%)
Aphthous ulceration and other oral lesions (20%)
Liver disease
  chronic active hepatitis (3%)

---

small bowel and biopsy, which shows histological features of inflammation with granuloma formation. The affected portions of bowel, which are not always contiguous, are thickened and inflamed; narrowing of segments causes intestinal obstruction and, because inflamed areas become attached to other parts of the bowel, fistulas develop with malabsorption.

Non-enteropathic features may occur in both colitis and Crohn's disease. Various skin lesions including erythema nodosum and pyoderma gangrenosum (multiple, sterile pustules with black over-lying skin) occur, as do recurrent oral aphthae. The oral lesions of Crohn's disease are more extensive with linear ulcers and heaped margins, plus a 'cobble-stoned' appearance of the mucosa. Acute iritis and conjunctivitis occur in some as does an arthritis resembling ankylosing spondylitis. The non-enteropathic features, with the exception of joint disease, accompany exacerbations of the bowel disorder.

Treatment of ulcerative colitis and Crohn's disease confined to the colon is initially conservative — corticosteroids orally or topically (by enema), according to the extent of the disease. Failure to respond to medical treatment, or perforation, acute dilatation of the colon, stricture formation and the development of carcinoma are indications for surgery, the whole colon and the rectum being removed (panproctocolectomy) and an ileostomy fashioned. The operation is very successful, many patients showing great improvement in general health.

Crohn's disease involving the small intestine is more difficult to treat, particularly by surgery, since the disease may skip portions of bowel and resection of diseased segments can be followed by new lesions appearing in the anastomosis. The symptoms are either acute or chronic abdominal pain, with diarrhoea and episodes of obstruction. Surgery is required for stricture and sometimes for fistula, but resections are limited and by-pass procedures avoided. Medical treatment consists of oral corticosteroids or ACTH, often in combination with immunosuppressive drugs such as azathioprine. Specific vitamin deficiencies may develop because of malabsorption and are treated by parenteral therapy. Prolonged parenteral feeding may sometimes be necessary; in a few instances for more than a year.

Other diseases of the large bowel

Diverticular disease of the colon is frequently asymptomatic, being discovered by contrast X-rays (barium enema) as protrusions of mucosa due to high intraluminal pressure which are diffusely spread throughout the bowel, particularly in the sigmoid region. Symptoms are more common with increasing age and consist of intermittent, colicky lower abdominal pain with constipation and incomplete rectal emptying. Bleeding can occur and is often heavy. Other complications include obstruction, perforation, with peritonitis and local abscess formation, and fistula formation between bladder and/or vagina and the colon.

Asymptomatic diverticular disease does not require treatment but those patients with symptoms are advised a high fibre diet, the refined food of Western society being an important aetiological factor in the disorder. Surgical resection is the treatment of choice in complicated cases, sometimes with a short-term proximal colostomy to aid healing of the anastomosis. An alternative operation is longitudinal division of the circular muscle of the colon.

Carcinoma of the colon is the commonest tumour of the bowel and may occur anywhere in the large bowel, the site determining the presenting features. Carcinoma in the ascending colon and caecum often presents with iron deficiency anaemia and, in some patients, diarrhoea with a palpable mass. Lesions in the descending, pelvic, and sigmoid colon usually present as change in bowel habit and obstruction. Perforation and peritonitis occurs most often with sigmoid growths. Diagnosis is made by barium enema and colonoscopy if radiography fails to distinguish carcinoma from Crohn's and diverticular disease.

Surgical treatment of carcinoma of colon involves resection of half of the large bowel (hemicolectomy) together with the draining lymph nodes. Attempts are made to restore bowel continuity but sometimes a permanent colostomy, through which faeces are passed, is required. Results of surgical treatment are good particularly if the carcinoma has not penetrated the full thickness of bowel wall (66% 5-year survival after radical excision).

Carcinoma of rectum presents with change in bowel habit and bleeding with defaecation. Some patients present with painful tenesmus, others with dysuria and frequency, due to involvement of the bladder. Surgical resection usually involves the anal canal with a permanent colostomy, although high lesions may sometimes allow restoration of bowel continuity.

◀ Change in bowel frequency, consistency of stools, and bleeding require full investigation including barium enema and fibreoptic examination of the entire large bowel

The acute abdomen

Acute abdominal pain is probably the most common medical emergency and often a difficult diagnostic problem which depends on history and clinical findings, with only a few simple laboratory tests. The differential diagnosis is made difficult by extra-abdominal causes including pneumonia, myocardial infarction and diabetic ketoacidosis mimicking true intra-abdominal emergencies.

Intra-abdominal causes for pain may be inflammation of organs such as the appendix, gallbladder, Fallopian tubes and pancreas. Obstruction of bowel by strangulated hernia, of biliary tract and ureter by stone

Table 6.7. Acute abdomen pain

Abdominal causes
    inflammatory lesions — appendix, diverticulitis,
        pancreas, gallbladder, Fallopian tubes
    obstruction — bowel, ureter, bile ducts
    perforation — peptic ulcer, colon
    haemorrhage — ruptured spleen, tubal pregnancy
    torsion — ovarian cyst, bowel (large)
    vascular — ruptured aortic aneurysm, embolism of
        arteries (valvular heart disease)
Extra-abdominal causes
    thoracic — pleurisy and pericarditis
    metabolic — diabetic ketoacidosis, lead poisoning,
        porphyria
    neurological — tabes dorsalis, herpes zoster (lower
        thoracic segments)

---

cause acute colicky pain. The pain of perforation of the stomach, duodenum and small bowel is usually of sudden onset. Bleeding from a ruptured spleen, Fallopian tube pregnancy, or a leaking abdominal aneurysm may also cause acute abdominal pain. Torsion (twisting) of the bowel or an ovarian cyst can present as pain of sudden onset and, in the former, with symptoms of intestinal obstruction.

Acute appendicitis may occur at any age, although rarely in early childhood or in the elderly. The typical features are central abdominal pain, followed by nausea or vomiting and anorexia; the pain then moves to the right lower quadrant. Other intra-abdominal conditions can mimic acute appendicitis including perforated peptic ulcer, acute cholecystitis, Crohn's disease of the terminal ileum, pyelonephritis, acute salpingitis and tubal pregnancy in the female, and gastro-enteritis in the child. The treatment, having established the diagnosis, is immediate appen-dicectomy except where the symptoms have subsided, the patient is too ill, or when the appendix has perforated with the formation of an inflammatory mass (appendicular abscess). Operation is deferred in the case of appendicular abscess for 3 months, provided that symptoms improve with conservative therapy (fluid diet and bed rest).

Acute intestinal obstruction may be mechanical, due to hernia and adhesions following previous surgery, or neurogenic–paralysis or inhibition of peristalsis which may be caused by drugs, electrolyte imbalance and peritoneal infection. Mechanical obstruction in the small bowel or colon may be acute or chronic, according to the speed of onset of symptoms. The typical features, whatever the site, are colicky abdominal pain which doubles the patient up; abdominal distension, particularly with large intestinal lesions; constipation; and vomiting, which occurs early in high (small bowel) obstruction but may be absent with colonic lesions.

The causes of small intestinal obstruction are usually hernia, adhesions, Crohn's disease and intussusception (telescoping of the bowel), the latter being commonest in the young. The most frequent cause of large intestinal obstruction is tumour, although diverticular disease may do so and, less commonly, adhesions and sigmoid volvulus (twisting of the colon).

The treatment of intestinal obstruction depends on the speed of onset, a chronic lesion allowing detailed investigation and elective surgery where necessary. Acute obstruction requires urgent surgery after rapid preparation.

Preoperative preparation consists of gastric aspiration, and fluid and electrolyte replacement by intravenous infusion. Severe dehydration and potassium depletion with alkalosis may occur, with secondary renal failure.

The principles of surgery for obstruction are to define the cause, determine how much of the liberated intestine is viable, and how much should be resected. Small intestine can usually be resected with immediate anastomosis; large bowel lesions may require a temporary proximal colostomy.

Adynamic (neurogenic) small bowel obstruction is treated conservatively by gastric aspiration and intravenous fluid and electrolyte infusion. The underlying cause such as hypokalaemia, peritonitis or pancreatitis must also be treated; drug therapy (ganglion-blocking agents, now rarely used in the treatment of hypertension) should be withdrawn and antidotes given.

Diseases of the liver and biliary system

7

The functions of the liver are numerous and can be summarized as —

1. Storage. The liver stores glycogen, fat, probably proteins, vitamins and substances concerned in blood formation and regeneration.
2. Synthesis. The liver synthesizes the plasma proteins, fibrinogen, prothrombin and heparin.
3. Formation and destruction of red blood cells (potential).
4. Detoxicating function. The liver exerts a protective action by conjugation of toxic substances absorbed from the bowel or their complete destruction.
5. Metabolism. The liver has a major role in the metabolism of carbohydrate, fat and protein. The liver has the only immediately available reserve of blood glucose (glycogen), and responds sensitively to changes in blood concentration, taking up glucose when the level is high and releasing it when low. The liver also regulates the withdrawal of fat from stores and produces ketones from the dissimilation of fatty acids.
6. Bile secretion. Hepatic cells secrete bile continuously into bile capillaries from which it passes via the hepatic and bile ducts into the duodenum.

Jaundice

Bilirubin enters the plasma following breakdown of haem in the reticuloendothelial system and is removed on passage through the liver, where it is conjugated with glucuronic acid prior to biliary excretion. Excess

◄ Plasma bilirubin may be slightly increased without jaundice being clinically apparent

118

accumulation of bilirubin in the blood is recognized by a yellow appearance of the skin and mucosa (jaundice). Recognition of jaundice varies according to whether the patient is seen in natural or artificial light. Biochemical tests of liver function may show elevation of bilirubin which cannot be detected clinically.

Jaundice may be due to accumulation of *unconjugated bilirubin*, which occurs with over-production (e.g. haemolysis), and failure of uptake or impaired conjugation by hepatic cells. Unconjugated bilirubin is lipid-soluble so that it is not excreted in the urine, which remains normal in colour. However, some bilirubin will be taken up and conjugated by the liver, so that bile enters the bowel, giving the stool its normal colour. During its passage through the bowel, bilirubin is broken down by the action of colonic bacteria producing soluble substances, including urobilinogen which is reabsorbed and excreted in urine and bile.

◀ Pale stools and dark urine suggest obstructive jaundice, dark stools and yellow urine suggest haemolysis

Jaundice also occurs when there is *absent or impaired biliary flow* into the bowel (*cholestasis*), due to obstruction of the major ducts or disease of finer radicles of the biliary tree within the liver. In biliary obstruction the conjugating mechanism remains intact, but conjugated bilirubin is regurgitated into the bloodstream and, being water-soluble, is filtered by the kidney and appears in the urine, which is dark. The stools become pale due to reduced amounts of conjugated bilirubin in the bile. Bile salts are retained in obstructive jaundice, causing intense itching (pruritus).

A third class of jaundice (hepatocellular), due to diffuse parenchymal disorders, such as hepatitis and

Table 7.1. Classification of jaundice

Prehepatic jaundice: due to excessive red cell breakdown (haemolytic jaundice)

Hepatic: due to diffuse liver disease (cirrhosis or hepatitis) or failure of the liver to transport or conjugate bilirubin (congenital enzyme defects)

Obstructive jaundice: impaired or absent biliary flow which may be intrahepatic (due to drugs, hepatitis or cirrhosis) or due to blockage of the common bileduct by stone or pancreatic tumour. Associated pruritus

---

cirrhosis, is due to failure of bilirubin transfer from blood to bile combined, in some instances, with cholestasis, due to damage to the biliary tree.

Signs and symptoms of liver disease

The signs of liver disease result from failure of its metabolic functions. The most common is *jaundice*, with or without itching, and changes in urine and stool colour. Jaundice may be the only abnormal finding in patients with liver disease, particularly viral hepatitis, and other acute disorders (e.g. drug-induced hepatic damage). Chronic liver disease (cirrhosis of the liver, chronic hepatitis and alcoholic liver disease) may present other features of failure of function.

Table 7.2.   Signs and symptoms of liver disease

Jaundice (with or without itching and change in stools)
Bleeding tendency
Pigmentation (melanin) — particularly obstructive
Spider naevi and palmar erythema
Fluid retention (dependent oedema and ascites)
White nails (hypoalbuminaemia)
Confusion, loss of interest, impaired memory, flapping
   tremor, in extreme cases coma (hepatic encephalopathy)
Features suggesting Cushing's syndrome (alcoholic liver
   disease)
Dupuytren's contracture and parotid enlargement
   (alcoholism)

A *bleeding tendency* develops in severe liver disease, due to failure of synthesis of clotting factors and in a few instances reduced numbers of platelets (*see* Chapter 8). There may be bruising, occasionally purpura, excessive bleeding after dental extractions and spontaneous haemorrhage from the gastrointestinal tract — a serious complication of liver disease.

Fluid retention can also occur in liver disease, usually associated with hypoalbuminaemia, due to reduced hepatic synthesis. Ascites, however, may occur in spite of a normal serum albumin, due to obstruction of portal venous blood flow through the liver (portal hypertension). Renal retention of salt and water, because of failure of the liver to inactivate aldosterone, is an additional factor in hepatic oedema.

Glucose intolerance is common in patients with hepatic cirrhosis and is due to insulin resistance. Complications of diabetes are unusual, however, and hyperglycaemia or glycosuria is usually a chance finding.

Endocrine disturbances due to hepatic disease occur more frequently in the male. Hypogonadism with small testes, diminished potency and infertility are the result of failure of the liver to inactivate oestrogens. Feminization can develop in chronic liver disease, the male breast increasing in size and truncal hair distribution showing a feminine pattern. Other features thought to be due to the effects of oestrogen are spider naevi that occur on the arms, face, neck and upper thorax and erythema of the palms. However, palmar erythema may also be seen with rheumatoid arthritis, thyroid disease and, sometimes, without obvious cause.

Some patients with alcohol-induced liver disease are suspected of having *Cushing's syndrome*. Plasma corticosteroid levels may be high, due to decreased inactivation by the liver, and fall to normal when alcohol consumption is moderated (*see* Chapter 9).

Patients with acute and chronic liver disease are unduly *sensitive to many drugs*, particularly sedatives and analgesics. Diminished metabolic rate, reduced extraction by the liver during the first pass of the drug through the circulation, altered volume of distribution due to fluid retention and reduced protein binding, due to hypoalbuminaemia, are some of the factors that make prescribing difficult.

◄ Patients with acute and chronic liver disease are unduly sensitive to many drugs

Failure of the liver to detoxify ammonia and other enterogenous waste products (amino acids and phenols) may cause *neuropsychiatric disturbances (encephalopathy)* in end-stage chronic liver disease and acute fulminating hepatic failure. Most of these toxins are derived from bacterial breakdown of protein in the gut which, in part, explains hepatic encephalopathy following gastrointestinal bleeding in some patients with cirrhosis.

The early features of encephalopathy are irritability, lack of concentration, loss of interest and impaired memory. A coarse, slow flapping tremor of the outstretched hands may be the only sign at this stage, followed by confusion, drowsiness and coma. In addition to gastrointestinal bleeding, infection and injudicious prescribing of sedatives may all precipitate encephalopathy.

Osteoporosis and osteomalacia may develop in patients with chronic liver disease, causing bone pain and spontaneous fractures. Several factors are involved in the development of bone disease including poor diet, malabsorption and failure of the liver to convert vitamin D to active metabolites (*see* Chapter 12).

Viral hepatitis

The term 'viral hepatitis' refers to infections caused by at least four different viruses — hepatitis A (infectious hepatitis), hepatitis B (serum hepatitis) and non-A, non-B hepatitis, of which there are at least two kinds. The clinical illness caused by each virus is similar but can be differentiated by laboratory tests. Mild forms of hepatitis occur, without the patient appearing jaundiced, the diagnosis being made only if blood tests are done, by chance, during the illness.

The usual clinical picture of hepatitis begins with mild fever, nausea, upper abdominal discomfort and loss of appetite, lasting for 4–5 days before jaundice becomes clinically obvious, although urine tests (for urobilinogen) during this phase are positive. Once jaundice becomes apparent the nausea, abdominal pain and anorexia usually cease. The stool and urine are usually of normal colour. In a few patients, however, the fine radicles of the biliary tree are affected causing an obstructive picture. The severity of jaundice varies, although in most patients the colour fades within two weeks. Almost every patient goes on to make a complete recovery, only a few (usually virus-B, possibly non-A, non-B virus) progressing to chronic liver disease or acute fulminating hepatic failure.

Hepatitis A is endemic throughout the world and a high proportion of infected patients are asymptomatic. The usual incubation period is 28 days and the disease has a low mortality, patients being mildly incapacitated for a few weeks. There is no evidence of progression to chronic liver disease.

◄ The clinical illness due to infection with hepatitis virus A, virus B and virus non-A, non-B is similar

Hepatitis A is spread by the faecal-oral route and outbreaks occur where there is poor sanitation, with food and water contamination. Epidemics of infection occur in school children and their families; sporadic cases may follow eating raw and partly cooked shellfish. The diagnosis can be confirmed by finding hepatitis A antibody in the patient's plasma, the prevalence of which in healthy adults (blood donors) varies from 25 to 40% in countries such as Switzerland and U.S.A., and in excess of 90% in Israel and Yugoslavia. Carriers are not known.

Immunoglobulin may be given to prevent or attenuate the clinical illness; it has been given prophylactically. The virus has been grown in tissue culture and this major step provides the means of producing a killed or live vaccine.

◄ There is no evidence that hepatitis A virus infection progresses to chronic liver disease or is followed by a carrier state

Table 7.3.   Groups likely to develop hepatitis B or become a carrier

Patients requiring frequent blood products by transfusion or
    injection (haemophiliacs, some haemodialysis patients)
Long-stay patients (mental handicap)
Impaired immune mechanisms
    natural
    acquired (patients on steroids or azathioprine)
Staff of haemodialysis units or mental institutions
Drug abusers
Prostitutes
Homosexuals
Those from endemic areas (Africa and Asia)

Hepatitis B has its effects in every field of clinical practice, medical and dental, and is associated with progression to chronic active hepatitis, cirrhosis and, in some areas of the world, primary liver cancer. Incubation is 60–180 days. Infection may be followed by a persistent carrier state, particularly in residents of long-stay hospitals, patients requiring repeated transfusions of blood (or its products) such as the haemophiliac, those with immune deficiency, and patients on haemodialysis. The carrier state also occurs in drug abusers, homosexuals and prostitutes.

There are three serological markers of hepatitis B in the serum:

a. surface antigen — Australia antigen and later the surface antibody.
b. core antigen — located in the core of the virus (Dane particle).
c. E antigen — which correlates with number of virus particles in serum.

Carrier states may be detected, by persistence of surface antigen for more than six months, in 5–10% of those who have had a clinical infection.

Although originally thought to be transmitted only by blood transfusion, or its products, there is evidence that the virus is infective by mouth and that saliva, serous and urogenital discharges can be the source of infection. Transmission may result from accidental innoculation of minute amounts of blood during dental procedures or use of instruments that have become contaminated.

◀ Hepatitis B is infective by mouth and may also be spread by intimate contact and the sexual route

The clinical illness is often more serious with virus-B than virus-A. Massive necrosis leading to fulminating hepatic failure occurs in some patients and chronic hepatitis and cirrhosis develop in a few.

The disease can be controlled by hepatitis B immunoglobulin, which may also be given post-exposure following a single event or in haemodialysis units, when preventive hygienic measures cannot be implemented. Active immunization is possible with a killed vaccine, prepared from subunits of the surface antigen, which appears to be safe and effective.

Non-A, Non-B hepatitis virus infections usually follow transfusions of blood, or blood products, although sporadic cases occur. The illness is often subclinical, although a few fulminating cases have been described and there is a risk of chronic active hepatitis and cirrhosis.

A carrier state for non-A, non-B virus has been found but, unlike virus-B, clustering of cases in families has not. There is no evidence of transmission by personal contact or the sexual route. Short and long incubation period forms occur, which are probably due to at least two serologically different forms of the virus. A specific immunoglobulin is not yet available nor, since the virus has not been cultured, is a vaccine.

◀ Non-A, non-B hepatitis virus is not transmitted by personal contact, but a carrier state and progression to chronic hepatitis does occur

Chronic hepatitis

Chronic hepatitis is a chronic inflammatory reaction in the liver, continuing without improvement for six months or more. Two forms are recognized on the basis of histological appearances in the liver: chronic persistent hepatitis, a benign condition, and chronic active hepatitis, which may progress to cirrhosis, in which the architecture of the liver is distorted.

◄ Chronic persistent hepatitis is a benign condition but chronic active hepatitis often progresses to cirrhosis

Chronic persistent hepatitis may follow virus B and virus non-A, non-B infections; acute alcoholic liver damage; be associated with inflammatory bowel disease; and may be a chronic drug reaction to paracetamol, aspirin, methyldopa and other drugs. The patient usually has few symptoms other than fatigue, discomfort over the liver and alcohol intolerance. The diagnosis is sometimes made when hepatitis B antigen is found in the blood of a donor or during routine examination. The signs of chronic liver disease — spider naevi, palmar erythema and oedema — are not seen. Cirrhosis does not develop; since the prognosis is excellent, treatment is not necessary. However, some patients are a risk to the dentist and others because of the carrier state.

◄ Chronic persistent hepatitis may follow acute alcoholic hepatitis, occur with Crohn's disease, complicate methyldopa therapy and follow virus B hepatitis

Chronic active hepatitis may be associated with persistent hepatitis B virus infection and can follow non-A, non-B virus infection. The same clinical and histological picture follows hepatic drug reactions to methyldopa, isoniazid, paracetamol and other drugs; alcoholic hepatitis may also present the same features. In some patients, usually women at puberty and menopause, the cause is not known, but there are immunological changes and LE cells may be found in the blood; this type is called 'lupoid hepatitis'.

◄ Chronic active hepatitis may follow virus B and virus non-A, non-B hepatitis, complicate drugs including paracetamol, occur in alcoholics, and may be associated with LE cells in the peripheral blood

Hepatitis B antigen-positive chronic active hepatitis should be suspected in hospital staff who have contact with blood, homosexuals, drug abusers who share needles and syringes, and immigrants of African, Chinese and Mediterranean origin. The condition is sometimes diagnosed in apparently healthy individuals and rarely follows blood transfusion. Physical examination is usually normal, jaundice and features of liver failure developing late in the illness. The asymptomatic patient is treated only if there is biochemical evidence of progression, or worsening of the histological

◄ Hepatitis B antigen-positive chronic active hepatitis affects the 25–50 age group, particularly homosexuals, immigrants or those who have lived in China and Africa, and drug abusers

appearance after an interval of six months. Predniso-lone and azathioprine are sometimes given to induce immunosuppression, although there is no good evi-dence that this prevents progression to cirrhosis.

Alcoholic liver disease

In the U.K. alcohol accounts for 45–65% of all cirrhosis; in France and U.S.A. the incidence is probably higher. Females are more susceptible than men to a given alcohol intake. Non-cirrhotic liver damage due to alcohol is twice as common as cirrhosis.

Fat accumulation in the liver is the commonest effect of excessive alcohol consumption and represents metabolic overload, since ethanol cannot be stored; these changes are completely reversible. Cell damage by alcohol is idiosyncratic, dependent on the indi-vidual's response, which may be related to HLA

◀ Non-cirrhotic liver damage due to alcohol is twice as common as cirrhosis

◀ Although cell damage caused by alcohol is idiosyncratic there are 'safe' upper limits for alcohol consumption, being higher in the male

Table 7.4. Alcoholic liver damage

'Safe upper limits
    40 g/day males
    20 g/day females
(1 bottle spirits
    240 g alcohol)
Pathological changes in liver
    normal
    fatty change }Reversible
    acute hepatitis
    chronic hepatitis
    cirrhosis
    liver tumour (hepatoma)

Table 7.5. Alcohol withdrawal compared with encephalopathy and Wernicke's syndrome

	Withdrawal	*Encephalopathy*	*Wernicke's*
Consciousness	Alert	Drowsy	No change
Tremor	Fine, fast	Slow, flapping	Gross ataxia
Pulse	Fast	Normal rate	Fast
Anxiety	Yes	No	No
Speech	Fast, incoherent	Slurred	Slurred
Hallucination	Yes	No	Yes

Table 7.6. Alcohol abuse: signs and symptoms

Social
disruption of families
poor work performance, repeated job changes
frequent drunkenness
violent behaviour, towards spouse and children
repeated accidents
Neuropsychiatric
amnesic attacks
fits
tremulousness
night sweats
depression
loss of libido

antigens. Immunological mechanisms may also play a part in the development of cirrhosis.

The clinical features of alcoholic liver disease vary widely from the incidental finding of abnormal biochemical tests or liver enlargement to features of established cirrhosis. Dupuytren's contracture and parotid swelling may occur with both alcohol-induced fatty liver and cirrhosis. Jaundice can also be the presenting feature; the pattern being that of small bile vessel obstruction, haemolysis or hepatocellular damage. Ascites and bleeding from the gastrointestinal tract due to portal hypertension are sometimes the initial presentations. Neuropsychiatric disturbances also occur but it is important to differentiate hepatic encephalopathy from Wernicke's syndrome (due to vitamin B_1 deficiency) and the effects of alcohol withdrawal.

◀ Clinical features of alcoholic liver disease do not correspond with the degree of damage

Alcohol abuse

Recognition of alcohol abuse is important if anything is to be done to help patients control drinking habits. Even when cirrhosis is established, life expectancy can be prolonged by abstinence.

Apart from signs of chronic liver disease the other features that suggest alcohol abuse are behavioural, mental and physical changes. The abuser often causes family breakdown; has a poor work performance and frequent job changes; may be violent in behaviour, even to children; and is prone to frequent accidents. Episodes of amnesia, tremulousness, night sweating, loss of libido and seizures can be physical features of alcohol abuse.

Agencies such as local councils on alcoholism and Alcoholics Anonymous have much to offer both patient and family, in addition to regular follow-up by physicians or G.Ps. Re-education of the patient, particularly concerning his drinking habits, and rehabilitation with return to employment, if possible, are crucial.

Other damage caused by alcohol

Apart from the liver disease, other organs can be damaged by alcohol.

Neuropsychiatric manifestations are common including tremor of the outstretched hands and with intention, grand mal seizures and peripheral neuropathy. Grand mal seizures of late onset (40–60 years of age) are always regarded with suspicion if there are other features of alcohol abuse (*see* Chapter 11). Peripheral neuropathy affects the legs more often and

Table 7.7.   Alcoholic damage (other than hepatic)

Neuropsychiatric
     mixed sensory/motor peripheral neuropathy
     grand mal seizures
     tremor
     pre-senile dementia
     subdural haematoma following injury
Cardiac
     atrial fibrillation
     cardiomyopathy
     (vitamin B_1 deficiency — beri-beri)
GIT tract
     gastritis
     pancreatitis
     abdominal pain
     diarrhoea and malabsorption

severely than the arms and is usually of a mixed motor-sensory type, which can be so disabling as to prevent the patient from walking (*see* Chapter 11). Some patients have folic acid deficiency and in these there is improvement with folate supplements; in some patients damage seems to be due to a 'toxic' action of alcohol and recovery takes place, slowly, with total abstinence.

Mental changes, presenile dementia and encephalopathy due to vitamin deficiencies occur in some alcoholics. Because they are prone to accidents the incidence of subdural haematoma is high in alcoholics (*see* Chapter 11).

Alcohol can damage heart muscle (cardiomyopathy) and cause disturbances of cardiac rhythm presenting as heart failure. Other substances in alcoholic beverages (apart from ethanol), such as cobalt salts, can cause cardiac damage. Vitamin B_1 deficiency occurs in some alcoholics and may also result in cardiac failure.

Gastrointestinal complications of alcohol damage include gastritis, often mistaken for peptic ulcer, diarrhoea and malabsorption. Acute and chronic relapsing pancreatitis can also complicate alcohol abuse.

Cirrhosis of the liver

Apart from chronic active hepatitis and alcohol liver damage the other causes of hepatic cirrhosis in the U.K. are rare metabolic diseases: iron overload (haemochromatosis) or deposition of copper in the liver, as well as in the CNS (Wilson's disease). Protein malnutrition is a more important cause in under-developed countries. In many patients the cause is unknown (cryptogenic)

Cirrhosis can be suspected on clinical grounds because of numerous spider naevi, palmar erythema, fluid retention and jaundice but, ultimately, diagnosis depends on the histological demonstration of disturbed liver architecture. Liver biopsy may be impossible because of persistent coagulation defects.

The management of cirrhosis consists of treating the cause, where possible, and complications such as gastrointestinal haemorrhage, fluid retention, hepatic encephalopathy and disturbances of glucose metabolism. Haemochromatosis may be treated by regular venesection and iron chelating drugs (desferriox-amine); Wilson's disease by chelation of copper with penicillamine; and chronic active hepatitis with steroids and azathioprine.

The prognosis for cirrhosis depends on development of hepatic encephalopathy. Unless the episode is precipitated by an alcoholic debauch or gastrointestinal haemorrhage the patient survives six months or less after developing encephalopathy.

Obstructive jaundice

Impaired or absent biliary flow may be due to obstruction of the major bile ducts and of the finer radicles of the biliary tree. Jaundice is usually of gradual onset, associated with itching, pale stools and dark urine. The degree of jaundice can vary and there may be pain, due to gallstones, or weight loss with carcinoma of pancreas.

Apart from jaundice the other signs are scratch marks, pigmentation (in chronic cases) and bruising, or other evidence of easy bleeding.

Whatever the cause of biliary obstruction there are several important complications, which worsen as the period of obstruction lengthens. Gradual destruction of liver cells may occur with fibrosis and nodular regeneration — the changes of biliary cirrhosis. Bone disease (osteomalacia and osteoporosis) develops due to failure of absorption of vitamin D and impaired conversion to its metabolically active form. Bone pain and pathological fractures may occur; in a few, secondary hyperparathyroidism develops.

Table 7.8. Complications of obstructive jaundice

Liver cell damage — may progress to cirrhosis
Bleeding — failure of vitamin K absorption
Metabolic bone disease — vitamin D malabsorption
Repeated infections of biliary tract
Pigmentation (melanin)
Raised blood lipids (with xanthelasma)

Failure of vitamin K absorption impairs synthesis of several blood clotting factors with easy bruising and frank bleeding. Intramuscular and intravenous vitamin K_1 must be given prophylactically before surgery, however minor.

◀ Vitamin K_1 should be given to all patients with obstructive jaundice before any form of surgery

Two other complications of biliary obstruction are infection in the biliary tree, sometimes complicated by septicaemia, and secondary melanin pigmentation of the skin.

Precise diagnosis of the site of obstruction, using various imaging techniques, is essential before attempting surgical correction of the lesion. Surgery is needed for stones, strictures (usually following previous surgery for stone) and neoplasm of the biliary tree and pancreas. In addition to vitamin K therapy adequate hydration is ensured to prevent renal failure that can occur with biliary tract disease, possibly due to bacterial toxins. Intra-hepatic obstruction cannot be treated surgically and only supportive measures (injections of fat-soluble vitamins) are possible — except in viral hepatitis, when corticosteroids may be helpful.

◀ Biliary tree obstruction may be within the liver (due to cirrhosis, hepatitis and drugs) or extrahepatic (gallstones, carcinoma of pancreas or bileducts and pancreatitis)

Gallstones

It is estimated that between 10 and 15% of the adult population in U.K. have gallstones and in the younger patient they are twice as common in the female, particularly before the menopause. The stones may be formed of cholesterol (often solitary) or pigment (bilirubin); mixed forms occur (cholesterol, calcium and pigment).

Pigment stones in U.K. patients occur with chronic haemolytic anaemias, but in the Far East infection of bile and *Ascaris* worms have an important role. The pathogenesis of cholesterol-rich stones is less well understood but it is possible that changes in bile composition result in supersaturation and subsequent crystallization with stone formation.

◀ Colic and jaundice are symptoms of gallstones but fatty food intolerance, 'dyspepsia', burping and abdominal discomfort occur with equal frequency in patients with and without calculi

Jaundice and colic due to passage of a stone are the typical symptoms of cholelithiasis. Fatty food intolerance, 'dyspepsia', burping, vague abdominal discomfort and acid reflux into the mouth occur with equal frequency in patients with and without gallstones.

The diagnosis of stones is made by radiography and imaging techniques such as ultrasound. Up to 30% of gallstones are radio-opaque. Translucent stones are usually made of cholesterol.

Gallstones that do not cause symptoms are usually left untreated and in patients considered unfit for surgery (having radiolucent stones) a bile acid (CDCA), given orally over a period of months, may cause dissolution of the stone.

When stones impact in the lower biliary tree it may be possible to remove them using a fibreoptic instrument passed into the duodenum via the mouth. After cutting the sphincter around the duct calculus can be removed or crushed.

Gallstones causing jaundice, pain or acute inflammation of the gallbladder (cholectystitis) are usually treated surgically. Cholecystectomy is performed with great attention to the extrahepatic biliary system, which can be irreversibly damaged by the surgeon, leading to stricture or leaking of bile after the operation. The common bile duct is explored during operation if the patient has been jaundiced. Operation can be complicated by bile leak and by suppuration in the biliary tree.

Pancreatitis

Inflammation of the pancreas may be acute, show a relapsing course of acute symptoms, or it can be chronic.

Acute pancreatitis may complicate gallstones, drug therapy (steroids, diuretics, paracetamol) and alcohol abuse. The presenting features are acute abdominal pain, profuse vomiting and, in the severe or fulminating form, profound shock with renal failure and severe metabolic disturbances (electrolytes and calcium). The basic principles of management are treatment of shock, relief of pain and attempts to reduce pancreatic secretion, by emptying the stomach of acid through a naso-gastric tube. There is little place for surgical intervention, although laparotomy may be inadvertently performed in the mistaken diagnosis of perforated ulcer, cholecystitis or ruptured aortic aneurysm. The disease must also be differentiated from myocardial

◀ Up to half the cases of pancreatitis in U.K. are due to gallstones, whereas in U.S.A. and France alcohol abuse is a more important cause

infarction, intestinal strangulation or mesenteric arterial embolism, in patients with atrial fibrillation.

Chronic pancreatitis usually presents with repeated attacks of pain (some patients have none), weight loss, malabsorption and diabetes mellitus. It is usually related to alcohol abuse and gallstones, but may complicate hyperparathyroidism. Medical treatment consists of the management of acute attacks, insulin for diabetes, and correction of malabsorption by giving pancreatic enzymes with food. Surgery may be helpful for severe chronic pain, by relieving obstruction of pancreatic or bile ducts, removing the gland or the sympathetic nerve ganglia receiving pain fibres from the pancreas.

◀ Severe pain in chronic pancreatitis is difficult to treat and narcotic addiction is a real risk in such patients

Problems of hepatic diseases for the dentist

It is important that the dentist should recognize the patients who are likely to be carriers of hepatitis B. Haemophiliacs, patients on haemodialysis, drug addicts, patients who have recently been jaundiced, and those with impaired immunity are likely carriers and should be referred for screening tests before dental treatment is undertaken. Even so, 'high risk' patients are treated unknowingly by dentists.

If the patient is known to be a carrier the dentist and helpers should wear gloves, face masks and spectacles, and use disposable instruments. All syringes and needles used for local anaesthesia should be discarded and high-speed hand pieces should not be used.

Table 7.9. Management of 'high risk' carrier undergoing dental treatment

Dental surgeon and assistants should wear gloves
Use disposable instruments when possible
Wear face mask and spectacles
Treat patient at end of session
Avoid using high-speed drills
Dispose of needles and syringes used for LA or GA
Autoclave non-disposable instruments (formaldehyde for
    heat-sensitive instruments)
Wipe down all surfaces (chlorine)

Non-disposables should be sterilized immediately and all working surfaces wiped down with disinfectant solutions.

The prescribing of drugs for patients with liver disease can cause some problems for the dentist, in particular alterations in drug metabolism (conjugation and oxidation), as a result of which the individual may be excessively sensitive to sedatives and analgesics. Barbiturates, phenothiazines and benzodiazepines should be given with caution in patients with hepatic disease.

Table 7.10. Problems of drug prescribing in patients with hepatic disease

---

Drug transport
    reduced plasma protein increases free drug in plasma
    affects salicylates, anticoagulants, sulphonamides,
        hypoglycaemics and doxycyline. Small doses re-
        quired
Drug diffusion
    fluid retention increases volume of distribution
Drug metabolism
    oxidation impaired (propranolol)
    reduction impaired (corticosteroids)
    conjugation impaired (sulphonamides, barbiturates)
Drug elimination
    impaired if secreted in bile (rifampicin)
Alcoholic liver disease
    interaction between alcohol and drugs (barbiturates and
        benzodiazepines)

Reduced albumin concentration will affect the plasma levels of drugs that are carried by the protein in plasma; reduced doses of sulphonamides, doxycycline and salicylates are needed. Fluid retention affects the action of drugs because of altered distribution volumes. Impaired absorption of fat-soluble vitamins and some antibiotics can occur in patients with obstructive jaundice.

The patient with alcoholic liver disease provides the additional problems of poor compliance with prescriptions and altered brain sensitivity to certain drugs (opiates and benzodiazepines). Alcohol also interferes with drug metabolism, particularly the coumarin anticoagulants, benzodiazepines and barbiturates. The effects of short-acting barbiturates used for general anaesthesia are unpredictable in the alcoholic; the stage of excitement is enhanced in some patients.

Blood and reticulo-endothelial diseases

8

The formed elements of the blood comprise the red cells, white cells and platelets. From birth haemopoiesis is normally restricted, with the exception of lymphocytes, to the marrow of the long bones and flat bones (such as the pelvis and sternum).

Red blood cells (erythrocytes) are derived from the erythroblast series in the bone marrow, which, as they mature, acquire haemoglobin and lose their nucleus, by extrusion, before entering the circulation. Iron, folic acid, vitamins B_{12} and C, thyroxine and trace elements, such as cobalt, are essential for red cell production.

White blood cells (normal $3 \cdot 50\text{--}11 \cdot 8 \times 10^9$ cells/litre) belong to one of three series; the granulocytes, lymphocytes and monocytes. The cytoplasm of granulo-

Table 8.1.   Basic haematological investigations

Red cell count	$3 \cdot 8\text{--}5 \cdot 50 \times 10^{12}$ cells/litre
Packed cell volume (PCV)	$0 \cdot 35\text{--}0 \cdot 54$ (fraction of unity)
Haemoglobin concentration	$12 \cdot 0\text{--}16 \cdot 5$ g/decilitre
Mean corpuscular volume (MCV)	78–96 fl (femtolitre)
Mean corpuscular haemoglobin concentration (MCHC)	31–36 g/dl
Mean corpuscular haemoglobin (MCH)	32–36 pg (picogram)
White cell count	$3 \cdot 5\text{--}11.8 \times 10^9$ cells/litre
neutrophils	$1 \cdot 4\text{--}7 \cdot 8 \times 10^9$/litre (40–75%)
eosinophils	$0 \cdot 02\text{--}0 \cdot 12 \times 10^9$/litre (1–6%)
basophils	$0 \cdot 01\text{--}0 \cdot 02 \times 10^9$/litre (less than 1%)
lymphocytes	$1 \cdot 2\text{--}3 \cdot 5 \times 10^9$/litre (20–45%)
monocytes	$0 \cdot 2\text{--}0 \cdot 9 \times 10^9$/litre (2–10%)
Platelets	$150\text{--}350 \times 10^9$/litre

cytes contains granules that can be stained with dyes (haematoxylin and eosin), being derived from a common precursor, the myeloblast. The neutrophil granulocyte is the most abundant white cell (40–75% of the total); it is a phagocyte, ingesting and destroying bacteria and inflammatory tissue. Eosinophils (1–6% of total) also have a phagocytic function — consuming antigen–antibody complexes, and found especially in the mucosa of the respiratory and alimentary tract. Basophil granulocytes (less than 1% of total) play a role in antigen–antibody reactions.

Lymphocytes, the second most abundant white cell (20–45%), are, functionally, of two kinds — the B lymphocyte, responsible for antibody production, and the T lymphocyte, responsible for cell-mediated immunity. The two types of lymphocyte can be distinguished by their cell surface characteristics: B cells having surface immunoglobulin, T cells being capable of attachment to foreign cells (sheep erythrocytes). The thymus influences the maturation of T cells; B lymphocytes are dependent on the bone-marrow. Monocytes (2–10%), which appear like large lymphocytes, are phagocytes, scavenging all particulate matter.

Platelets are produced by giant cells (megakaryocytes) in the bone-marrow and usually number $120–400 \times 10^9$/litre. Their function is the early arrest of bleeding from damaged capillaries and small blood vessels.

Most blood cells have a short life in the circulation, platelets having a span of 8–14 days; granulocytes only 3–4 days; red cells 120 days; but some lymphocytes may survive in the blood for many years. Most cells are removed from circulation by the lymphoid tissue and spleen. Red cell haemoglobin is broken down to iron, protein and porphyrin; the latter being converted by a series of enzyme-controlled steps to bilirubin, which is excreted by the liver (*see* Chapter 7).

Anaemia

The normal haemoglobin concentration of blood is 12·0–16·5 g per decilitre and the red cell count

$3·80-5·50 \times 10^{12}$ cells/litre. When whole blood is spun down in a centrifuge cells occupy 35–54% of the total ($0·35-0·54$ expressed as fraction of unity, the usual reference value for packed cell volume or haematocrit).

From the haemoglobin concentration, red cell count and haematocrit certain indices are derived — mean corpuscular volume (MCV: 78–96 femtolitre), and mean corpuscular haemoglobin concentration (MCHC 31–36 g/decilitre). These indices are helpful in deciding the likely cause of anaemia.

Anaemia is a reduction of haemoglobin below the normal for the patient's age and sex. This may be due to reduction in red cell numbers and/or haemoglobin content. The symptoms of anaemia are similar whatever the cause: fatigue, lassitude, headache, faintness, breathlessness and palpitations. The similarity to the symptoms of heart disease is the result of change in cardiac function due to reduced oxygen-carrying capacity of the blood. Some patients have specific symptoms, such as paraesthesiae in the hands and feet (vitamin B_{12} deficiency) or difficulty with swallowing, due to an oesophageal web in some patients with iron deficiency. In other patients there may be gastrointestinal symptoms (dyspepsia or diarrhoea) due to the underlying cause for anaemia or there may be a history of frank, heavy blood loss (e.g. epistaxis, trauma or surgery).

◀ Symptoms due to anaemia are non-specific and similar to those of heart disease. Other symptoms are usually due to the underlying cause

In older patients, severe anaemia may precipitate heart failure and angina pectoris, particularly those with ischaemic or hypertensive heart disease. Reduced oxygen-carrying capacity can also precipitate symptoms of ischaemia in other parts of the body — claudication in the legs and transient stroke.

◀ Anaemia may precipitate the symptoms of cardiac ischaemia and heart failure, especially in the elderly and those with coronary and hypertensive heart disease

Table 8.2. Causes of iron deficiency

Increased physiological requirement — growth, menstruation, pregnancy
Pathological blood loss — uterine (menorrhagia), gastrointestinal loss
Nutritional defect — low iron diet, inhibitors in diet (eggs, alkalis, tea)
Malabsorption — coeliac disease etc., postgastrectomy, achlorhydria

Table 8.3. Causes of microcytosis

MCV less than 78 fl
    Iron deficiency
    Thalassaemia
    Rare — lead poisoning
    Rare — defect in haem synthesis (sideroblastic anaemia)

The most common anaemia in clinical practice is that due to *iron deficiency*, surveys showing a prevalence of 15–20% in women, during reproductive life, in Western Europe. The normal dietary requirement is very small, since only 1–2 mg of iron are lost each day, although there is a physiological increase in requirements during growth, menstruation and pregnancy.

◀ Iron deficiency anaemia occurs in 15–20% of women in reproductive life in European countries

Negative iron balance can develop because of increased physiological requirement, pathological loss (bleeding from bowel, uterus and kidneys), nutritional defect (poor diet and inhibitors in food) and failure of absorption (coeliac disease, post-gastrectomy). These factors deplete iron stores and, if the compensatory increase in small bowel absorption is exceeded, overt iron deficiency appears.

The characteristic haematological features of iron deficiency are reduced MCV and MCHC, the red cells appearing on microscopy to be smaller than normal (microcytic) and paler (hypochromic).

Special features in the history of iron deficiency are age (infants develop true nutritional deficiency); sex (females in the reproductive age range are particularly

Table 8.4. Causes of macrocytosis

MCV greater than 96 fl
    alcoholism
    liver disease
    hypothyroidism
    blood regeneration (following haemolysis or bleeding)
    myeloma
Commonest
    megaloblastic anaemia (vitamin B_{12} and folate
      deficiency, drugs)

prone); race (worm infestations being a common cause in Africans); diet (large amounts of cereals, tea and eggs or small consumption of meat and fish being contributory); drugs (aspirin, steroids and anti-rheumatics can cause blood loss); recent growth spurt; gastrointestinal symptoms; and urogenital complaints.

The tongue is smooth and atrophic in up to half the patients with overt iron deficiency, and angular stomatitis (usually in the edentulous) occurs in almost a quarter. Koilonychia occurs in up to 40% of patients but post-cricoid web formation due to mucosal atrophy in the pharynx occurs in less than one in ten.

◀ Smooth tongue, angular stomatitis (particularly in the edentulous), and nail changes may be present in patients with iron deficiency

History and examination usually give a clear indication of the cause of iron deficiency but, if no clues are found, further investigation of the whole gastro-intestinal tract is necessary. Discovery of the under-lying cause is essential to treatment, since prescribing iron does no more than treat symptoms.

Parenteral iron therapy (either intramuscular or intravenous) is rarely necessary except when rapid response is required such as in the later stages of pregnancy. Refractory iron deficiency suggests three alternatives, failure to take oral therapy, continuing blood loss or malabsorption.

Anaemia can occur in association with *chronic disorders*, particularly neoplasia, infection, renal disease and collagen disorders, such as rheumatoid arthritis and systemic lupus. The red cells are usually normal in size (normocytic; MCV normal) and stain normally (normochromic; normal MCHC). The possible mechanisms for this form of anaemia include shortened red cell survival, impaired bone-marrow response, defective iron transport and reduced erythro-poietin production by the kidney. The anaemia responds once the underlying illness has been success-fully treated.

◀ Most chronic illnesses such as infections, malignancy, renal disease, rheumatoid arthritis and other collagen diseases are accompanied by moderate anaemia

Deficiency of vitamin B_{12} and folic acid, as well as drugs that interfere with DNA replication (cytotoxic drugs), cause anaemia associated with change in the morphology of the bone-marrow erythroblast. These cells are larger than normal (megaloblasts) and circulating red cells are large (macrocytes), staining deeply (hyperchromia).

Megaloblastic anaemia due to vitamin B_{12} deficiency is rarely dietary (vegans). It may occur with coeliac

Table 8.5. Causes of vitamin B$_{12}$ deficiency

Inadequate intake
    vegans; some Asian women in pregnancy
Malabsorption
    lack of intrinsic factor (pernicious anaemia)
    total or partial gastrectomy
Small bowel disease
    Crohn's disease; removal of the terminal ileum
    stagnant contents (small bowel by-pass and diverticula)
    tapeworm (Finland fish tapeworm)

---

disease and Crohn's disease (*see* Chapter 6) but is usually due to pernicious anaemia, of autoimmune origin, in which gastric atrophy impairs intrinsic factor formation. Intrinsic factor (IF) is necessary for absorption of dietary vitamin B$_{12}$ by binding with it and facilitating uptake in the ileum.

Vitamin B$_{12}$ deficiency may follow partial gastrectomy. Failure of absorption occurs in spite of normal amounts of IF in coeliac disease, fish tape-worm infestations of the small bowel, bacterial overgrowth in the upper jejunum, and with drugs such as metformin (an oral hypoglycaemic agent) or anticonvulsants (primidone).

Apart from the symptoms of anaemia vitamin B$_{12}$ deficiency may present with paraesthesiae in hands and feet, difficulty in walking, and falling over in the dark — symptoms due to neuropathy and spinal cord involvement. Glossitis and angular cheilosis can cause discomfort before anaemia is severe. The tongue characteristically has a 'beefy' red, smooth, glazed appearance.

◀ The tongue in vitamin B$_{12}$ deficiency is characteristically 'beefy' red, smooth and glazed in appearance

◀ Paraesthesiae in the feet, difficulty in walking and falling over in the dark may be the symptoms of vitamin B$_{12}$ neurological damage

The skin has a lemon-yellow tint due to mild haemolytic jaundice. Purpura and bleeding due to thrombocytopenia occur less commonly.

The diagnosis of vitamin B$_{12}$ deficiency is made on the appearances of the blood film and bone-marrow, assay of its blood levels and measurements of absorption, using radioactive-labelled vitamin (Schilling test). After initial treatment with enough vitamin B$_{12}$ to correct anaemia and replenish stores, monthly maintenance doses are given indefinitely in patients

Table 8.6. Folate deficiency

Inadequate intake
    old age, poverty, alcoholism
Malabsorption
    coeliac disease
    Crohn's disease
Excess demands
    pregnancy and lactation
    malignant disease (myeloma)
    chronic disease (tuberculosis, rheumatoid arthritis)
    haemolysis (sickle cell disease, thalassaemia)
Drugs
    anticonvulsants, barbiturates
    alcohol
    ? the oral contraceptive

---

with pernicious anaemia. The underlying cause is treated in other cases, if possible.

Folate deficiency is usually the result of inadequate dietary intake in the poor, the elderly, those who live alone and in alcoholics. Fresh green vegetables and fruit, liver, yeast and nuts contain folic acid which is destroyed by overcooking. Folate deficiency may also occur in malabsorption states, when there is increased utilization (pregnancy), chronic haemolysis and inflammatory disorders. Drugs such as anticonvulsants, barbiturates, the oral contraceptive and trimethoprim can also cause folate deficiency, often in the context of a poor diet.

There are no specific symptoms or clinical features of folate deficiency, the diagnosis being made on the blood and bone-marrow appearances, confirmed by assay of serum and red cell folic acid.

Treatment of folate deficiency with 5 mg folic acid by mouth each day for four months is usually effective, but may have to be continued if the underlying cause is irreversible (e.g. Crohn's disease). Folic acid therapy can increase seizure frequency in epileptics treated with anticonvulsants.

Haemolytic anaemia occurs when the lifespan of red cells is so shortened that the bone-marrow cannot maintain normal numbers in the circulation. Premature red cell destruction occurs if there is abnormality of

◄ Inmates of institutions, old people living alone and alcoholics are particularly at risk of developing folate deficiency

Table 8.7. Causes of haemolytic anaemia

Genetically determined disorders
    spherocytosis
    haemoglobinopathies (HbS and thalassaemia)
    abnormal energy pathways — glucose-6-phosphate
      deficiency
Acquired disorders with antibodies to red cells
    haemolytic disease of newborn
    autoimmune anaemia — drugs, SLE, RA or viral
Acquired disorders without antibodies
    drugs
    infection
    renal failure

the cell membrane (spherocytosis is one example; damage by immunoglobulins in immune haemolytic anaemia is another); where there is excessive trauma (turbulence with prosthetic heart valves); and with physically abnormal haemoglobin (sickle cell disease and thalassaemia).

The clinical features of haemolysis differ according to cause although all patients have signs and symptoms of anaemia and mild jaundice. Some haemolytic disorders, particularly sickle cell disease, have periodic symptoms or 'crises', due to massive red cell destruction.

Glucose-6-phosphate deficiency is an X-chromosome-linked disorder with approximately 100 million affected individuals world wide. The deficient enzyme protects the red cell against damage caused by drugs with an oxidant action — sulphonamides, primaquine (an antimalarial) and phenacetin. Ingestion of the drug is followed by fever, malaise and passage of dark urine due to intravascular haemolysis. Similar episodes may follow the ingestion of fava beans (broad bean) in those from Mediterranean areas. The disorder is particularly common in Orientals and Greeks, sometimes presenting as jaundice in the neonatal period. The diagnosis is established by a simple enzyme assay. Affected individuals are advised to avoid provocative drugs and foodstuffs.

The sickling disorders occur because haemoglobin S differs from normal HbA such that during hypoxia its molecules form linear stacks which deform the red cell. The resultant sickle cell shape causes haemolysis, increased blood viscosity, small blood vessel occlusion, and tissue infarction. The heterozygous form (HbA and HbS; sickle cell trait) is asymptomatic unless the individual is exposed to marked hypoxia (e.g. during general anaesthesia and in unpressurized aircraft). The homozygous form (the individual receiving the gene for HbS from both parents) causes an incapacitating disease, due to chronic anaemia, from early life. The child develops a typical appearance with bossing of the skull, upper dorsal kyphosis and long limbs. Death occurs before the end of the second decade.

Crises may occur in both homozygote and heterozygote, taking several forms, although the most typical presentation is with severe back and limb pain, fever and prostration. Infarction of abdominal organs, lungs, brain and bones causes typical features with residual damage. These episodes can be related to infection, hypoxia and acidosis, sufferers having a particular susceptibility to pneumococcal and *Salmonella* infection. Crises can occur more frequently during pregnancy.

◄ Crises in sickle cell disease may be precipitated by infection, hypoxia and acidosis

Diagnosis depends on awareness that any patient of Afro-Asian origins may have the trait. A rapid screening test for sickling can be performed; the haematological values are often normal in the trait. It is essential to screen any susceptible patient undergoing general anaesthesia.

There is no specific treatment for sickle cell disease or any of the other haemoglobinopathies. Folic acid supplements and early treatment for infections are important, plus oxygen and rehydration during a crisis.

The thalassaemias are a group of genetic disorders of haemoglobin synthesis occurring predominantly in Mediterranean regions, the Middle and Far East. They have, however, been recognized in every racial group. The abnormalities occur in the globin peptide chains. The haematological features vary from severe anaemia with gross abnormalities of size and shape of red cells to mild iron deficiency, in those with small amounts of abnormal haemoglobin (persistence of the fetal form HbF; and HbA_2).

◄ Heterozygous forms of thalassaemia present with mild anaemia which becomes worse during pregnancy and with intercurrent illness

Red cell membrane abnormalities cause haemolysis as a result of increased fragility and destruction in the spleen. *Spherocytosis* is the most common of these disorders, being inherited as an autosomal dominant, presenting as haemolytic crises, gallstones and chronic leg ulcers.

Haemolysis due to antibodies against red cells can occur in the newborn (Rhesus haemolytic disease), with drugs (methyldopa and mefenamic acid), with lymphoma, chronic leukaemia, systemic lupus erythematosus, and infection with mycoplasma, measles or mumps. Severe anaemia may occur in acquired haemolytic disease but there are not specific features other than those of any underlying disorder.

A variety of diseases can be associated with haemolysis, without antibody formation, including liver disease, renal failure, infection (both protozoan, e.g. malaria, and bacterial) and malignancy (particularly stomach).

Red cells, granulocytes, monocytes and platelets are produced in the bone-marrow from a single parent cell (the 'uncommitted' stem cell) which can be damaged by chemicals or vitamin deficiencies as well as being affected by congenital disorders. The subsequent *aplastic anaemia* is due to reduction in bone-marrow cellularity with agranulocytosis, thrombocytopenia and a reduced monocyte count; the numbers of lymphocytes in peripheral blood are maintained or increased.

Aplastic anaemia may follow high-dose therapeutic radiation or cytotoxic drugs, given for leukaemia and disseminated malignancy. Other drugs may cause

Table 8.8.   Treatment of aplastic anaemia

General
    isolation
Transfusions
    red cells
    platelets, for clinical reasons, e.g. bleeding, not to
      increase the numbers
    white cells
Antibiotics
Prevention of infections
    usually endogenous (from skin and mouth)
    oral toilet, antiseptic and antifungal mouth washes
Androgens and corticosteroids

bone-marrow damage (chloramphenicol and phenyl-butazone) as well as benzene and other chemicals, including DDT. Hepatitis B may, occasionally, be complicated by severe anaemia.

The usual presenting feature of bone-marrow aplasia is a bleeding tendency with frank haemorrhage or purpura. Bacterial and fungal infection occurs frequently, particularly in the mouth, and is an important cause of mortality; it can be the presenting feature. The commonest cause of death is bleeding.

◄ Aplastic anaemia usually presents as a frank bleeding tendency

The primary aim of treatment of aplastic anaemia is to keep the patient alive until spontaneous recovery occurs or bone-marrow transplantation can be carried out. Severe agranulocytosis necessitates isolation in special units to prevent infection. Red cell, platelet and white cell transfusions, as well as steroids and anabolic hormones, have been tried with variable success.

Myeloproliferative diseases

Proliferation of the precursor cells in the bone-marrow causes a group of diseases called 'myeloproliferative disorders'. Although proliferation of red cell, platelet, leucocyte and fibroblast precursors results in distinct disease entities, there are features in common and transition from one form to another occurs.

Polycythaemia rubra vera (PRV) is a chronic condition in which there is over-production of red cells

Table 8.9. Polycythaemia

Primary		
Secondary		
	hypoxia	high altitude
		congenital heart disease
		chronic pulmonary disease
	tumours	renal carcinoma, cysts,
		hydronephrosis
		bronchogenic carcinoma
	stress and dehydration (relative rather than true	
		polycythaemia)

causing an increase in haematocrit. Diagnosis depends on exclusion of polycythaemia secondary to chronic hypoxaemia, stress and dehydration.

PRV may be asymptomatic but commonly presents with headaches, dyspnoea, dyspepsia, flatulence and bleeding episodes (epistaxis and gastrointestinal haemorrhage). Symptoms of vascular insufficiency (visual disturbances and claudication) are common and itching may follow a bath. Gout occurs in PRV and secondary polycythaemia.

PRV can be treated by repeated venesection, which eventually causes iron deficiency with sore tongue and angular stomatitis; with cytotoxic drugs; and with radioactive phosphorus (^{32}P). Transformation to chronic myeloid leukaemia and myelofibrosis occurs, although death is usually due to vascular complications or haemorrhage.

Myelofibrosis is the result of proliferation of fibroblast precursors in the bone-marrow, blood-forming cells being replaced by fibrous tissue. The usual presentation is as anaemia, weakness and abdominal pain due to giant splenic enlargement. The patient may be known to have previously had or been treated for PRV. There may be purpura due to thrombocytopenia. There is no satisfactory treatment for the disease, which usually follows a progressive course over 3–5 years. Frequent blood transfusions are needed. Terminally, there may be transformation to chronic myeloid leukaemia.

Essential thrombocythaemia is a rare disorder in which, despite very high platelet counts, there is a bleeding tendency, usually from the gastrointestinal tract. Purpura is rare, however, and episodes of thrombosis may occur.

◄ Polycythaemia rubra vera presents with a wide variety of symptoms, few of which are due to altered blood viscosity

The leukaemias

The leukaemias are disorders of white cell production characterized by abnormal and excessive proliferation of leucoblasts, leading to increase in the number of white cells in the peripheral blood. Excessive leucoblast proliferation leads to anaemia, agranulocytosis and thrombocytopenia; death is usually due to infection or haemorrhage.

Table 8.10.   Diagnosis of acute leukaemia

History
    short, multiple symptoms which may mimic other
        diseases
Signs
    anaemia, haemorrhage, infection
    tissue infiltration: gums and skin: particularly AML
    enlarged lymph nodes, hepatosplenomegaly, sometimes
        testes (ALL)
Peripheral blood
    blast cells
Bone-marrow
    essential for diagnosis and assessing remission

The leukaemias are conventionally classified as 'acute' and 'chronic' according to the speed of onset and the appearance in the peripheral blood of blast cells. Chronic leukaemias are more insidious and may sometimes be diagnosed by chance blood counts; they are also typified by few blast cells in the peripheral blood except in the terminal phase.

Acute leukaemia is classified according to the proliferating cell line, lymphoblastic (ALL), myeloblastic (AML) and monocytic. The clinical features are similar in all three although enlargement of lymph nodes is more typical of lymphoblastic leukaemia. Onset may be acute or insidious and may mimic other conditions, particularly acute viral infections and infectious mononucleosis. There may be a vague history of a 'flu-like' illness with fever, malaise and symptoms of anaemia. Spontaneous bleeding may occur from the gums with purpura; throat and mouth ulceration occurs, which may be complicated by systemic infection. Although primarily a disease of bone-marrow or lymphatic tissue other organs may be infiltrated, including the gums, skin, nervous system and, occasionally, bone.

The presence of large numbers of blast cells in the peripheral blood confirms the diagnosis, although a bone-marrow biopsy is essential. There is usually a normochromic, normocytic anaemia, thrombocytopenia, and a variable white cell count from 5 to 100 $\times$ 10^9 cells/litre (90% blast and other immature cells).

Acute lymphoblastic leukaemia frequently infiltrates the CNS and treatment involves not only attempts to induce remission with combination drug therapy (e.g. vincristine, prednisolone and doxorubicin) but also cranial irradiation and injections of methotrexate into the CSF. Maintenance combination therapy is essential, consisting of methotrexate and mercaptopurine. These principles of management have achieved marked improvement in duration of complete remission in specialized children's units.

Acute myelogenous leukaemia has a poorer prognosis, since the specific antileukaemic effect of the drugs available to treat the condition is small. Combinations of drugs, such as daunorubicin and arabinoside C, may achieve remission. Supportive therapy with blood transfusion, control of infection, treatment of haemorrhagic tendency, and correction of electrolyte problems may be necessary. Attempts to boost the patient's own defence mechanisms are sometimes used when chemotherapy has failed. Bacterial antigens, such as BCG, and the patient's own irradiated leukaemic cells may prolong the survival, which is normally less than one year.

Chronic lymphatic leukaemia (CLL) is characterized by a progressive accumulation of malignant lymphocytes in the lymphatic and reticular systems with a steady rise in lymphocytes in blood and bone-marrow.

The disease occurs in the later years of life, affecting men more often than women, being asymptomatic in up to 15%. Symptoms are insidious in onset with fever and weight loss. There may be anaemia, thrombocytopenia and infections. The lymph nodes are often markedly enlarged and there may be infiltration of the skin. Antibody production is impaired in patients with CLL and they are prone to bacterial and viral infections (*see* Chapter 17).

The diagnosis is confirmed by blood count (total numbers may exceed 1000×10^9/litre) and bone-marrow smear. Treatment is delayed until the patient has symptoms when chemotherapy (mustine, chlorambucil or cyclophosphamide), radiotherapy or corticosteroids may be given. The overall prognosis for CLL is good, 50% of patients surviving 5 years; some for 15–20 years until they die of an unrelated disease.

◄ More than half the children with ALL will be alive and well 5 years after diagnosis

◄ AML has a more acute onset than ALL, occurring in an older age group and having a poorer prognosis

◄ CLL is often asymptomatic, being discovered because of enlarged lymph nodes or an abnormal blood count

Chronic myeloid leukaemia (CML) is also more common in males but occurs in a younger age group; a childhood variant also occurs. The presenting features are usually due to anaemia or marked splenic enlargement, with abdominal pain and distension. Haemorrhage may occur due to thrombocytopenia; gout can be a complication.

Diagnosis is made on the appearances of blood and bone-marrow; cytogenetic studies of the white cells sometimes showing a characteristic chromosome (Philadelphia). Treatment usually consists of chemotherapy (busulphan, hydroxyurea), radiation to the spleen and, in a few patients during remission, an elective splenectomy. The quality of life is improved by these measures but survival is not greatly prolonged, death occurring from haemorrhage, infection or a terminal transformation to acute myelogenous leukaemia.

◀ Treatment of CML improves the quality of life but does not significantly prolong the survival

Agranulocytosis

Failure of granulocyte production by the bone-marrow may occur as an isolated disorder or, more commonly, in association with failure of red cell and platelet production (pancytopenia). Agranulocytosis is most often due to drug therapy (chloramphenicol, phenylbutazone, oxyphenbutazone and amidopyrine) but may follow virus infections (hepatitis B). Certain chemicals (benzene) and irradiation may also cause agranulocytosis although usually as part of pancytopenia.

◀ Agranulocytosis is usually due to drug therapy

Fever, throat and mouth ulcers with pyogenic and fungal infections are the typical presenting features. The diagnosis is made on blood and bone-marrow appearances, the latter being difficult to obtain.

There is no satisfactory treatment for agranulocytosis; corticosteroids, white cell transfusions, folic acid and anabolic steroids having been used with varying success. Prevention of infection is a most important part of general treatment by skin sterilization and frequent mouth washes with antiseptic and antifungal agents. The patient is best managed at home or in isolation.

◀ Agranulocytosis and aplastic anaemia may be difficult to differentiate in some cases from AML, myelosclerosis and bone-marrow infiltration by carcinoma

Haemorrhagic diseases

Patients with severe haemostatic defects bleed excessively and spontaneously and do not present a major
diagnostic problem. Mild defects, however, may only
be unmasked by trauma, such as dental extraction,
when there may be difficulty in deciding whether the
bleeding is the result of generalized haemostatic
disorder or local problems.

Bleeding following trauma is controlled by three
inter-related factors (*Fig.* 8.1):

   a. The reaction of the blood vessel to injury.
   b. Formation of a platelet plug at the site of injury.
   c. Coagulation of blood.

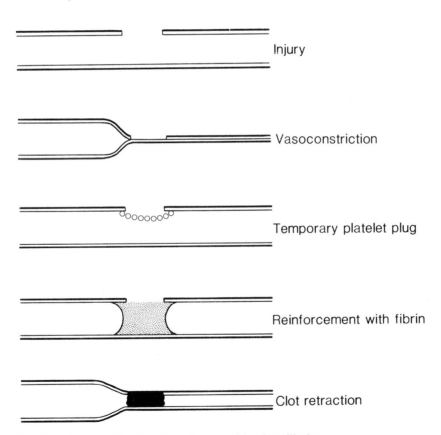

Fig. 8.1. Arrest of bleeding from damaged blood capillaries.

When a blood vessel is severed there is, initially, vasoconstriction; platelets adhere to the subendothelial connective tissue so as to form an unstable plug, which is made firm, within a few minutes of injury, by fibrin.

Blood coagulation is a series of complex steps resulting in the formation of a fibrin clot. Activation of the process may occur through intrinsic or extrinsic pathways, the latter being faster and stimulated *in vivo* by damaged endothelium and extravascular tissues. Clotting by the intrinsic pathway begins with activation of a circulating factor (XII) by foreign surfaces, such as a prosthetic heart valve and the subendothelial layers of blood vessels.

Abnormal bleeding may be caused by —
a. Defective blood vessels
b. Thrombocytopenia
c. Abnormality of platelet function
d. Defects in blood coagulation
e. Excessive breakdown of fibrin (fibrinolysis).

Acquired defects are more common in clinical practice.

A generalized haemostatic defect can present as bleeding from multiple sites or spontaneously including purpura, haematomas, large bruises and haemorrhage into joints (haemarthroses). Coagulation defects pre-

◀ In coagulation defects the bleeding time is normal but the *in vitro* clotting time is prolonged

Table 8.11.   Blood coagulation

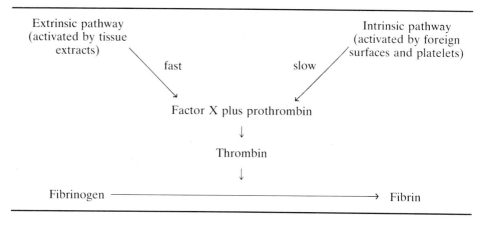

sent with joint, muscle and gastrointestinal haemorrhage; platelet/capillary defects with skin, nose and
uterine bleeding.

Inherited disorders present in infancy and childhood
(although haemophilia may first be diagnosed at or
beyond the age of 50). There is usually a story of
bleeding with trauma, previous operations or dental
extractions. A positive history of family bleeding
disorder suggests an inherited haemostatic defect.
Careful history-taking normally helps to decide
whether a bleeding disorder is congenital or acquired.

Bleeding due to vascular disorders, thrombocytopenia or platelet dysfunction starts within seconds
of injury and continues for hours; recurrence is uncommon once it has stopped. Post-traumatic bleeding
in coagulation defects can be delayed, sometimes
by several hours, and recur during the subsequent four
or five days.

◄ Thrombocytopenia
and vascular disorders
present with prolonged
bleeding time but clotting
time is normal

Precise diagnosis of a generalized bleeding disorder
depends on laboratory tests including bleeding time,
platelet count, prothrombin time, clotting time and,
where suspected, assay of the coagulation factors and
tests of platelet function.

Table 8.12.   Clinical features of coagulation defects and platelet/capillary disorders

	Coagulation defects	*Platelet/capillary defect*
Bleeding from cuts and scratches	Uncommon, not severe	Usually profuse
Bruising	Large	Usually small
Bleeding into joints	In severely affected patients	Rare
Nose bleeding	Unusual	Common
Gastrointestinal bleeding	Rare unless patient has peptic ulcer	Common
Blood in urine	Common	Not usual
Bleeding after surgery (including dental extraction)	Delayed up to 12 hours	Immediate, at the time of surgery
Effect of pressure at bleeding site	No effect on bleeding	Controlled by pressure

Vascular defects causing abnormal bleeding

Vascular disorders present with easy bruising and spontaneous bleeding, the underlying defect being either in the vessels themselves or in the connective tissue supporting them. A diagnosis of vascular defect is made after thrombocytopenia and platelet function defects have been excluded.

The most common inherited vascular disorder causing abnormal bleeding is *hereditary telangiectasia*, characterized by multiple capillary and arteriolar dilatations in mucous membranes (nose and mouth) and skin. Bleeding usually begins in early adult life and becomes progressively worse, since the lesions become more numerous with age. There is no treatment other than local measures (pressure and cautery) and oestrogens, which act by causing squamous metaplasia of the mucosa.

◄ The dilated blood vessels of hereditary telangiectasia blanch on pressure and become larger and more numerous with age

Acquired vascular defects causing bleeding include senile purpura (mainly on extensor surfaces of the arms and due to changes in connective tissue with age), scurvy, Cushing's disease, corticosteroids, other drugs and infections.

Thrombocytopenia

Decreased platelet production, increased destruction, and pooling in an enlarged spleen result in thrombocytopenia which presents with easy bleeding, purpura, epistaxis and uterine bleeding, heavy enough to cause

Table 8.13.   Thrombocytopenia

Failure of production
    bone-marrow aplasia
    drugs and chemicals
    marrow infiltration (carcinoma, myeloma)
    megaloblastic anaemia
Reduced survival of platelets
    idiopathic thrombocytopenic purpura
    acute infections
    SLE
    drug sensitivity
Platelet pooling in an enlarged spleen

anaemia. Thrombocytopenia may be acute, chronic or induced by drugs.

Acute thrombocytopenia in children is often related to preceding infection (rubella). The onset of purpura, bruising and bleeding is sudden. Although the mechanism is not clearly understood, it is thought that platelets are destroyed by antigen–antibody complexes. The condition is self-limiting.

Chronic thrombocytopenia is often primary (idiopathic thrombocytopenic purpura, ITP) but may be secondary to systemic lupus, Hodgkin's disease and CLL. In ITP platelets are coated with autoantibody, being destroyed in liver and spleen. Symptoms are more gradual in onset, iron deficiency anaemia occurring in the female especially, because of heavy uterine bleeding.

Steroids may increase the platelet count temporarily but in nearly 70% splenectomy is necessary. After a symptom-free interval of several years, signs of systemic lupus appear in some patients (*see* Chapter 12).

Drug-induced thrombocytopenia occurs as the result of combination with plasma proteins to form an antigen and subsequent antibody formation. Antigen–antibody complexes attach to platelets causing their destruction. Recovery follows withdrawal of the drug with the platelet count rising within 1–2 weeks. Steroids may be required if bleeding is severe.

Excessive bleeding in spite of normal or increased numbers of platelets suggests a disorder of function, which may be inherited or acquired. Failure of ADP production by platelets is one example of inherited functional disorder. Acquired defects occur in patients taking aspirin, with myeloproliferative disorders or renal failure.

Coagulation disorders

Inherited deficiency of each of the coagulation factors has been described, but in clinical practice only haemophilia (A and B) and von Willebrand's disease are important numerically, and these are still relatively rare. Haemophilia A is about five times more common than B and both are transmitted as sex-linked recessive traits. Von Willebrand's disease is transmitted as an autosomal dominant. Other inherited coagulation disorders are thought to be autosomal recessive.

Haemophilia A results from synthesis of an abnormal factor VIII (antihaemophilic globulin: AHG) with reduced biological activity. Severely affected patients bleed heavily and spontaneously, whilst those moderately affected may not bleed except following surgery or trauma.

Characteristically, bleeding in severe haemophilia occurs into muscles and joints, the latter leading to permanent crippling because of fibrous ankylosis, unless treated promptly. Post-traumatic bleeding presents as large, spreading haematomas which can compress structures such as nerves, blood vessels, even the airways in the neck and mediastinum.

Treatment is given when bleeding occurs or operation contemplated, but the general principles of management of a life-long disability are avoidance of injury, with social and psychological care. The defect is treated by intravenous injections of factor VIII concentrates, the amount given varying according to whether bleeding is spontaneous (AHG given to achieve a plasma level 20% of normal) or surgery is contemplated (factor VIII increased to 50% of normal). Many sufferers now treat themselves with factor VIII concentrates as soon as bleeding is suspected, which has, in recent years, reduced the incidence of haemarthrosis and need for hospital admission.

Haemophilia B is due to impaired production of factor IX (Christmas factor), causing a similar but milder bleeding tendency. Factor VIII concentrates also are effective in controlling bleeding and preparing

◀ Factor VIII concentrate is given when bleeding occurs in haemophilia A or when surgery is contemplated

Table 8.14.   Factor VIII (AHG) levels and severity of bleeding level (% of normal)

50–100	No bleeding manifestations
25–50	Bleeding excessively after serious accidents and major surgery
5–25	Excessive bleeding after dental extractions
1–5	Sometimes bleed spontaneously
0	Bleeding with trivial injury and spontaneously into joints and muscles

Table 8.15.   Blood products used to treat haemophilia

Fresh whole blood
Fresh frozen plasma
Cryoprecipitate
Frozen — dried human AHG
Frozen — dried animal AHG (bovine and porcine)

patients for surgery. Factor IX is not thermolabile, unlike factor VIII, and patients suffering from haemophilia B can be treated with stored whole blood, although this is avoided because of the risk of minor blood group incompatibility.

Von Willebrand's disease is characterized by a prolonged bleeding as well as prolonged clotting time. In addition to a low factor VIII level there is a defect in platelet function. It appears that reduced factor VIII production is responsible for the abnormal platelet function. The disease, which occurs in both sexes, causes a mild bleeding tendency and is treated by infusion of factor VIII concentrates.

◄ Von Willebrand's disease is associated with a prolonged bleeding time and a mild coagulation defect

Acquired coagulation disorders are more common in clinical practice, being due to multiple clotting factor deficiencies. The most frequent is vitamin K deficiency, causing impaired synthesis of several coagulation factors by the liver. Because vitamin K is fat-soluble, deficiency can occur with malabsorption (coeliac disease etc.), potentiated by antibiotics. Bile salts are essential for fat absorption and vitamin K deficiency with bleeding disorder can occur in patients with biliary tract obstruction (*see* Chapter 7). Intramuscular or intravenous vitamin K_1 corrects the problem.

Derangement of the coagulation mechanism is common in patients with liver disease and is partly due to defective synthesis of clotting factors. Thrombocytopenia also occurs with portal hypertension because of splenic pooling of platelets. A third factor is increased fibrinolytic activity. Bleeding with liver disease is usually mild to moderate, sometimes called 'pseudo-haemophilia'. Severe haemorrhage may occur from oesophageal varices and in patients in the terminal phase of liver disease. Vitamin K_1 corrects the coagulation defect in part, but fresh frozen plasma and

◄ Bleeding in liver disease is due to defective synthesis of several clotting factors and thrombocytopenia, in some cases anti-fibrinolytic agents may be needed to prepare the patient for surgery.

Patients *on anticoagulant therapy* may require dental treatment and can pose problems for the dentist. The important principles of management of these patients is to ensure proper haemostasis by use of sutures and to avoid, if possible, any change in anticoagulation, unless a prothrombin time measured before treatment is excessively prolonged (more than twice control values). There is no indication for reversal of anticoagulant effect with vitamin K, nor any adjustment of dose, unless the patient is advised by the anticoagulant clinic. Reversal of anticoagulation in patients with heart disease and prosthetic valves can result in fresh thrombus, complicated by embolism or interference with prosthesis function.

Multiple myeloma

Multiple myeloma is a disseminated malignancy of plasma cells occurring in the middle aged and elderly. The disease causes bone destruction, marrow failure and excess production of immunoglobulins.

The commonest presenting symptom is bone pain, most often in the thoracic and lumbar spine, but occasionally in the ribs, limb girdles and mandible. Pathological fractures can occur in the ribs and spine causing truncal pain and neurological symptoms if there is spinal cord compression. Anaemia, thrombocytopenia and agranulocytosis develop because of plasma cell infiltration of the bone-marrow predisposing to bleeding and infection. The predisposition to infection is also due to impaired production of normal immunoglobulins.

◄ Bone pain and pathological fracture is the commonest presenting symptom of myeloma

Renal failure occurs in patients with myeloma for several reasons including renal rubular damage caused by small proteins, raised serum calcium and uric acid, and infection.

The diagnosis of myeloma is made on the basis of excess plasma cells in bone-marrow smears, an abnormal immunoglobulin in the blood, and evidence of bone destruction. Treatment consists of chemotherapy, with radiation therapy, corticosteroids, and drugs to reduce raised serum calcium and uric acid. Phenylalanine mustard (melphalan), vincristine and cyclophosphamide are each effective in achieving and prolonging remission.

Localized plasma cell neoplasms can occur either in association with multiple myeloma or in patients without abnormal immunoglobulin production. The usual presentation is as a polypoid or sessile mass in the soft tissues of the nose and upper respiratory tract, mouth or pharynx; more than one tumour may occur at the same time. Treatment consists of local radiotherapy and that for the multiple myeloma, if present.

◄ Localized plasma-cytoma is an indolent form of myeloma presenting as a swelling in the mouth, pharynx, upper and lower respiratory tract

The lymphomas

Hodgkin's disease

Hodgkin's disease is a malignant disease of the lympho-reticular system in which there is steady, progressive involvement of lymphatic sites and eventual infiltration of other organs (liver, lung and bone-marrow). The disease can occur in any age group and is more common in men.

◄ The usual presentation of Hodgkin's lymphoma is as painless cervical lymphadenopathy

The usual presentation is as painless cervical lymphadenopathy, although any nodes may be affected. Occasionally the initial lymphatic enlargement is in the mediastinum, liver or spleen. Very rarely extra-lymphatic deposits in the dura, lungs and skin are the initial presentation. Systemic symptoms including fever, sweating, weight loss, malaise and pruritus follow the appearance of enlarged nodes. Anaemia, purpura and jaundice may develop later in the illness.

Diagnosis is made by lymph node biopsy. The extent of the disease must be established, since this will dictate the subsequent treatment and gives some idea as to prognosis.

Involvement of a single lymph node group (stage I) or two or more groups on the same side of the diaphragm (stage II) are treated by irradiation, which achieves 5-year survival rates in excess of 80%. Radiation damage to the lungs, pericardium, kidneys, bowel and spinal cord can follow but is rare.

When lymph nodes on both sides of the diaphragm are involved (stage III) or when there is disseminated involvement of more than one extra-lymphatic site (stage IV), patients are treated with combination chemotherapy, consisting of steroids and cytotoxic drugs, in six courses over a period of 6 months. Five-year survival rates of 75% can be achieved in this way and it is possible that a proportion of these patients will be cured.

Non-Hodgkin lymphoma

These lymphomas include those previously classified as lymphosarcoma, reticulum cell sarcoma, giant follicular lymphoma etc. They resemble Hodgkin's disease clinically, but do not have the same histological appearances, nor do they follow the same progression. They may occur in various sites such as the gastro-intestinal tract and CNS.

Accurate histological diagnosis is important in deciding treatment and prognosis. Multiple drug régimes are of benefit in some patients whereas others need to be managed in the same way as for acute leukaemia.

◄ Five-year survivals in excess of 70% are achieved by combination chemotherapy in patients with Hodgkin's lymphoma

Thyroid disorders and disturbances of calcium metabolism are the most common endocrine problems encountered in clinical practice and have some importance for dentists. Rarer endocrine disturbances that have important features for the dentist are acromegaly and adrenal disorders, particularly hypoadrenalism (Addison's disease).

All endocrine glands secrete hormones into the blood flowing through them. Hormones have effects on cells in distant organs in the body and their release is controlled by a process of negative feedback. The hormones control the development and metabolic activity of the 'target organs'.

The gonads, thyroid and adrenal cortex are largely under the control of the anterior pituitary gland which, in turn, is controlled by peptides released from the hypothalamus into the hypothalamic-pituitary portal veins. Negative feedback is via the hypothalamus which responds to variations in blood hormone levels.

Many hormones can be assayed by biological or chemical means; these are essential for optimal management of endocrine diseases and can be used in screening programmes (diagnosis of neonatal hypothyroidism). Fasting, drug therapy, intercurrent illness, time of day and, in the female, the menstrual cycle are among the factors that affect hormone levels.

Certain symptoms suggest that a patient is suffering from endocrine disorder. Tiredness may have an endocrine basis and usually worsens throughout the day unlike non-organically caused tiredness which is more pronounced earlier in the day. Adrenal, pituitary and thyroid disorders can cause tiredness.

◀ Tiredness of recent origin which worsens during the day should suggest an organic cause

Weight loss may be due to many other disorders, such as occult carcinoma, pulmonary tuberculosis and malabsorption, but it occurs in many patients with diabetes mellitus, adrenal insufficiency, hyperthyroidism and anorexia nervosa, although the latter is a disorder with secondary endocrine dysfunction. Obesity may also have an endocrine basis, but being overweight is usually the primary problem. Weight gain may occur secondary to hypothyroidism, Cushing's syndrome, ovarian cysts and hypogonadism.

Delay in puberty may be due to endocrine disease, although non-endocrine disease such as malabsorption and chromosome disorders can also be responsible. In most cases there is no clear cause for the problem, particularly where there is a family history of delayed puberty. Juvenile hypothyroidism, Cushing's syndrome and pituitary failure due to tumour may all interfere with puberty.

◀ The patient who complains of being overweight has seldom been found to have an endocrine cause

Thyroid diseases

Goitre

The term 'goitre' is used to describe any enlargement of the thyroid. It occurs four times more frequently in women, particularly during puberty and pregnancy. Goitres in the younger patient are usually diffuse; in the older patient, again particularly in the female, the enlargement is irregular, or nodular.

The patient or a relative may notice a goitre or it may be noted incidentally by a health-care professional,

Table 9.1.　Causes of goitre

Iodine deficiency
Idiopathic
Physiological — puberty
　　　　　　 — pregnancy
Graves' disease
Hashimoto's disease
Drugs and foodstuffs causing enlargement (goitrogens)
Thyroiditis
Disturbances of thyroid hormone synthesis
Tumours

such as a dentist. A brief history should be taken to assess whether the gland is under- or over-active and whether the enlargement has been rapid, a feature of malignancy. Drugs can cause goitre, particularly cough medicines, and there may be a family history of enlarged glands.

Most patients with goitre have no evidence of systemic disorder but some show signs of hyperthyroidism. Goitre is not an invariable feature of hypothyroidism. Tender goitres may indicate thyroiditis or anaplastic carcinoma, and lymph node enlargement in the neck suggests malignancy. Solitary nodules may be benign or malignant, clinical examination being of little help in making the distinction. Large multinodular goitres may extend behind the sternum and can, occasionally, be wholly retrosternal, causing compression of the trachea with stridor and wheezing; the jugular veins may be distended but not pulsatile. Hoarseness associated with goitre is an important sign indicating recurrent laryngeal nerve paralysis, a feature of malignancy, unless there has been previous operative damage.

Investigation of goitre includes tests to determine the level of thyroid function and the cause of the enlargement, including thyroid autoantibodies, thyroid radioisotope scanning, radiokinetic studies of function and thyroid biopsy.

Management of goitre depends on cause; goitre with thyroid dysfunction requiring treatment to achieve euthyroidism (normal levels of serum thyroid hormones); *euthyroid diffuse goitre* usually requires no therapy except when it is very large and cosmetically embarrassing, when thyroxine will reduce the size after several months' treatment. The *euthyroid multinodular goitre* may also be treated by thyroxine but this is successful in less than a third and surgery is often recommended, although the nodules may reappear in the remnant. The *solitary nodule* is usually treated by surgical exploration and, if a papillary or follicular carcinoma is found, total thyroidectomy is followed by radioiodine ablation. Poorly differentiated carcinoma is usually treated by radioiodine therapy and has a poor prognosis; medullary carcinoma is also treated by total thyroidectomy and investigation performed to find possible associated parathyroid and adrenal tumours. Finally, *thyroiditis*, if painful, is usually treated with

◄ Rapid enlargement of the gland, weakness of voice and unilateral pain extending up to the ear are features that suggest thyroid cancer

◄ Medullary carcinoma of thyroid may be associated with neurinomas on the lips, in the mouth or on the eyelids

steroids for a few weeks; other forms are treated with thyroxine.

Hyperthyroidism

Hyperthyroidism or thyrotoxicosis results from an excess of circulating thyroid hormone(s) (T4 — thyroxine — and/or T3 — triiodothyronine) and arising either from diffuse hyperplasia and hypertrophy of the gland (Graves' disease) or from single or multiple 'toxic' nodules of the thyroid (Plummer's disease). Thyroiditis may also be associated with hyperthyroidism, particularly in North America, and well differentiated carcinoma can also be functionally overactive.

Table 9.2. Graves' disease and toxic nodular goitre compared

	Graves' disease	*Toxic nodular goitre*
Gland	Diffuse, fleshy	Nodular, irregular, asymmetrical
Age	Younger	Older
Eye signs	Common	Rare
Cardiac problems	Uncommon	Common, masking thyroid problem
Autoimmune disease (including pernicious anaemia)	Common	Uncommon

Hyperthyroidism is a common disorder, especially in the female (male : female ratio 1 : 5 to 10). The onset is gradual, rarely rapid, symptoms being for the main part non-specific, affecting particularly the cardiovascular, neuromuscular, gastrointestinal and reproductive systems. The features vary with age, cardiovascular signs and symptoms predominating in the older patient, behaviour changes and abnormal movement of the limbs in the child.

The degree of ocular involvement varies in Graves' disease but usually amounts to mild lid retraction. In more severe cases the eye is very prominent (proptosis) with oedema of the conjunctiva (chemosis) and paralysis of eye movements. Loss of vision is a rare complication. The degree of associated hyperthyroid-ism is variable and ophthalmic signs may occur in the absence of overt systemic disorder.

Sudden life-threatening increase in severity of the disease may occur in some patients during thyroid surgery in an inadequately prepared patient. 'Thyroid crisis' may also occur after other forms of surgery, if the hyperthyroidism has not been recognized, and in association with respiratory tract infections.

The diagnosis of hyperthyroidism depends on clinical awareness, but is always confirmed by biochemical tests, since distinction from anxiety state in a young person can be difficult. Occult tuberculosis, carcinoma and diabetes mellitus can also produce features that simulate hyperthyroidism. Generally, measurement of serum T4 with reference to its binding proteins, which may be affected by pregnancy, drugs and other illness, is all that is necessary to confirm hyperthyroidism; serum T3 may help in difficult cases.

The treatment of hyperthyroidism may be by drug therapy, radioactive iodine or surgery. The choice is often arbitrary and can be dictated by the skill and experience of a surgeon as well as the age and preference of the patient. Drug therapy with beta-adrenergic blockers, in the short term, and carbimazole and thiouracils, for 2–3 months, are often used in preparation for surgery. Long-term therapy with the thionamides has the major disadvantage that the disease will recur in 50% of patients, usually within a few months of stopping treatment.

Surgery aims to cure hyperthyroidism by removing the bulk of functioning thyroid tissue. Recurrent laryngeal nerve damage and removal of the parathyroid glands are rare complications, but hypothyroidism may follow, over a 10-year period, in up to 30%.

Radioiodine controls hyperthyroidism by destroying functioning thyroid cells but it is difficult to predict the amount of tissue that will be damaged by a given dose. The incidence of hypothyroidism following such treatment is high (about 50–60% after 20 years) but otherwise there are no serious side effects, neither cancer nor leukaemia following radioiodine therapy. Because of the theoretical risk of genetic damage the use of iodine 131 is restricted to post-menopausal women, except in U.S.A. where it has been given to children.

Deficiency of circulating thyroid hormone results in slowing of all body functions (*hypothyroidism*). In severe forms deposition of mucinous substances in the skin and other tissues results in a typical facial appearance (myxoedema). There are many causes of hypothyroidism including destruction of the gland by surgery, irradiation and thyroiditis; defects of hormone synthesis and failure of development.

Hypothyroidism is insidious in onset, the symptoms being non-specific and often attributed to functional or non-organic disease. The disorder may present to any specialist in internal medicine and to general and dental surgeons.

◄ Because the onset is insidious and variable the diagnosis of hypothyroidism is only made if clinicians are alert to the possibility, particularly in those previously treated for hyperthyroidism

The skin is usually dry, scaly and thickened. There is often a malar flush and scalp hair is coarse and brittle, with balding. The pulse is slow and there may be oedema of the legs, with normal venous pressure. Goitre is uncommon but when present suggests iodine deficiency, defects in hormone synthesis or auto-immune (Hashimoto's) thyroiditis.

◄ Hypothyroidism in a child or juvenile may be associated with macroglossia

The diagnosis is usually confirmed by a low serum T4 and a raised TSH, if the disorder is primarily of thyroid origin.

Treatment with thyroxine is usually well tolerated but may precipitate myocardial ischaemia, particularly in the older patient. The adequacy of replacement therapy can be judged by measurement of serum TSH.

Hyperparathyroidism

Increased secretion of parathormone may occur either in association with chronic renal failure or as the result of an adenoma of one of the four parathyroid glands. Primary hyperparathyroidism is four times more common in women.

There is a wide spectrum of presenting complaints of primary hyperparathyroidism and 15% of patients are asymptomatic. Nearly half present with renal stones and less than 1 in 10 with bone problems. Occasionally there are other endocrine associations such as thyrotoxicosis, and adenoma of an adrenal.

◄ Biochemical screening and dental X-rays sometimes detect asymptomatic patients with hyperparathyroidism

The diagnosis is made on the clinical features, the finding of a raised serum calcium and exclusion of other

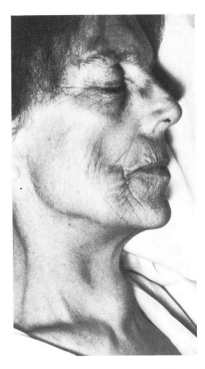

Fig. 9.1. Thyroid nodule. Midline swelling in neck which moved on swallowing. Middle-aged female who presented with congestive cardiac failure. Thyroid function tests confirmed hyperthyroidism.

causes of hypercalcaemia. Measurements of serum PTH are difficult to interpret, since levels may be in the normal range or undetectable with grossly elevated serum calcium.

The dentist may be made aware of hyperparathyroidism because of bone disease affecting the mandible. Radiographs may show a 'moth-eaten' appearance of the jaws, with loss of the lamina dura. Cystic radiolucencies can occur in the mandible as part of generalized bone disorder (osteitis fibrosa cystica) but is rare. Other bones that may be involved include the phalanges, which show sub-periosteal resorption of the cortex and cystic radiolucencies.

Giant-cell epulides may be seen in the mouths of patients with hyperparathyroidism. These lesions are not diagnostic of the disease and there may be no obvious cause.

Treatment of hyperparathyroidism consists of surgical removal of the adenoma, although location may be difficult and time consuming, even after multiple PTH assays obtained by neck vein catheterization. Failure to find an adenoma suggests that there is another cause for hypercalcaemia such as malignancy (bony metastases, myeloma and raised serum calcium without metastases), vitamin D intoxication, sarcoidosis and, rarely, thyrotoxicosis.

Table 9.3.   Clinical features of hyperthyroidism

General health — weight loss, sweating and heat intolerance
Cardiac — palpitations, dyspnoea, angina, atrial fibrillation,
            heart failure
Gastrointestinal — vomiting, diarrhoea, palmar erythema,
            spider naevi
Ocular — prominent eyes, diplopia, grittiness, lid retraction
Psychological — emotional lability, nervousness, tremor,
            psychosis
Other endocrine effects — amenorrhoea, loss of libido
Goitre — diffuse or nodular

Adrenal diseases

Cushing's syndrome

Cushing's syndrome results from increased circulating levels of either endogenous or exogenous cortisol. Spontaneous Cushing's syndrome is uncommon and may be of either pituitary or adrenal origin. It is four times more common in women and may occur in children, in whom adrenocortical carcinomas are more common.

By contrast, iatrogenic Cushing's syndrome is common, usually due to high doses of corticosteroids needed to treat inflammatory of immunological disorders. Sometimes, excessive replacement therapy is given to patients with hypoadrenalism.

The major clinical features of Cushing's syndrome are obesity, hypertension, excessive bruising, muscle

◀ Alcoholic patients may show features typical of Cushing's syndrome which resolve when alcohol intake is stopped

weakness, back pain, diabetes mellitus, psychiatric disturbance, menstrual disturbance and, in children, growth retardation. Alteration of fat distribution contributes to the moon face and protuberant abdomen as well as the large fat pads in the supraclavicular region.

Hypertension and fluid retention, induced by excess cortisol, and ischaemic heart disease are the main causes of morbidity and mortality in Cushing's syndrome. Excessive bruising occurs either spontaneously or at the site of minor trauma and results from loss of collagen supporting the blood vessel wall. Back pain results from osteoporosis and fractures may occur in any bone, particularly the vertebrae, either spontaneously or following minor trauma. Mild diabetes mellitus can complicate Cushing's syndrome and is a result of the actions of cortisol on carbohydrate metabolism.

Endogenous Cushing's syndrome may be due to excess ACTH production by the pituitary, an autonomous adenoma or carcinoma of the adrenal, or ectopic production of ACTH by oat cell carcinoma of bronchus or carcinoid tumour. It is usually possible, except with benign tumours, to distinguish the ectopic ACTH syndrome. Screening tests involve measurement of cortisol in urine and plasma, before and after an oral steroid (dexamethasone) which normally suppress cortisol levels and production; suppression does not occur with Cushing's syndrome.

Treatment depends on the cause. Adrenal tumours are removed since many, especially the larger ones, are malignant. When the cause is ectopic ACTH production the treatment is that of the primary lesion and

Table 9.4. Clinical features of Cushing's disease and ectopic ACTH by carcinoma

	Cushing's disease	*Oat cell carcinoma*
Sex	Mostly female	Mostly male
Pigmentation	Uncommon	Common
Speed of onset	Slow	Rapid
Oedema	Rare	Common
Weight loss	Rare	Common
Course	Years. Death due to hypertension, infection	Days to weeks. Death due to carcinoma

recurrences. Excess ACTH production by the pituitary (Cushing's disease) is treated by attempts to remove the tumour either by the transphenoidal route or by implantation of a radioactive substance (yttrium-90) into the sella.

Hypoadrenalism

Primary hypoadrenalism (Addison's disease) is an uncommon disease caused by destruction of the adrenal cortex. There is a variety of pathological causes, the most common being autoimmune disease and tuberculosis or surgical removal, either for malignant disease (female breast) or for Cushing's syndrome. There is an association between autoimmune adrenal disease and Hashimoto's disease, pernicious anaemia and ovarian failure.

The clinical features are non-specific and depend on the chronicity and severity of the disease. Pigmentation of the skin and buccal mucosa is caused by the direct action of ACTH on melanocytes, lowered cortisol production acting by negative feedback to increase ACTH production. Exposed areas, skin creases, scars, any part of the buccal mucosa and the tongue may be affected. Lassitude and weakness with anorexia, nausea and vomiting are invariably present but are non-specific and often misinterpreted. Profound falls in blood pressure on standing (postural hypotension) can often result in faints and injury.

◄ Skin pigmentation in Addison's disease preferentially affects exposed areas, pressure areas, flexure parts of joints, recent scars and the buccal mucosa

Table 9.5. Causes of pigmentation

Causes of buccal mucosal pigmentation
    Idiopathic
    Racial
    Small bowel polyps

Causes of generalized melanin pigmentation
    Malignant disease
    Chronic infections (tuberculosis)
    Malabsorption
    Neurofibromatosis (freckled appearance)
    Polyostotic fibrous dysplasia (large areas of pigmentation
      with normal skin)

The condition must be differentiated from a wide variety of psychiatric disorders. Similar skin pigmentation may occur with malignant diseases, tuberculosis, liver disease, malabsorption and chronic renal disease. Mouth pigmentation is usually racial or idiopathic; patchy pigmentation on the lips occurs with small bowel polyps. Localized melanin pigmentation may occur in naevi, with neurofibromatosis and rare bone disorders such as polyostotic fibrous dysplasia. Pigments other than melanin can cause similar appearances including iron deposition in haemochromatosis, silver, and haemosiderin in some bleeding diseases (*see* Chapter 15).

Diagnosis depends on awareness of the disorder. Confirmation is obtained by measurements of plasma cortisol and demonstration that ACTH fails to cause increase in the level. X-ray of the abdomen may reveal calcification in the adrenal glands if the disorder is due to previous tuberculous disease. Clinical and serological evidence of autoimmune disease, such as Hashimoto's thyroiditis or pernicious anaemia, and a family history of insulin-dependent diabetes mellitus are found in some patients.

Treatment consists of replacement of the amount of cortisol normally secreted (approximately 20 mg/day) in morning and evening doses. A dose of 30 mg per day is rarely needed although patients are advised to double the dose and seek medical advice if they are ill (respiratory infections) or likely to undergo significant stress. A few patients require a steroid (fludrocortisone) with more powerful salt-retaining properties than cortisone with a close check on blood pressure, which is usually low when the patient is undertreated and rises with overtreatment.

◀ Patients with Addison's disease are advised to double the dose of steroid and seek medical advice if they feel ill or suffer significant stress. They should also carry a steroid card

Careful regulation of steroid medication is required for any surgical procedure, however minor. Dental treatment under general anaesthesia requires adjustment of the dose — doubling of the amount on the day of the procedure — or 100 mg hydrocortisone sodium succinate intramuscularly 1 hour before the operation. Signs of undertreatment are faintness, particularly on standing, nausea and vomiting; a temporary increase in dose of cortisone for 24 hours, followed by the normal replacement amount, is required.

Adrenal medulla

Like the sympathetic nerves the adrenal medulla can synthesize, store and secrete noradrenaline and adrenaline, which are released in response to hypotension, hypoglycaemia and other environmental stresses. Functioning tumours may derive from the sympathetic nervous tissue in the medulla (phaeochromocytoma), the excess release of catecholamines causing paroxysmal or persistent hypertension.

Phaeochromocytoma occurs in less than 1% of hypertensive patients. It may be associated with neurofibromatosis (von Recklinghausen's disease) or other endocrine tumours, particularly medullary carcinoma of the thyroid and hyperparathyroidism (multiple endocrine adenomatosis — MEA type 2).

Typical features of phaeochromocytoma are intermittent episodes of hypertension, often associated with palpitations, apprehension, excessive sweating and flushing with headaches. In some patients the rise in blood pressure is sustained and may be asymptomatic. In the paroxysmal form the disorder can be difficult to distinguish from anxiety states and hyperthyroidism.

Diagnosis depends on the demonstration of increased formation of catecholamines and their excretion in the urine. Treatment involves removal of the tumour after previous localization by CT scanning or ultrasound. The risk of induction of anaesthesia and removal of the tumour is considerable, causing severe paroxysms of hypertension with life-threatening arrhythmias. Chemical blockade of adrenergic receptors is essential before and after the operation.

Pituitary disorders

Tumours in the pituitary fossa are usually adenomas from the anterior lobe although craniopharyngioma, derived from the pouch of Rathke, may occur and metastases from carcinoma, other cerebral tumours and granulomas may involve the gland. Endocrine disturbances can occur with over- or under-secretion of one or more of the hormones produced by the gland. In addition pituitary tumours may cause insidious loss of vision, paralysis of ocular movements and pupillary abnormalities.

The commonest nonhormone-secreting pituitary tumour is the slowly growing chromophobe adenoma which presents either as visual disturbance or hypopituitarism. The most common functioning tumours are those causing acromegaly (eosinophilic tumours); the prolactinoma, secreting excessive amounts of prolactin with associated changes in breasts and menses in the female, and libido and sexual function in the male; and basophil neoplasm associated with Cushing's syndrome. Tumours can also develop after bilateral adrenalectomy for Cushing's disease, and are associated with deep pigmentation of the skin and buccal mucosa (Nelson's syndrome).

◄ Skin and mucosal pigmentation may occur with pituitary tumours that develop after bilateral adrenalectomy for Cushing's disease

Hypopituitarism

The clinical picture is determined by the hormone(s) affected and the stage in growth and development when hypopituitarism develops. Growth hormone (GH) deficiency in childhood results in severe retardation of longitudinal growth, with delay in bone and epiphysial closure; in adults deficiency of GH results in a tendency to hypoglycaemia. Deficiency of gonadotrophins may lead to delayed puberty, failure of epiphysial closure and the development of eunuchoid skeletal proportions; deficiency developing after puberty is characterized by infertility, secondary amenorrhoea and loss of secondary sexual characteristics.

Deficiency of thyrotrophin causes hypothyroidism which may impair growth in childhood; in the adult the features are similar to primary hypothyroidism, but are less dramatic. ACTH deficiency causes few problems, since aldosterone secretion from the adrenal gland is not under pituitary control, and the blood pressure and electrolyte problems of primary adrenal failure do not occur. The major clinical features of ACTH lack are a tendency to spontaneous hypoglycaemia and pallor of the skin, due to impaired pigmentary response.

The commonest causes of hypopituitarism are tumours (primary and secondary), granulomas (such as sarcoidosis and syphilis), infarction (due to tumour, or necrosis following delivery in the pregnant woman due

◄ Infarction of pituitary tumours presents with severe headache, vomiting and neck stiffness, which may be followed by 'cure' of a secreting adenoma

to heavy bleeding — Sheehan's syndrome), trauma and developmental causes (often associated with disorders of sensation of smell, colour vision, and hearing).

Diagnosis can be made by assessing the secretion of all pituitary hormones, as well as imaging techniques to determine the size of the sella turcica and visual fields to assess the extension of any tumour.

Treatment depends on the cause. Removal of tumours can be achieved by the transfrontal route or transphenoidally, if small. Radiotherapy may be used as an adjunct to surgery, and in some centres yttrium implantation is used. Replacement therapy is in accord with the needs of the individual patient. Dexamethasone in doses of 0·5–0·75 mg daily is often preferred (mineralocorticoid replacement being unnecessary) with advice to double or quadruple the dose during intercurrent illness or with 'stress' such as minor procedures. Thyroxine is given in doses of 100–150 μg/day. In children growth hormone replacement is effective but is available through a few centres only. Males are given testosterone by implants, lasting 3–6 months, and chorionic gonadotrophin if there is concern about infertility. In the female replacement therapy can be given with a cyclical oestrogen–progestogen combination; attempts to achieve fertility with various gonadotrophins are not without side-effects and require co-operation from the patient.

Acromegaly

Excessive growth hormone (GH) production leads to abnormal enlargement of most organs of the body (including the tongue). The clinical features of acromegaly include thick, lined, redundant, greasy, sweaty skin, prognathism, a bulbous nose and splayed teeth. Apposition of teeth no longer occurs and the bite is often reversed, so that chewing may be difficult.

Involvement of mucosa and cartilage of the respiratory tract leads to obstruction of the paranasal sinuses and narrowing of the larynx, with voice changes and risk of obstruction during anaesthesia. The hands and feet are broad. Cardiac involvement is common, with raised blood pressure in a third of cases. Heart failure is a common cause of death.

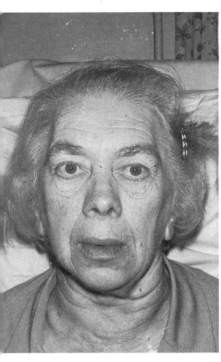

Fig. 9.2. Acromegaly with multinodular euthyroid goitre.
Note the coarse features.

Exuberant overgrowth of bone occurs around large joints, together with cartilage overgrowth, and a degenerative arthritis affecting the knee, shoulder and hips develops. There is often muscular weakness and there may be compression of peripheral nerves, for example, at the wrist leading to paraesthesiae in the hand and weakness of grip (carpal tunnel syndrome). A few patients with acromegaly have renal stone associated with hypercalcaemia and half of these have a parathyroid tumour.

Frank diabetes mellitus occurs in 1 of 5 patients with acromegaly, since GH is an insulin antagonist, and remission usually occurs when the hormone levels have been reduced to normal by treatment. Goitres occur in one-third of acromegalics (Fig. 9.2) and a few patients become frankly thyrotoxic. The goitre is multinodular and may contribute to upper airways obstruction caused by mucosal and cartilaginous changes in the larynx.

Diagnosis of acromegaly depends on awareness of the condition and most investigations are usually confirmatory. The specific diagnostic test is the measurement of plasma GH following a glucose load during which, in a normal patient, there is suppression of levels; in acromegaly, suppression does not occur or there is a rise in GH levels.

Treatment of acromegaly depends on the presence of visual symptoms caused by pressure of the tumour on the optic chiasma (*see* Chapter 11). In such patients, transphenoidal surgery is performed and may be done preserving pituitary function. Radiotherapy and implantation of yttrium may also be effective for these tumours, although only when it is contained within the sella. The dopamine agonist, bromocriptine, is frequently used for acromegaly and other functioning pituitary tumours. However, GH levels are controlled in only half of the patients with acromegaly treated with the drug and reduction in tumour size is not universal: in some growth of the adenoma has occurred.

◀ A large tongue, spaced teeth, prognathism and a reversed bite, with difficulty in chewing, are the important oro-facial features of acromegaly

◀ Patients with acromegaly may have insulin-dependent diabetes and one-third have associated goitre, which can be toxic

Marfan's syndrome (*see* Chapter 16)

This is a generalized disorder of connective tissue affecting the cardiovascular, skeletal and ocular systems. It is inherited as an autosomal dominant and affected individuals are tall, thin and have long extremities. The span is greater than height and the length of the lower half of the body is greater than the upper. The fingers are long (arachnodactyly) and there may be kyphoscoliosis with pigeon breast or pectus excavatum. The face is long and narrow, the palate is high-arched and the jaw usually protrudes. There may be hypermobility of joints, although this is not invariable, with 'double-jointedness' of the knees, especially, and dislocation of the hips, patella and toes. Dislocation of the lens occurs in 70% and there is often severe myopia.

The most important abnormalities in Marfan's syndrome are those affecting the heart and major blood vessels. There is disruption of the elastic fibres of the aortic media and an increase in collagen, with subsequent progressive diffuse dilatation of the ascending aorta and weakening of the aortic valve ring, leading to aortic valvular incompetence that progresses to left ventricular and subsequently congestive heart failure. Heart failure and rupture of the aorta are the most common causes of death although infective endocarditis may develop on the abnormal valve. The average age at death in a large series of patients was 32 years.

Marfan's syndrome presents clinical features that are similar to the condition of homocystinuria, an inborn disorder with abnormal collagen (*see* Chapter 16). The joints are not, however, hyperextensible and in contrast to Marfan patients there is osteoporosis.

◀ Marfan's syndrome can be distinguished from homocystinuria by the absence of mental retardation, but there is a risk of infective endocarditis on the abnormal aortic valve in both

Diabetes mellitus

Diabetes mellitus is a state of chronic blood glucose elevation often accompanied by other clinical and biochemical abnormalities. The clinical features vary from a totally asymptomatic to a rapidly lethal form. The term 'diabetes mellitus' is comparable to 'anaemia' and 'hypertension', highlighting an identifiable feature, indicating therapeutic actions, but only suggesting possible causes since this is not a single disease entity.

A raised fasting blood glucose (more than 8 mmol/litre) or a postabsorption level in excess of 11 mmol/litre are a clear indication that the patient has diabetes mellitus. If the blood glucose level is equivocal a single measurement made 2 hours after a 75 g oral glucose load establishes the diagnosis if this is above 12 mmol/litre. An oral glucose tolerance test, performed in the morning, after 3 days of an adequate carbohydrate diet, comprising blood samples taken fasting and at 1 and 2 hours after a 75 g glucose load is often used. If capillary blood glucose is greater than 7 mmol/litre (fasting) and 11 mmol/litre at 2 hours the diagnosis is established, provided that drugs and physical states that affect glucose tolerance have been excluded.

Although the exact levels of blood glucose necessary for diagnosis are emphasized this is seldom a real problem in clinical terms, particularly when symptoms of thirst, polyuria with glycosuria and weight loss are present, when a single measurement is usually all that is required.

Because diabetes is not a single disease entity it is classified according to whether it is primarily a disturbance of insulin production or secondary to other disease that affects glucose tolerance. Alternatively, primary and secondary diabetes can be classified as 'insulin dependent' (IDDM) or 'non-insulin dependent' (NIDDM). Genetic susceptibility seems to play a more important part in NIDDM, almost all affected identical twin pairs being concordant for the disease compared with about 50% for IDDM.

Secondary diabetes may occur in association with diseases of the pancreas, hormonal disorders (such as hyperthyroidism), drugs (corticosteroids and diuretics) and as part of rare genetic syndromes (affecting carbohydrate and/or lipid metabolism).

The management of diabetes has three principal aims — to restore the disturbed metabolism to normal, to prevent or delay the progress of short- and long-term complications and to provide the patient with the knowledge, motivation and means to care for himself. If the patient is obese, dietary restriction alone is the first line of management, whereas if the patient is thin and has conspicuous thirst and polyuria, and has ketones in the urine, there is a clear indication for insulin therapy. Oral hypoglycaemics are usually prescribed in the older patient who has been obese but in whom, in spite of reducing weight, blood glucose remains increased.

◀ Thirst and polyuria in a non-obese patient are usually an indication of the need for insulin

There are many insulin preparations of varying degrees of purity (purity meaning that 'contaminants' have been removed, rendering the preparation less immunogenic, and avoiding antibody formation). They are of pork or beef origin. Most newly diagnosed patients are stabilized on purified preparations, usually pork insulins, unless there are religious objections. By variations in the physical state of the insulin, duration of action can be altered from short duration and onset of effect (soluble or regular insulin) to intermediate and long duration (insulin zinc suspensions). Optimal

◀ Best control of diabetes can be achieved by two doses of insulin per day

control of blood glucose is achieved by multiple daily dosage (usually twice daily because it is flexible, easily understood and controlled by the patient).

Oral agents have a small but established place in diabetic management and are either sulphonylureas, with actions primarily on insulin release, or biguanides with a mixture of actions on glucose absorption and its hepatic and peripheral metabolism. Sulphonylureas may interact, with enhanced metabolic effects, with other sulphonamides, aspirin, anticoagulants and beta-adrenergic blockers (*see* Chapter 16). Some patients are intolerant of the sulphonylureas and may develop mucocutaneous reactions. Biguanide therapy is rarely used as the sole drug in treating diabetes, being given to improve control achieved by sulphonylureas.

Dietary management of the diabetic patient depends on the patient's habitual food patterns, with spacing of meals and qualitative and quantitative variations according to economic factors and personal fads. Bread, potatoes, rice, cereals, pasta and some fruits form the basis of the normal carbohydrate intake, which is restricted and fat consumption is kept at low levels. Needs of the diabetic child have to be reviewed as they change with age, growth and activity.

Hypoglycaemia may occur in any diabetic patient controlled with insulin or oral therapy. The usual explanations are delayed meals, unusual physical exertion, misread dosage of insulin and, very rarely, the inadvertent intravenous injection of insulin. There are important warning signs of hypoglycaemia, due largely to catecholamine release, consisting of pallor, sweating, shakiness, a forceful heart beat and a feeling

◄ Patients with diabetes are usually taught to recognize the symptoms of hypoglycaemia and to avoid episodes by small changes in insulin dosage and food intake to cope with changes in life-style

Table 9.6. Coma in a diabetic

	Dehydration	Hyper-ventilation	Blood pressure	Skin	Blood glucose
Hypoglycaemia	0	0	Normal	Cold, clammy	Low
Ketoacidosis	+++	+++	Normal or low	Warm	High
Other comas (syncope, stroke, seizures)	0 to +	0 to +	Variable	Normal	Normal

of apprehension. Later features are disturbance of behaviour, judgement or consciousness, due to cerebral glucose lack. The speed at which the symptoms progress varies with the preparation used, being more rapid with pork insulin.

Most patients can cope with early hypoglycaemia themselves by taking readily available carbohydrate such as four or five lumps of sugar or glucose tablets; another person may provide a sweetened drink. If the patient is unable to drink, because of falling consciousness level, it may be necessary to give 20–50 ml of 10% glucose solution intravenously and, if recovery is slow or there is difficulty with intravenous injection, 1 mg of intramuscular glucagon.

Preparation of the diabetic patient for minor surgery, which will result in missing of more than one meal, involves modification of insulin dosage or discontinuation of oral therapy. It is most important to avoid hypoglycaemia which, in most patients, requires giving only 50% of the usual dose of insulin together with intravenous glucose. It is rarely necessary to give supplementary insulin, or intravenous glucose, after dental surgery since the diabetic patient will usually be able to return to normal activity and take glucose-containing fluids shortly afterwards. If there is delay, it is important that blood glucose levels should be monitored. To achieve optimum diabetic control any procedure should be as early in the day as possible.

◄ Patients with stable insulin-dependent diabetes require approximately 50% of their usual insulin dose on the day of minor surgery

Long-term diabetes leads to important vascular complications affecting vessels of various sizes; major arteries are damaged by atheroma; terminal arteries and arterioles in the heart and kidneys may be involved; and smaller vessels and capillaries in the retina and kidneys are also damaged with decreasing function of those organs. Peripheral nerves may also be affected with motor, sensory and autonomic symptoms. The lens and the skin can also be affected.

These disorders develop with increasing frequency as the duration of diabetes lengthens and some are probably related to poor blood glucose control, particularly the microvascular and neuropathic complications. Not all long-standing diabetics develop these problems and genetic or racial factors may be important.

Diabetic retinopathy occurs in about 80% of insulin-dependent diabetics after 15–20 years. In developed countries diabetic retinopathy is the commonest cause of blindness between ages 30 and 64 years. Photocoagulation of the abnormal blood vessels using the xenon arc and the argon laser is used in an attempt to arrest the course of sight-threatening forms of the disease.

◄ Although it cannot be prevented entirely by photocoagulation, blindness can be reduced in the diabetic

Diabetic neuropathy, particularly in its asymptomatic form, occurs commonly in diabetics (*see* Chapter 11). It occurs as a symmetrical, sensory 'glove and stocking' form with numbness of the feet and hands, affecting the reading of Braille in the blind diabetic. The major hazard is that trauma may be unnoticed and be followed by sepsis. Some peripheral neuropathies affecting the hands, feet and trunk may be very painful. Single cranial nerves may be affected, particularly the IIIrd, VIth, VIIth and XIIth nerves, often of rapid onset, with recovery after several months. Involvement of the autonomic nerves occurs in a few diabetics with unpleasant symptoms including diarrhoea, postural hypotension, urinary retention and incontinence due to overflow, facial sweating associated with eating, and impotence. Respiratory arrest during or after anaesthesia or after any respiratory depressant can occur, and cardiac denervation with tachycardia and loss of cardiovascular reflexes may be the reasons for sudden unexplained death during anaesthesia, respiratory infections and hypoxia.

◄ Mononeuropathy due to diabetes may affect oculomotor, facial and hypoglossal nerves, but recovery does occur

◄ Autonomic neuropathy associated with diabetes may be complicated by cardiac denervation and the risk of sudden death during anaesthesia

Renal disease may complicate diabetes; a glomerular lesion causing proteinuria, oedema formation and gradual deterioration of renal function. Renal failure progresses at a slower rate but after ten years of proteinuria most diabetics are likely to be in the terminal stage. Renal damage usually occurs in the insulin-dependent diabetic, and the disease becomes more difficult to control. Management of the renal failure is as for glomerulonephritis and other causes of CRF (*see* Chapter 10).

◄ Fluid retention, causing peripheral oedema, is the first sign of diabetic involvement of the kidney, with associated problems of drug excretion and toxicity

Coronary, cerebral and peripheral arterial disease is the major cause of chronic ill health and premature death in both forms of diabetes. The reasons for the increased susceptibility to atheroma and hypertension are not known. Angina and myocardial infarction occur frequently, the mortality for the latter being twice as high as for the non-diabetic. The risks of general anaesthesia in the diabetic with coronary heart disease are greater than in the healthy patient, particularly if there is coincident autonomic neuropathy.

Infections of any kind, including dental abscess, may precipitate uncontrolled diabetes with ketone formation and acidaemia. This syndrome (*ketoacidosis*) may also occur with inadequate insulin dosage, delayed diagnosis of new diabetics, following myocardial infarction and after trauma. Lack of insulin causes increased release of fatty acids from adipose tissue which are converted to ketone bodies in the liver. Ketone bodies are not harmful in themselves but, being organic acids, they dissociate producing hydrogen ions, with a fall in blood pH and hyperventilation. Increased glucose production is associated with marked polyuria and accompanying losses of sodium and potassium.

Ketoacidosis is usually of gradual onset with symptoms of weight loss, fatigue, thirst and polyuria over a period of weeks. Vomiting, leg cramps and abdominal pain may occur in children. Most patients

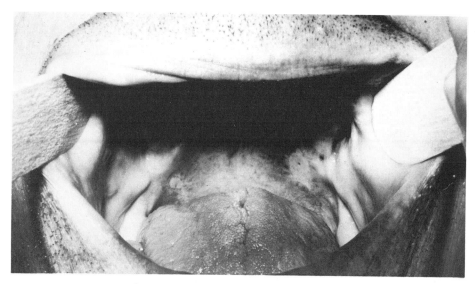

Fig. 9.3. Bilateral ulceration on the soft palate in diabetic on recovery from episode of ketoacidosis.

are drowsy when seen; an unconscious patient has a very poor prognosis. The patient is usually dehydrated, hyperventilating and has the smell of acetone in the breath. There is tachycardia, warm skin and sometimes fever.

Treatment requires correction of fluid and electrolyte disturbance and insulin either intramuscularly or by continuous intravenous infusion. The precipitating factor should be established and antibiotics given if there is suspicion of infection. Early recognition is very important since the mortality is up to 10% in expert units.

Growth and development of children

Between birth and adolescence there are three major changes — physical growth, sexual development and emotional development — which are all closely related such that gross abnormality of one can affect the others. The dentist should be able to recognize whether the child is as developed as his/her age and, if there is marked disparity, report the findings to the patient's parents and family doctor.

Repeated measurements of height and weight are only a crude measure of development and physical fitness. Physical proportions also change at different stages of development representing growth of individual tissues at varying rates. The nervous system develops most rapidly in infancy, corresponding with which the head is large at this stage representing one-quarter of total length. The gonads grow slowly until the onset of puberty when sexual development is accompanied by a characteristic 'pubertal spurt' of growth, the head representing approximately one-seventh of total length and proportions becoming slender as opposed to the squat appearance of the infant.

Assessment of development can also be made by radiological examination, the centres of ossification and fusion of epiphysis being used to show whether osseous development is delayed or advanced for age. Dentition provides limited confirmatory evidence, the individual variations in age of eruption of teeth being considerable.

In the older child it is important to note evidence of onset of puberty which appears in both sexes at about 11 years of age. In girls the spurt in growth occurs as the breasts start to enlarge at about 12 years of age and menarche (the start of the menstrual cycle) at 13 years. Boys grow later, beginning their spurt about two years after girls but add more to their pre-pubertal height.

Single measurements of height are of little value and must be repeated after a minimum period of 3–4 months and at the same interval for at least one year. A child who is short for his age may be healthy, and it is just as possible to be of average height and be ill. If a child is small for his parents, looks normal and has a low growth velocity it is likely that the cause is either endocrine deficiency or a general disorder such as cardiac, respiratory, gastroenterological or renal disease. If the child has an abnormal appearance it is likely that the cause is a chromosome abnormality or bone disorder.

The underlying condition causing short stature is treated wherever possible, though this can only achieve maximal effect at the time of diagnosis and cannot increase it.

Children who are tall for their parents may be so because of early puberty. If the child is of normal appearance and the velocity of growth is increased growth hormone excess (gigantism) and hyperthyroidism are possible. An abnormal appearance of the tall child usually suggests Marfan's syndrome or homocystinuria and the genetic abnormality — Klinefelter's syndrome.

Delay in puberty is most often physiological. In boys short stature is the usual explanation for delay but, in girls, is often accompanied by chromosomal abnormalities and failure of gonad development (Turner's syndrome). Absence of pubertal change by the age of 14 is not uncommon in boys, but pathological cause will be found in most girls of this age. Among the causes for late puberty are gonadotrophin deficiencies, emotional causes, testicular and ovarian disorders and abnormalities of adrenal hormone synthesis.

Precocious puberty is more likely to be pathological in boys, the reverse being true for delayed puberty. The causes are also hypothalamic, pituitary, gonadal or adrenal disorder.

Renal diseases

10

The kidney serves important excretory functions, clearing plasma of protein waste products; maintains fluid, electrolyte and acid-base balance; controls arterial blood pressure; and has important endocrine functions in producing erythropoietin, dihydrocholecalciferol and some prostaglandins.

The glomerulus filters up to 170 ml of urine per minute, measured by using substances, such as inulin, which are not secreted or absorbed by the tubules. Plasma creatinine is a good guide to glomerular filtration in most patients, except in those with border-line renal function, and can be used to assess the steady loss of kidney function in patients with chronic renal failure.

In passing through the tubules glomerular filtrate is concentrated, its pH changed and numerous substances (phosphate, amino-acids, uric and other acids) are excreted into or absorbed from the fluid. The only tubular functions that can be easily tested are concentration and acidification (for detection of congenital disorders such as renal tubular acidosis).

Table 10.1. Normal values for renal function

Sodium	135–145 mmol/l	Low in pre-renal failure
Potassium	3·5–5·0 mmol/l	High in late chronic renal failure
Chloride	96–106 mmol/l	High in congenital tubular disease
Bicarbonate	23–29 mmol/l	Low in chronic renal failure
Urea	2·5–7·0 mmol/l	High in CRF, sodium depletion
Creatinine	60–130 μmol/l	High in CRF
GFR (age 20)	100–170 ml/min	
male (age 50)	90–140 ml/min	Low in renal failure
female (age 70)	70–115 ml/min	

185

Patients with impaired renal function often react abnormally to certain drugs and customary doses can result in serious toxic effects. Many drugs are eliminated by the kidney and their clearance from plasma is proportional to the glomerular filtration. Other drugs may be affected because the metabolic transformation rate is modified by renal failure. Protein binding of drugs may be decreased in renal disease, either because of reduced plasma protein concentration and/or competition for binding sites with accumulated waste products of similar size molecules, thus causing a higher fraction of free drug in the plasma, greater pharmacological action and increased incidence of side-effects. Distribution of drugs may also be affected by renal failure, the associated anaemia and fluid retention resulting in different distribution volumes and concentration of drugs.

◄ If possible it is best to use drugs unaffected by kidney disease in patients with renal failure and to use drugs with a wide margin of safety

It is not easy to prescribe drugs in patients with renal failure. It is best to use drugs the distribution, metabolism and elimination of which is unaffected by kidney disease as well as those drugs with a wide safety margin between therapeutic and toxic concentrations.

◄ When prescribing a drug for a patient with renal failure it is practice to either reduce the dose per interval or increase the interval

Hypertension may be a consequence of renal disorder but it can also play a part in the pathogenesis of renal disease. There is an increased incidence of hypertension in patients with intrinsic renal disease and this probably accelerates the deterioration in kidney function. In most patients the hypertension is caused by salt and water retention, and can be controlled by sodium restriction and diuretic therapy. In a few patients increased renin production may play a greater role in the cause of raised blood pressure. The cardiac and neurological complications of raised blood pressure due to renal disease are as frequent as in essential hypertension (*see* Chapter 3).

Anaemia becomes more marked as renal failure progresses, the reduction in red cell numbers being due, largely, to reduced production of erythropoietin by the kidney. It is possible that some accumulated waste products may cause bone-marrow suppression.

Presenting symptoms of renal disease

Patients with renal disease may present with symptoms

that arise from the urinary tract or, more commonly in renal failure, with symptoms related to the general, cardiovascular, musculoskeletal and neurological effects of disturbed kidney function. In some patients the renal disease is discovered by chance.

Pain in the loin may be due to stone, obstruction of drainage from the kidney and to infection. Renal colic may also complicate renal stone formation and is a severe pain radiating from the loin to the iliac fossa and genitalia, lasting several hours and associated with sweating and vomiting. The passage of a stone down the ureter to the bladder is the usual cause of renal colic, although it may occur with blood clot and necrotic bits of kidney substance.

◀ Loin pain in renal disease is usually due to stone in the pelvis, obstruction to drainage or infection

Pain during and immediately after passing urine (dysuria) is usually due to bladder infection, but may be due to trauma. Frequency of urination, urinary incontinence (enuresis), passing of blood in the urine (haematuria) and retention of urine are other symptoms that may occur with disease of the bladder and urethra.

◀ Dysuria implies irritation of the bladder or urethra, usually due to infection

◀ Retention of urine is usually due to obstructive, neurological or psychological causes

The systemic symptoms of renal disease are largely those due to impaired kidney function, although some are the consequence of heavy protein loss in the urine. Fluid retention causing oedema of the legs and the face, after overnight resting in bed, occurs in both nephrosis and in renal failure. Gastrointestinal symptoms are common in severe renal impairment, consisting of nausea, vomiting, abnormal taste and, as a near terminal event, hiccoughs. The anaemia that accompanies chronic renal failure produces the usual symptoms of lassitude, breathlessness and faintness. Generalized itching of the skin may sometimes be a presenting feature, and oral ulceration occurs in patients who

Table 10.2. Manifestations of chronic renal failure

General — Lethargy and irritability
Gastrointestinal — Anorexia, nausea, vomiting, hiccough
Cardiovascular — Raised BP, fluid overload and depletion
Skin — Itching, purpura
Blood — Anaemia, abnormal platelet function
Musculoskeletal — Growth failure, bone pain, proximal myopathy
Neurological — Headaches, seizures, neuropathy (dialysis patients)

become severely dehydrated. Bone pain in the lumbo-sacral region and the thighs occurs, particularly in children, the patient often having a rolling gait due to a proximal myopathy.

Many patients come to medical attention because their renal disease is discovered by chance, proteinura or haematuria being discovered at routine medical examination.

Chronic renal failure

Chronic renal failure (CRF) often affects relatively young people and because of this and the large costs of renal replacement therapy in medical, technical and fiscal terms causes moral and political problems.

The signs and symptoms of end-stage CRF are the same whatever the underlying cause, except when the

Table 10.3.   Chronic renal failure

Glomerulonephritis	1 in 3
Pyelonephritis	1 in 10
(obstruction ureteric reflux)	
Polycystic disease	1 in 10
Diabetic renal disease	1 in 10
Raised blood pressure	1 in 12
Drugs (analgesic abuse)	1 in 50

Table 10.4.   Causes of glomerulonephritis

Antiglomerular basement membrane antibody 5%
Immune complex disease 80% +
    Acute
       drugs, toxins, foreign serum proteins
       bacterial (streptococci)
       virus (ECHO and influenza virus)
    Chronic
       bacterial (infective endocarditis)
       protozoan (malaria)
       virus (hepatitis B)
       tumour and lymphoma antigens
T cell dysfunction — minimal change glomerulonephritis

renal disease is part of a systemic disorder such as SLE, diabetes and amyloid disease when the patient may present other features of the underlying problem.

The commonest cause of CRF is chronic glomerulonephritis, accounting for a third of all cases, whilst diabetes, polycystic disease and pyelonephritis each account for one in ten.

Glomerulonephritis has many forms and several causes, all of which present with proteinuria, haematuria and the presence of formed elements (cells and casts of tubules) in the urinary sediment. Renal biopsy is necessary in most patients to establish the exact form of glomerulonephritis and the possible cause. A few cases of glomerulonephritis are due to antibody against glomerular basement membrane, either arising spontaneously or after a viral infection; but most are due to deposition of immune complexes in glomerular vessels. Immune complex deposition in the glomerulus occurs acutely with drugs, foreign proteins, bacterial infections (usually streptococci), and with viruses (ECHO virus and influenza). Chronic immune complex disease may occur with bacterial endocarditis, malaria, viruses (hepatitis B), SLE, and with tumours (Hodgkin's lymphoma and carcinoma).

The symptoms of CRF usually appear when 90% of kidney tissue has been destroyed. The cause of the symptoms has not been identified, but it is not the raised blood urea. It is now thought that molecules of certain size, which can be removed by dialysis, cause the multisystemic effects of CRF. As kidney function worsens the ability to compensate for variations in salt and water intake is lost and severe dehydration can occur following episodes of vomiting or diarrhoea, whilst fluid overload can occur with intravenous infusion. Remaining functional units of the kidney (nephrons) develop an increase in excretory rate, which partly compensates, although any episode of fluid loss has to be treated urgently.

◀ Renal impairment is often well advanced before any symptoms occur

Severe anaemia which does not usually respond to iron, vitamin B_{12} or folic acid can occur in many patients with CRF. Blood transfusion has to be given with caution because of the risk of deterioration in renal function and fluid overload. Bleeding due to platelet defect and thrombocytopenia occurs from the bowel, or following trauma such as dental extraction.

In some patients, CRF may be due to reversible factors including urinary tract obstruction, hypertension and chronic urinary infection. It is important to search for treatable and preventable causes once the diagnosis has been made. The possibility of analgesic abuse causing kidney damage has always to be borne in mind, particularly in middle-aged women with mild psychiatric disturbance, since further deterioration in renal function can be prevented by stopping the drugs.

◀ An important preventable cause of CRF is analgesic abuse, often used for chronic pain and frequently associated with mild psychiatric disturbance

Specific curative treatment for CRF is, however, rarely available, and once the diagnosis is made the patient's kidney function is monitored carefully and complicating factors, such as raised blood pressure, urinary infection and dehydration, are corrected and all drug prescriptions carefully reviewed. It may be necessary to control fluid intake, particularly in those with oedema, and dietary restriction of protein (to 40 g/day) is enforced in the later stages of the disease. Plasma phosphate levels rise, as renal function worsens, and is the initiating factor in bone disease (renal osteodystrophy). The plasma phosphate level can be controlled with aluminium hydroxide and dietary control of phosphate/calcium (*see* Chapter 12).

When renal function falls to 10% of normal or less, suitable patients must be given renal replacement therapy (peritoneal dialysis, haemodialysis or renal transplantation). *Peritoneal dialysis* is established by inserting a stiff silastic catheter into the peritoneum, permitting pre-warmed fluid to be run into the cavity (in aliquots of approximately 2 litres), which is allowed to 'dwell' and is then drained, all over a period of 1 hour. Peritoneal dialysis can be used as an acute measure to control acute renal failure or, in specialized units, the patient with CRF may have dialysis in this way for 40 hours per week. The patient undergoing chronic ambulatory peritoneal dialysis (CAPD) may lead a normal life between dialysis periods and this technique controls the biochemical features of renal failure. Some complications, such as peripheral neuropathy, seem less common with CAPD. The osmolality of the dialysis fluid can be raised above that for plasma by alterations in glucose concentration, allowing more fluid to be removed with each dialysis, and the blood acid-base balance altered by adding lactate — which is

◀ The quality of life in end-stage renal disease can be improved by peritoneal dialysis, haemodialysis and kidney transplants

metabolized to bicarbonate in the liver — to the dialysate.

Haemodialysis is more efficient than PD, but requires access to the circulation by a shunt or fistula between an artery and vein, in the leg or forearm. Haemodialysis is used in acute renal failure, where there is increased catabolism of protein, as with infections, and in chronic renal failure. In CRF dialysis must be performed 2–3 times per week for a total period of 8–30 hours. Haemodialysis can be performed in the patient's home, although it causes stress on the rest of the family, problems being exacerbated except in strong family units. Patients undergoing chronic haemodialysis may gain employment but are usually not able to work to the full or overtime. Survival is good, 70–80% of patients being alive three years after starting this therapy.

Renal transplantation is the major alternative to haemodialysis and, when successful, restores a patient to virtual normality, without the tedium of dialysis, for up to 30 hours per week. Transplantation is indicated: when the patient requests a change, after a long period on dialysis; when dialysis fails; when social circumstances, such as family support, poor housing and employment are against dialysis; and in the younger patient. Rejection and infections are the commonest complications suffered by transplanted patients. Most patients require life-long treatment with immuno-suppressive drugs (usually prednisone and azathio-prine), which increases the incidence of herpes (zoster and simplex) infections, fungal infections of the mouth and pharynx with *Candida*, which may spread down the gastrointestinal tract, and bacterial infections. Raised blood pressure, obesity and avascular necrosis of the head of the femur, the head of the humerus and the bones of the foot may also occur in these patients. Bone-marrow suppression caused by azathioprine results in anaemia; thrombocytopenia and agranulo-cytosis may also cause problems.

Survival after transplantation is improving, some patients, both male and female, becoming fertile. A little under half have a functioning kidney at three years after transplantation of a cadaver kidney, and nearly two-thirds have good renal function when the

◀ Haemodialysis is more efficient than peritoneal dialysis and 70% are alive after 3 years on home dialysis

◀ Successful renal transplantation enables the patient to lead a normal life and restores fertility, which chronic dialysis does not

◀ Gram-negative and virus infections are more common in the transplanted patient and are the most frequent cause of death because of impaired cell mediated and humoral immunity, as well as non-specific mechanisms (disturbed anatomical barriers)

◀ 70% of patients with live donor grafts are alive 3 years after operation, as are approximately 50% of those who received cadaver kidneys

graft is from a living related donor, where there is close matching of the major histocompatability antigens.

Nephrotic syndrome

Nephrotic syndrome is characterized by reduced serum albumin concentration and oedema resulting from protein loss in the urine, the amount varying from 3 to 10 g and more per day. The cause of the protein loss is damage to the glomerulus, either by idiopathic glomerulonephritis or as a consequence of systemic disorders, such as SLE, diabetes mellitus, myeloma, some carcinomas and lymphoma.

The increase in permeability of the glomerulus is partly compensated for by reabsorption by the tubules of proteins 'leaked', but this is limited. The different proteins lost varies according to the glomerular disease; in some, the smaller molecules are lost and the larger retained; in others, this selectivity does not occur. The liver has considerable capacity to increase protein synthesis so as to replace the smaller amounts lost, but when proteinuria exceeds 10 g/day compensation is exceeded, plasma albumin falls and body protein stores are depleted.

Table 10.5.   Causes of nephrotic syndrome

Idiopathic
    minimal change renal disease (children)
    proliferative glomerulonephritis
    membranous renal disease
    focal glomerulosclerosis
Associated with other disease (usually membranous nephro-
      pathy)
    SLE and RA
    drugs (penicillamine, gold, tolbutamide)
    infections (syphilis, malaria, leprosy, hepatitis B)
    carcinoma, lymphoma
    diabetes mellitus
    myeloma

As plasma albumin falls plasma volume shrinks inducing salt and water retention and some degree of renal impairment; as a consequence of these changes, as well as reduced plasma oncotic pressure, oedema develops. The oedema of nephrotic syndrome is mobile, being most prominent in the face, around the eyes, in the morning and in the legs once the patient has been up and about. Ascites often occurs in children.

Protein depletion has systemic effects since albumin, apart from its oncotic effects, also acts as a carrier protein for hormones (thyroxine and corticosteroids). Nephrotic syndrome is sometimes associated with goitre. Other transport proteins are lost including transferrin, causing iron deficiency and, in some instances, anaemia. Loss of immunoglobulins (IgG) increase vulnerability to infection, and thrombus formation may be promoted because of loss of thrombolytic factors. Serum calcium is also lower than normal, partly because of reduced plasma albumin, partly because a vitamin D metabolite is lost in the urine. The concentration of some plasma proteins may be increased, because the molecules are too large to be filtered through the glomerulus, especially those which carry cholesterol. There is a suggestion that the subsequent hyperlipidaemia causes an increased incidence of ischaemic heart disease in younger patients with nephrotic syndrome.

Treatment of nephrotic syndrome consists of 'loop-acting' diuretics, such as frusemide, and a high protein diet (90 g per day). Treatment of the glomerular lesion with corticosteroids and immuno-suppressive drugs, such as cyclophosphamide, is beneficial in a few patients, particularly those with minimal changes on microscopy. The disease progresses, in many patients, to CRF and requires kidney replacement treatment.

◄ The oedema of nephrotic syndrome is more prominent about the face, neck and upper limbs in the morning and in the legs once the patient is up and active

◄ Loss of transport proteins in nephrotic syndrome may be associated with anaemia; loss of immunoglobulins with increased vulnerability to infection

Renal calculi

A urinary calculus consists of crystals of salts or acids that are sparingly soluble. The chemical composition of stones varies according to the age of the patient; cystine stones are commoner in the young and occur in both sexes; uric acid stones occur mainly in men over the age of 40; infected stones occur most often in females and can be related to pregnancy; and calcium stones are more common in males of all ages.

The usual presentation is with renal colic as the stone passes down the ureter. There may be haematuria, dysuria and sometimes the patient may be aware of passing 'sand' or 'gravel'.

The majority of stones are a mixture of calcium with oxalate and phosphate and, in 9 out of 10 of these patients, there is increased absorption of calcium from the gut together with increased urinary calcium excretion. Of the remainder primary hyperparathyroidism is the most frequent cause of calcium stone formation which can be cured by parathyroidectomy (*see* Chapter 9).

◄ 10% of patients with calcium stones have hyperparathyroidism which can be cured by surgery

Treatment of urinary calculus depends on the underlying cause, which may be correctable (hyperparathyroidism, recurrent infection, obstruction leading to urinary stasis). The general principles are those of relief of pain, high fluid intake, removal of stone causing urinary tract obstruction and prevention of recurrence. Drugs such as thiazide diuretics are beneficial in idiopathic hypercalciuria. Calculus may cause acute renal failure with cessation of urine formation but rarely CRF, except when persistent obstruction leads to dilatation of the ureter (hydronephrosis), infection and destruction of renal parenchyma.

Urinary tract infection

Infections of the urinary tract are a common problem in medical practice. Where there is not urinary tract obstruction infection does not progress to kidney scarring, raised blood pressure and renal failure. However, when there is reflux of urine backwards from bladder to ureter, due to incompetence of the valve mechanism at the vesico-ureteric junction, organisms ascend to the kidney, with consequent infection and renal scarring.

◄ Recurrent urinary tract infection suggests major underlying abnormality of the renal tract

Frequent episodes of infection require investigation of the urinary tract with an intravenous urogram and repeated urine culture to determine the pathogen, usually *E. coli*. If there is reflux from bladder to ureter, either surgical correction or long-term suppressive therapy with low doses of a suitable antibiotic is recommended.

◄ *E. coli* is the commonest causative organism of urinary infections occurring outside of hospital

Table 10.6. Factors associated with urinary tract infection

Pregnancy
Diabetes mellitus
Raised B.P.
Excessive use of analgesics
Genito-urinary abnormality and instrumentation of renal
    tract
Family history of renal disease

Urinary tract obstruction

Urinary tract obstruction occurs if the flow of urine is impeded at any point in its course from the calices of the ureter to the exterior. Initially glomerular filtration (GFR) will continue but, if the obstruction persists, eventually, the urinary tract dilatation no longer protects the kidney, filtration pressure is exceeded with fall in GFR.

There are many causes for urinary tract obstruction arising within the lumen (calculus, blood clot and tumour), within the wall (stricture following trauma and inflammation, as well as neurogenic causes) and

◄ Obstruction must be excluded in all cases of unexplained renal failure

Table 10.7. Causes of urinary tract obstruction

Within the lumen
    stone, blood clot, tumour
Within the wall
    stricture (inflammatory) — tuberculosis, gonococcal
    neurological (diabetes, MS, cord lesions)
    congenital malformations (urethra, ureter)
    trauma
From outside
    pressure by blood vessels (pelvi-ureteric junction)
    tumours in the pelvis
    prostatic hypertrophy

pressure from outside (by tumours, blood vessels and, in the male, the prostate). The symptoms of upper urinary tract obstruction are loin pain, often made worse by high fluid intake; whilst those of bladder outflow obstruction are hesitancy, diminished force of the urinary stream, dribbling at the end of urination and, finally, retention of urine, sometimes with overflow incontinence.

Diagnosis depends on radiological assessment of the site of obstruction, aided by ultra-sound, and by examination of the lower urinary tract with an optical instrument (cytoscope). Treatment is aimed at relieving obstruction and therapy for the underlying cause and any infection present. Operation for bladder outflow obstruction is usually performed when there is upper tract dilatation. When prostatic hypertrophy is the cause, after initial pain relief and bladder drainage, the gland is resected through the urethra or, occasionally, through the bladder.

Hereditary diseases of the kidney

Polycystic disease of the kidneys may present in infancy and adulthood. The infantile form may be obvious in the baby but may be first recognized in older children because of abdominal masses, which may be renal or hepatic. The child often looks abnormal, has a typical

Table 10.8.   Renal tubular disorders

Defects in renal tubular transport mechanisms
  Cystinuria — autosomal recessive — renal stones
  Hypophosphataemia — X-linked — rickets (vitamin D
    resistant)
  Renal tubular acidosis — dominant or secondary — renal
    stones — rickets
Defects in tubular response to hormones
  Diabetes insipidus — X-linked — polyuria, thirst
Secondary causes of multiple disorders
  Heavy metals — lead, gold
  Drugs — analgesics, aminoglycosides, out-dated
    tetracyclines
  Myeloma

---

appearance with low-set ears, broad flat nose and a small jaw (micrognathia). Progressive renal failure is invariable.

The adult form of polycystic disease of the kidney usually presents around the age of 40 and is a common cause of renal failure in adults. It may also present as haematuria, loin pain and raised blood pressure. Terminal renal failure may occur in some patients within 10 years of diagnosis, whilst other may have a normal lifespan.

There is a variety of renal tubular disorders which may be inborn errors of metabolism, affecting the transport of substances in the kidney and gut, as well as occurring with pyelonephritis and heavy metal (lead) poisoning. The age at onset of symptoms varies from infancy to adulthood, consisting of polyuria, thirst, bone pain (due to renal osteodystrophy), and renal colic due to aminoacid (usually cystine) stones. Diagnosis is made on the basis of biochemical abnormalities in plasma (acidosis) and urine (amino-aciduria and defects of concentration). Treatment consists of vitamin D and alkalies.

Neurological diseases 11

Disorders of the central nervous system are of importance to the dentist for many reasons: cranial nerve lesions which may present as oro-facial problems, such as weakness of muscles and non-dental facial pain; the effects of such diseases as Parkinsonism and multiple sclerosis on the face and mouth; and the problems of faints, fits and unconsciousness, that may occur due to brain disorders, and which can happen in the dental chair.

Structure and formation of the CNS

The central nervous system consists of the brain, brainstem, cerebellum and spinal cord. Structure and function are more intricately involved with each other in the CNS than in any other part of the body. The millions of neurones that make up the CNS tend to be grouped so that the nerve cells are grouped together (the 'grey matter'), as are the nerve fibres, which have a glistening appearance and are called the 'white matter'. Within the cerebellar and cerebral hemi-spheres the grey matter consists of a superficial outer layer, 'the cortex', in addition to the deeper grey areas found in the brainstem and spinal cord.

Within the cortex of both cerebral and cerebellar hemispheres there is localization of function and representation of the parts of the body within those areas. Higher psychical function is localized in the frontal lobes; vision in the occipital lobe; hearing in the superior aspect of the temporal lobe; motor function in the pre-central gyrus of the parietal lobe; sensory in the post-central gyrus; and speech in the dominant hemisphere, usually the left in right-handed individuals and the right in some, but not all, left-handers.

The *sensations* that are appreciated in all parts of the body may be divided into the cutaneous sensations of touch, pain, heat and cold, together with the sensation of pressure and movement arising from the tendons and joints, called 'somatic sensation'. The special senses, such as sight and hearing, have elaborate end organs for reception of the stimulus. Sensory information from the body passes from the periphery to brainstem and spinal cord and ascends to the thalamus, part of the deep grey matter of the cerebral hemispheres, and from there to the post-central gyrus in an orderly fashion, such that the contralateral (opposite) half of the body is represented upside-down. Sensation from the face is transmitted via the Vth cranial nerve, in a similar orderly fashion, to the descending nucleus of the trigeminal nerve (Vth) which sends information to the thalamus and thence to the sensory cortex on the contralateral side where it is represented the right way up, so that the neck area adjoins that for the top of the head. (*See Fig.* 11.1).

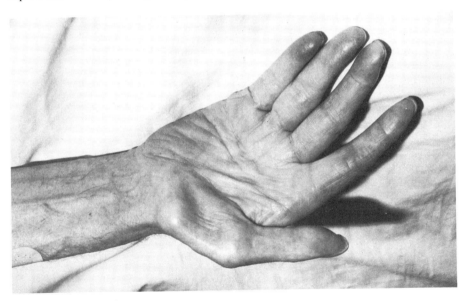

Fig. 11.1. Wasting of the small muscles of the hands. Lower motor neurone lesion due to motor neurone disease.

The *motor* area of the cortex occupies the pre-central gyrus and, like the sensory area, the opposite half of the body is represented upside-down. Fibres from the motor cortex pass through the internal capsule in an orderly arrangement with the head and face anteriorly placed and the lower limbs posterior. Via the cerebral peduncles the fibres then pass to the pons and those originating in the face areas of the cortex terminate at the motor nuclei of the Vth and VIIth nerves as well as the nuclei of the extinsic ocular and tongue muscles. Most of the remaining fibres cross to the opposite side at the lower end of the medulla, travelling down the spinal cord until they enter the spinal grey matter at the level appropriate to their origin in the motor cortex. A short neurone connects the upper motor neurone with the lower motor neurone, which originates in the anterior horn of the grey matter of the cord.

The motor system described has its effects on willed or skilled movements. Damage to the *upper motor neurone* (UMN) may occur at any point in its long pathway from the cortex to the connecting neurones in the spinal cord. The most frequent site for damage is in the internal capsule which produces weakness or paralysis of the limbs and face on the opposite side of the body (hemiparesis or hemiplegia, respectively) with stiffness (spasticity). Although there is loss of willed movement with an upper motor neurone lesion, involuntary movements may occur. In particular emotional movements of the face may be preserved and yawning may be associated with movements of a limb that cannot be moved voluntarily. Damage to the *lower motor neurone* (LMN), the final common pathway to the muscles, leads to complete paralysis with flaccidity of the muscles and wasting in the long term. Abnormal movements may occur in muscles paralysed following a LMN lesion, but are fine and dissociated (fasciculation) and are seen in the tongue with hypoglossal nerve damage.

Fibres from the motor cortex also form part of the *extrapyramidal system* and project to the cerebral grey masses, including the thalamus, from which there are connections with the cerebellum, the subthalamic nucleus, substantia nigra and the anterior horn cells. These fibres are concerned with positional adjustments of the body. Bending over to pick up a small object

◀ UMN has its effects on willed or skilled movements

◀ Involuntary movements, such as emotional expression in the face, are preserved in UMN lesions

◀ Fine, dissociated movements of paralysed muscles, fasciculation, is a feature of LMN lesions

requires skilled movements of the fingers but, if the person is not to fall, adjustment of the centre of gravity and maintenance of position must happen, which are the result of extrapyramidal activity. Disease of the extrapyramidal system does not cause paralysis but there is alteration of muscle tone, often feeling like a cogwheel when the hands or elbows are flexed and extended; there is poverty of spontaneous movements and falling forwards or backwards with minimal stimulus if the patient is standing still; in addition there are coarse spontaneous movements, particularly of the hands, called 'tremor', sometimes noted in the tongue and head (titubation).

◀ Maintenance of the position of limbs and the body by variation of muscle tone is the function of the extra-pyramidal system

The *cerebellum* controls movement whilst that movement is taking place. Control is exerted both before and when the movement is taking place and is achieved because of connections between the cerebellum and the motor cortex via the thalamus, and between specialized sensory organs in tendons and muscles and the cerebellum, which 'feed' the information needed for control. Disease of the cerebellum does not cause paralysis but chiefly manifests as lack of co-ordination of movements (ataxia) and tremor of the limbs during movement, not at rest, unlike that associated with extrapyramidal disease. In addition the tone of muscles is reduced in cerebellar disease, particularly in the limbs.

◀ The cerebellum controls movement whilst that movement is taking place

The *cranial nerves* are divided into twelve pairs although the first two, the olfactory (Ist) and optic (IInd), are purely sensory from specialized receptors. The *olfactory* nerves may be damaged in fractures through the anterior fossa of the skull, and by tumours or meningeal inflammation, causing impairment of the sense of smell. The sensory cortex may be damaged by tumour and there may be transient unpleasant olfactory sensations with reduced consciousness, called 'uncinate seizures' after the part of the temporal lobe which is the primary cortical area for this sensation.

Because of the length of the optic pathways damage may occur at many points from the *optic* nerve to the occipital cortex with resultant partial or total loss of vision and, because the fibres reflexly controlling pupillary size accompany the sensory fibres in part of the pathway, impairment of pupil response to light and accommodation stimuli may occur. Damage to one

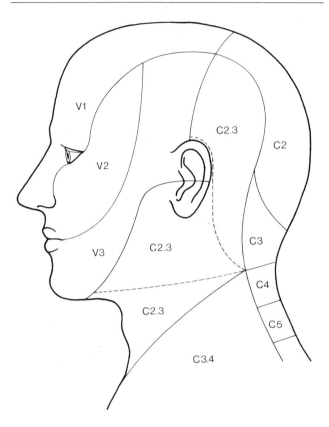

Fig. 11.2. Sensory innervation of face, head and neck.

optic nerve causes complete blindness in one eye, whereas lesions in the optic chiasma, usually caused by pituitary tumours, produce loss of the outer part of the field of vision in both eyes (bitemporal hemianopia). Posteriorly to the chiasma the fibres form the optic tract and may be intercepted by vascular lesions and tumours that invade the internal capsule, with defects in the contralateral halves of both visual fields (homonymous hemianopia), the patient noticing that he/she cannot see objects in that half of the field of vision without turning towards that side, and that driving a car becomes hazardous. Lesions at the beginning of the optic tract may interrupt the light reflex.

Paralysis of the external eye muscles is relatively common and may be due to skull fractures, meningeal inflammation, tumours, aneurysms of the intracranial arteries and generalized disorders, such as diabetes mellitus. The patient complains of double vision and there is usually an associated squint or strabismus. Squint may also be due to disease of the neuromuscular junction (myasthenia gravis). Most patients with squint do not have a cranial nerve lesion or disease of the neuromuscular junction (non-paralytic strabismus). Paralytic strabismus can be distinguished because there is a variable deviation of the axis of the eyes according to direction of gaze, whereas non-paralytic squint shows a constant deviation from the normal parallel optic axis. Double vision (diplopia) is not a symptom of non-paralytic squint.

◀ Paralytic squints show variation with position of gaze and are usually associated with diplopia

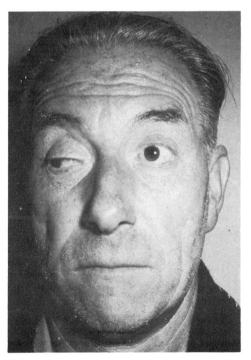

Fig. 11.3. R. third nerve palsy.
Note ptosis and deviation of eye outwards.

Paralysis of the *IIIrd cranial nerve* is associated with lateral deviation of the affected eye with associated drooping of the eyelid (ptosis) and usually pupillary dilatation due to parasympathetic nerve damage, the constrictor fibres accompanying the IIIrd nerve. Isolated damage to the *IVth cranial nerve* is unusual and cannot easily be detected when the other oculomotor cranial nerves are damaged. When the *VIth cranial nerve* is paralysed the eye fails to move laterally when the patient looks towards the side of the lesion.

◄ Paralytic squint may be caused by lesions of the cranial nerves supplying the extraocular muscles and disease of the neuromuscular junction

In addition to tumours, aneurysms, and diabetes mellitus paralytic squint may occur with hypertension, syphilis, cranial arteritis (*see* Chapter 12), blood disorders such as polycythaemia, myasthenia gravis and ophthalmic Graves' disease (*see* Chapter 9).

The *trigeminal Vth* nerve has both motor and sensory functions. Motor weakness is tested by forceful clenching of the jaw, when the muscles on the affected side are flaccid, or by opening the mouth when the jaw may deviate towards the affected side, because of weakness of medial pterygoid muscles. UMN lesions are not detected clinically since there is probable innervation from the motor cortex in both hemispheres.

The sensory functions of the trigeminal nerve are tested by response to touch, pain and temperature stimuli to the face, forehead and scalp as far as the vertex of the skull. Lesions affecting the first, or ophthalmic division result in loss of the blink reflex. Interruption of the sensory fibres causes loss of sensation in the territory of the affected branch and may be due to damage to peripheral branches by local lesions in the face and mouth. Damage within the skull may occur with fractures of the base of the skull, meningeal inflammation, tumours and diseases of the brainstem, such as infarction and multiple sclerosis. Irritation of the nerve fibres produces pain in the area supplied and is the cause of trigeminal neuralgia, although the underlying pathological cause is not known.

The *VIIth cranial nerve* has the function of mediating impulses to the muscles of the face, and an additional role as the pathway for taste and innervation of lacrimal and salivary glands. Facial palsy is a common cranial nerve lesion and may result from UMN or LMN lesions

Table 11.1.   Differentiation of UMN and LMN facial weakness

	UMN weakness	*LMN weakness*
Forehead wrinkling, eye closure	Intact	Involved
Emotional facial expression	Retained	Affected
Blink reflex	Retained	Affected
Lacrimation and taste	Unaffected	Affected
Tongue protrusion	Unaffected	Apparent deviation to normal side

(*see Table* 11.1). UMN facial paralysis usually occurs with weakness of the arm on the same side and with loss of speech (dysphasia) if the dominant hemisphere is affected. The likely causes for UMN lesions are cerebrovascular disease and tumours. LMN paralysis may be caused by a variety of conditions including cerebral tumours, vascular disease, diabetes, infections such as herpes zoster, middle ear disease and multiple sclerosis (*see Table* 11.2). The most frequent cause of facial paralysis is Bell's palsy, which is idiopathic and acute in onset. Transient facial paralysis may occur in dental practice following attempts to give an anaesthetic block to the inferior dental nerve.

LMN facial weakness may be associated with disturbance of taste and lacrimation. Loss of taste on the anterior two-thirds of the tongue occurs with many lesions of the facial nerve, particularly those central to the point at which the chorda tympani leaves it, in the middle ear.

The *VIIIth cranial nerve* is made up of two functionally different components: the vestibular nerve which transmits sensory information from the semicircular canals in the middle ear, and the acoustic nerve

Table 11.2.   Causes of LMN facial weakness

Bell's palsy — acute idiopathic
Vascular lesions — hypertension, syphilis
Diabetes mellitus
Multiple sclerosis
Middle ear disease — mastoiditis, chronic otitis media
Posterior fossa tumours
Herpes zoster — geniculate ganglion

which transmits information from the cochlea and the specialized sensory organ of Corti. Damage to the vestibular nerve fibres may occur in the middle ear or at any point during its course through the posterior fossa to the brainstem, usually by tumours, and may be associated with vertigo. Damage to the cochlear division is associated with loss of hearing, which also occurs with disease of the middle and inner ear (conductive deafness).

The *IXth* (*glossopharyngeal*) *nerve* is closely related to the vagus or Xth cranial nerve. It carries fibres subserving taste from the posterior third of the tongue and motor fibres to the pharynx. Because of intermingling of the fibres of the IXth and Xth nerves, pure glossopharyngeal nerve lesions are not easy to detect,

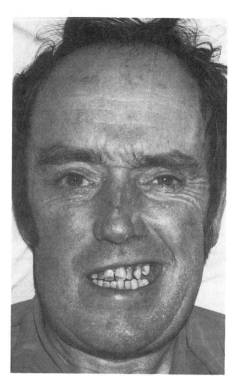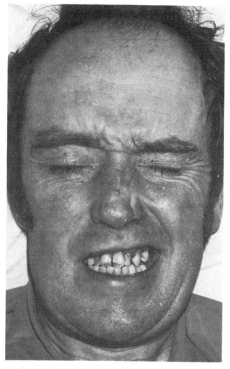

Fig. 11.4. R. Bell's palsy. Note absence of forehead creases on same side, absence of wrinkling around eye and incomplete closure of eye.

since testing of taste on the posterior part of the tongue is difficult. Paroxysmal pain may occur in the distribution of the nerve, which is usually severe (glossopharyngeal neuralgia) and, although uncommon, may require surgical interruption of the nerve to effect relief.

The *Xth cranial nerve, the vagus*, carries fibres of all types but is predominantly a visceral nerve concerned with the motor function of the larynx and pharynx, as well as autonomic effects on heart rate, size of the airways, mucus secretion and peristalsis of the bowel. The nerve has a long course and may be damaged at many points by trauma, enlarged lymph nodes and by aneurysms of the carotid artery and aorta. The most frequent lesion of the vagus is damage to the recurrent laryngeal nerves by tumour, by surgery or by aneurysms with consequent vocal cord paralysis, voice change and difficulty with expectoration of sputum. Lesions at a higher level in brainstem lesions (motor neurone disease and vascular disorders) may cause paralysis of larynx and pharynx with difficulty in swallowing and overspill of food and saliva into the trachea. UMN lesions of the vagus occur with bilateral damage, as in vascular disorders involving both hemispheres, occurring at an interval of some months and years. Occasionally transient slurring of speech (dysarthria) and difficulty with swallowing (dysphagia) complicate a stroke.

◄ Lesions of the vagus nerve in the brainstem cause paralysis of the larynx and pharynx with swallowing difficulty and overspill of food into the trachea

The *XIth cranial nerve, the accessory*, has motor function only and receives fibres from the medulla and from the third and fourth segments of the cervical portion of the spinal cord. Isolated lesions of the nerve are unusual and are associated with features of the Xth and XIIth cranial nerve lesions. The nerve supplies motor fibres to the sternomastoid and trapezius muscles and is responsible for movements of the head from side to side, lifting of the head from the horizontal and shrugging of the shoulders.

The *hypoglossal* or *XIIth cranial nerve* supplies motor fibres to the tongue and can be assessed by the mobility of the tongue. Weakness of one half of the tongue causes difficulty with protrusion in the midline, the tongue deviating towards the weakened side, which may show atrophy with a LMN lesion. Bilateral lesions are detected by difficulty in protrusion of the tongue

◄ Paralysis of half of the tongue is associated with loss of protrusion in the midline and deviation towards the weakened side

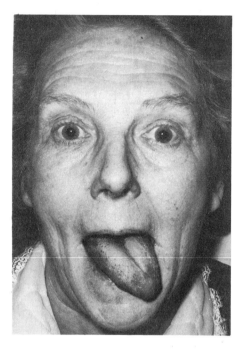

Fig. 11.5. L. hypoglossal nerve paralysis. Note deviation of tongue towards the affected side.

beyond the lips. LMN lesions are usually due to trauma, surgery, or pressure by enlarged lymph nodes in the neck, either malignant or, occasionally, tuberculous. Fasciculation of the tongue indicates that the lesion is in the LMN. Unilateral UMN lesions, acompanying a stroke, are usually transient; bilateral UMN hypoglossal lesions occur with pseudobulbar palsy, the tongue being small but not atrophic, although there is disturbance of swallowing and speech.

Symptoms and signs of neurological diseases

The symptoms of CNS diseases are few and the symptom-complexes that are encountered in clinical practice are likely to be due to many pathological processes.

Headache and facial pain are frequent features of CNS disorders and may be due to benign conditions such as migraine, or to more serious lesions such as cerebral tumours. Headache due to the latter is usually due to raised intracranial pressure, which also occurs with hydrocephalus (increased fluid and blood content of the brain) and with local pressure effects on blood vessels, dura and cranial nerves. The headache of raised intracranial pressure is worse on waking, may throb in time with the pulse, and is made worse by exertion, sneezing, lying or bending down. It is usually bilateral, both frontal and occipital, and associated with vomiting, with little preceding nausea, and deteriorating visual acuity. Occasionally patients have very high intracranial pressure without headache. Headaches due to the local pressure effects of tumours are generalized and when lateralized may not be on the same side. Lesions in the posterior fossa may cause pain in the neck referred to the face and throat.

◀ Headache, worse in the morning, vomiting and loss of visual acuity are the symptoms of raised intracranial pressure

Headaches may be vascular in origin and *migraine* is typical of disorder of this kind. The pain rapidly builds up to a throbbing sensation which may be generalized but is typically unilateral, hence the term 'hemicrania'. Attacks may last for up to 48 hours and, in the early stages, may be transiently relieved by pressure over the superficial temporal artery, which is often engorged and pulsating during the attack.

Double vision is usually a symptom of neurological disorder, particularly with strabismus, although monocular diplopia may be due to local eye disease. Non-paralytic or congential squints rarely cause diplopia.

Dizziness is a symptom that many patients have difficulty in describing accurately, but it is important to decide whether it is the sensation of light-headedness or faintness that is being described or true vertigo, which is the hallucination of movement, rotatory or swaying. Light-headedness may occur before syncope, or be associated with hypoglycaemia, hyperventilation and anxiety states. True vertigo indicates a lesion in the semicircular canal of the middle ear, the vestibular nerve, brainstem or, uncommonly, the temporal lobes (*see Table* 11.3) Pallor, sweating and vomiting are

Table 11.3. Causes of vertigo

Middle ear disease
Labyrinthine end organ lesions
Brainstem and vestibular branch of the VIIIth nerve lesions

common accompaniments of vertigo due to a peripheral labyrinthine lesion. Vertigo in some instances may be associated with hearing loss and *nystagmus* — jerking movements of the eye which may be exaggerated or provoked by the patient fixing his gaze on an object. Nystagmus may occur with central (brainstem) or vestibular nerve lesions and with disorders of the middle ear and semicircular canals (*see Table* 11.4). Nystagmus due to peripheral lesions is only present during vertigo, is brought out by fixing the gaze, and is unidirectional but not vertical. Central nystagmus is multidirectional, may be vertical, persists between attacks of vertigo, and is unaffected or abolished by fixation.

Transient loss of consciousness may occur in many neurological disorders and it is important to distinguish the two major causes, syncope and epilepsy. Syncope is defined as transient loss of consciousness caused by an acute decrease in cerebral blood flow, whilst an epileptic seizure is the result of an abnormal paroxysmal discharge of cerebral neurones, the number and location of which determine the features of the 'fit'. The distinction between seizure and syncope is not always easy, particularly if there has been no witness to an attack (*see Table* 11.5).

Table 11.4. Distinction between peripheral and central nystagmus

	Peripheral	*Central*
Both eyes	Yes	Can be, but may be greater in one eye
Direction	Unidirectional	Multidirectional
Persistency	During attacks vertigo	Persistent between attacks vertigo
Effects of fixation of gaze	Brought out	Abolished or unaffected
Vertical	Never vertical	May be vertical

Table 11.5. Distinction between epilepsy and syncope

	Epilepsy	Syncope
Colour	May be cyanosed	Pale and sweating
Pulse	Difficulty in palpation (because of convulsion)	Slow
Convulsions	Usual	Uncommon (except in elderly)
Urinary inconti- nence	Yes	Yes (if bladder full)
Tongue biting	Yes	No
Duration	Minutes or hours (post-ictal confusion)	Brief
Warning	None or sensory/motor	Noises in ear, visual loss
Provocation	None usually. May be alcohol, exertion, menses	Posture, coughing, pressure on neck in elderly

Loss of consciousness in syncope is usually gradual, accompanied by nausea, sweating and 'greying-out' of vision. The patient appears pale but recovers quickly once lying flat, and does not show confusion or neurological abnormalities. Twitching of the limbs and urinary incontinence may occur during syncope, particularly if the head is prevented from falling to the level of the heart, so that cerebral hypoxia occurs. Syncope usually occurs in response to strong emotional stimuli such as the sight of blood, or with standing for long periods or standing after prolonged sitting.

Generalized seizures may be associated with tongue biting, apnoea and widespread shaking movements of all limbs, the whole episode lasting two to three minutes and followed by confusion, which may last for hours. Minor seizures, or *petit mal*, are typically very

Table 11.6. Causes of syncope

Reflex (vasovagal) — haemorrhage, upright posture, hypoxia, emotion and pain
Respiratory — coughing, lifting weights
Cardiac — aortic valve disease, disturbances of cardiac rhythm
Loss of cardiovascular reflexes — diabetes, neuropathies, alcoholism, drugs (hypotensives, phenothiazines, levo-dopa)
Brainstem ischaemia — migraine, vascular diseases

brief, lasting a few seconds, consisting of involuntary jerking of limbs (myoclonus) which may also occur as the result of cerebral anoxia following cardiac arrest.

Transient loss of consciousness may also occur with non-neurological causes, particularly paroxysmal cardiac dysrhythmias which may also be associated with abnormal movements, as the result of cerebral hypoxia (*see Table* 11.6). Breath-holding in the young child may also cause central cyanosis with twitching.

Transient cerebral ischaemia is not normally associated with any impairment of consciousness, but syncope may occur although this is never associated with jactitation. Ischaemia of brain tissue rarely provokes epilepsy.

Table 11.7. Types of spontaneous involuntary movements

Tremor
Chorea
Myoclonus
Tics

Involuntary movements of the limbs, face and tongue without loss of consciousness may be a symptom or sign of neurological disorders of the central grey matter of the cerebral hemispheres, the basal ganglia (*see Table* 11.7). There are several types of spontaneous involuntary movements, the most frequent being *tremor*, a fast movement of the part affected, fingers or tongue, which is an up-and-down or forward-and-backward movement, often called 'sinusoidal'. Tremor may be present with the arms resting, when trying to maintain the position of the part affected or may occur only with movement (intention tremor). Resting tremor occurs with Parkinsonism and may be due to drugs, such as the phenothiazines. Postural tremor occurs with anxiety states, hyperthyroidism and alcohol (*see* Chapter 7). Intention tremor occurs with brainstem and cerebellar diseases such as multiple sclerosis, tumour and vascular lesions.

A less frequent involuntary movement is *chorea* in which there are continuous, randomly distributed and irregularly timed muscle jerks which may affect the face, may interrupt walking, and interfere with fine manipulations of the hands and with speech. The projected tongue pops in and out and the outstretched arms cannot be kept still. Chorea may complicate treatment with phenytoin and may rarely occur in young females on the contraceptive pill. It may occur in systemic disorders such as thyrotoxicosis and systemic lupus erythematosus; as well as with degenerative CNS disorders such as Huntington's chorea.

Myoclonus consists of brief shock-like movements of muscles, which may be a feature of *petit mal* and may occur with renal, hepatic and respiratory failure. *Tics*, although similar to myoclonus, are repetitive and can be controlled by the patient. The movements often involve the face (sniffing, blinking, lip-smacking) and are common in childhood, usually disappearing with maturity.

Sensory symptoms and signs may occur with diseases of sensory cranial nerves and the peripheral nerve trunks. The usual symptoms are numbness, tingling, and feelings of pins-and-needles in the face, hands and feet. When the legs are affected the patient may complain of a feeling of walking on cotton-wool.

Muscular weakness and wasting of muscle groups may be the features of both neurological and muscle disorders. The degree of weakness may vary from time to time and even during the course of a day, particularly in myasthenia gravis. The patient may notice difficulty in climbing stairs, stumbling while walking, weakness of hand grip, drooling from the mouth and, occasionally, difficulty with swallowing. Wasting is most obvious in the limbs, usually distal except when the spinal roots are predominantly affected when the proximal muscles are involved. The face and tongue may show wasting although, clinically, this is more difficult to detect particularly if there is bilateral involvement. Weakness without muscular wasting is a feature of UMN lesions, such as may follow 'stroke', with loss of voluntary but not involuntary movements, such as emotional changes in the face.

Vascular diseases affecting the CNS

The commonest disorders of the CNS are those due to vascular diseases (*see Table* 11.8). The underlying pathology of cerebrovascular incidents is varied and

Table 11.8.   Classification of stroke

Development
  completed
  progressive (may be subdural haematoma)
  transient ischaemia (may be embolic)
Underlying anatomy
  carotid artery
  vertebrobasilar artery
Vascular pathology
  atheroma
  hypertensive vascular disease
  embolism from heart or large vessels
  arterial disease other than atheroma, arteritis, syphilis

may be atheromatous degeneration of the cerebral vessels, hypertensive vascular disease, embolism from the heart or major arteries in the neck and thorax, and lesions such as arteritis, syphilis and aneurysm. Whatever the underlying vascular lesion the symptoms and signs are determined by the specific vessels involved, whether in the territory supplied by the carotid or the vertebrobasilar arteries.

The development of the stroke may vary from transient neurological disturbance, lasting less than 24 hours, to the progressive form evolving over hours and sometimes days, and the completed stage, where the disability is at its maximum within a few hours of onset. The development depends on the lesion in the brain that results from the vascular disease; haemorrhage into the substance of the brain being manifest as a completed stroke, often with deteriorating conscious level or coma from the onset; cerebral infarction may present as either the completed or progressive form; ischaemia is usually associated with transient signs and symptoms, although minor disability may persist.

Strokes in the territory of the cartoid artery produce contralateral weakness (hemiparesis), affecting the face and arm more than the leg in the case of middle cerebral occlusion, and the leg more than the upper limb if the anterior cerebral vessel is involved. If the dominant hemisphere is affected there may be speech disturbance, affecting comprehension and expression (dysphasia), and a lesion in either hemisphere following middle cerebral occlusion may cause loss of the contralateral half of the visual field (homonymous hemianopia), because of damage to the optic tract.

Strokes involving the vertebrobasilar artery have many different manifestations including diplopia, facial paraesthesia or numbness, dysarthria and ataxia. Swallowing may be affected because of weakness of bulbar muscles and there may be bilateral or alternate involvement of motor and sensory function in the limbs. Involvement of the posterior cerebral arteries causes hemianopia.

An important cause of stroke that is not directly due to the vascular pathology described is *subdural haematoma*. It is probably more common than thought and invariably follows head injury; unfortunately the history of trauma may not be obtained from the patient or his relatives. Bleeding occurs from the subdural veins producing features of a progressive stroke but with invariable depression of consciousness which is out of proportion to the severity of hemiparesis. There may be cranial nerve palsies, and differences in the size of pupils and symptoms that suggest raised intracranial pressure. The condition occurs most commonly in the young and the elderly. It is important to make an early diagnosis because the condition can be treated by craniotomy and removal of the clot.

Small *aneurysms* of the major intracranial arteries may arise at sites of congenital defects in the muscular coat, usually at the bifurcation of vessels. They may be symptomless, or present as life-threatening bleeding into the subarachnoid space, or by pressure effects on cranial nerves, usually those responsible for eye movements. The features of subarachnoid haemorrhage vary from sudden violent pain in the head or neck with vomiting and dislike of light (photophobia) to rapid onset of unconsciousness with death within 6 hours. The physical features are due to meningeal irritation with dislike of light, neck stiffness and transient stroke due to spasm of the blood vessel from which bleeding has occurred.

Subarachnoid haemorrhage due to aneurysm, without signs due to spasm, is often treated surgically, either by direct approach and clipping of the neck of the sac, or by carotid ligation in the neck. Where there is spasm surgery is delayed, but if the aneurysm is on the vertebro-basilar artery conservative management is advised.

Subarachnoid haemorrhage may also occur from angiomas of the brain, which are developmental abnormalities with precapillary links between arteries and veins. Epilepsy may also be a presenting feature of angioma, and some patients have classic migraine. Some angiomas may be associated with similar malformations in the skin of the head and neck, described as a port-wine naevus (Sturge-Weber syndrome, *see* Chapter 15).

Giant cell arteritis is a granulomatous inflammation of arteries that may present as stroke due to involvement of intracranial vessels. The disease is of importance for the dentist since the facial, maxillary and lingual vessels may be involved. Involvement of these extracranial arteries may give rise to tenderness of the vessels, pain in the face, jaw and mouth made worse by eating; there may be difficulty in opening the mouth and protruding the tongue, which may be painful and indurated, with glossitis, due to ischaemia. A more important complication is uniocular visual loss, which is irreversible in some instances. There may be associated systemic features including generalized muscle pains, anorexia, sweating, fever and general malaise. Diagnosis is made by biopsy of the superficial temporal artery, particularly a tender portion. Treatment with large doses of corticosteroids is dramatically effective and is continued in a small maintenance dose for a year or more. Episodes of retinal and cerebral ischaemia do not occur after steroid treatment for 3-4 days.

◀ A presenting feature of cranial arteritis may be pain in the face and jaw when chewing

Infective and inflammatory diseases of CNS

Meningitis, inflammation of the covering membranes of the brain, may be bacterial or viral in origin, and the disease may arise as the result of blood infection (bacteraemia or viraemia) or via direct spread from infection in the middle ear, the paranasal sinuses or following fractures of the base of the skull, which are associated with tears of the meninges. The bacteria that commonly cause meningitis are *Neisseria meningitides* (meningococcus), *Streptococcus pneumoniae* (pneumococcus), *Haemophilus influenzae* and *Mycobacterium tuberculosis*. A large number of viruses may cause meningitis, usually in a mild form, and inflammation of brain substance (encephalitis).

Whatever the cause the clinical features are those of meningeal irritation, and sub-arachnoid haemorrhage is only excluded by lumbar puncture and examination of the CSF. Features of meningitis, but with a normal CSF, may occur in children and young adults associated with intercurrent infections (meningism). Coma and neurological signs may arise from cerebral infarction due to venous occlusion, subdural collection of pus and cerebral abscess. Raised intracranial pressure may be produced by abscess formation or by cerebral oedema, secondary inflammation of the intracranial veins and venous sinuses.

Pyogenic meningitis is treated with the appropriate antibiotic given parenterally; injection into the CSF pathways being unnecessary. The mortality rate for bacterial meningitis is 10% (pneumococcal infections having the poorest prognosis), although it is higher in the tuberculous form which requires prolonged treatment with three antituberculous drugs. There is no specific treatment for viral meningoencephalitis, idoxuridine being given for the more severe forms such as that caused by herpes simplex, although most varieties improve with only general measures.

Brain abscess may complicate bacterial meningitis, but may also be caused by spread of sepsis from the middle ear or paranasal sinuses, by penetrating head injury and by blood-borne spread, particularly in patients with congenital heart disease. The first manifestation may be a single epileptic seizure or a self-limiting, meningitis-like illness with sterile CSF. Subsequently the manifestations are those of an expanding lesion, with progressive stroke, as may be expected with intracranial tumours and haematoma. After localization by CAT scanning, the treatment consists of antibacterials given parenterally and into the abscess cavity during procedures to excise or drain the lesion. Mortality remains high (30%) for cerebral abscess and is usually the result of rupture into the CSF pathways, or to cerebral infarction.

A further complication of meningitis is thrombosis,

due to inflammation, of the intracranial veins and venous sinuses, which may also complicate head injuries and disorders of blood coagulability. The clinical features consist of headache, fever and signs due to cerebral infarction. Thrombosis of the cavernous sinus is associated with lesions of the cranial nerves responsible for ocular movement and facial sensation.

Parkinson's disease and involuntary movements

No cause is known for the commonest disease of the basal ganglia, idiopathic paralysis agitans (Parkinson's disease). The pathological changes in the CNS are in the pigmented neurones of the brainstem, and are associated with a marked reduction in the amount of dopamine, which is the neurotransmitter at nerve terminals in the caudate nucleus and putamen of the thalamus. Although there are other biochemical abnormalities, such as reduced noradrenaline concentrations, the concept of dopamine deficiency has led to the introduction of treatment with levodopa.

Apart from resting tremor, which disappears with movement, the other main clinical features of Parkinson's disease are rigidity of muscles, a flexed posture with loss of stability, most obvious when the patient walks, and slowness of initiation and execution of movements (akinesia), of which the masked face and loss of blinking are typical features (*see Table* 11.9). Mental disturbances, mainly progressive intellectual deterioration, may occur in the later stages of the disease. Other symptoms and signs of Parkinson's disease are skeletal deformities of the hands that resemble rheumatoid arthritis, although there is no contracture; limitation of upward gaze of the eyes may

Table 11.9.   Clinical features of Parkinson's disease

Tremor — at rest, not made worse by movement
Rigidity — most marked axially but eventually affects limbs
Postural abnormalities — fixed posture, instability, small
    stepping gait
Akinesia — poverty of movements, facial immobility

occur, and episodes of prolonged upward deviations associated with facial flushing and sweating (oculogyric crises) can occur with post-encephalitis and drug-induced disease. Drooling of saliva and some difficulty in swallowing, with loss of weight, may also be features of the disorder.

Drugs (phenothiazines, reserpine, and butyrophenones), previous encephalitis, degenerative disorders, vascular disease of the CNS and head injury produce a syndrome like idiopathic Parkinson's disease.

There is no treatment that affects the underlying pathological changes of the illness, and the therapeutic aim is to maintain mobility without side effects. The drugs used are either anticholinergic in action, which may also cause dryness of the mouth, blurred vision and urinary retention, or dopaminergic, principally levodopa, alone or in combination with carbidopa or benserazide, which may cause nausea and postural hypotension.

Generalized involuntary movements (*see Table* 11.10) may also occur: in Huntington's chorea; as part of rheumatic fever (Sydenham's chorea) which may show recrudescence during pregnancy and with the oral contraceptive; with cerebral damage from anoxia or trauma during birth (athetoid cerebral palsy); and as

Table 11.10.　Involuntary movements

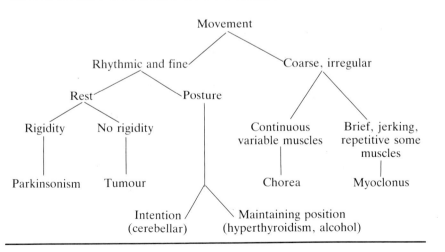

part of a rare disorder of copper metabolism, inherited as an autosomal dominant, with associated cirrhosis of the liver (Wilson's disease). A further common cause of generalized tremor is *benign essential tremor*, which is inherited as an autosomal dominant trait without any pathological or biochemical cause, as yet identified. The tremor is provoked by maintaining posture of the arms, but is not made worse by movement and is not present at rest, although the jaw, head and legs may be affected. Unlike Parkinsonism handwriting is not affected in benign essential tremor and the disorder is only slowly progressive, causing social inconvenience rather than disability.

Localized involuntary movements of the face, mouth and neck may be noted by the dentist. Unilateral, brief, irregular spasmodic contractions of the facial muscles (*hemifacial spasm*) may follow facial paralysis, or may be due to nerve compression by tumour or Paget's disease of bone, but can often be without obvious cause, affecting the middle aged and beginning with twitching around the eyes which subsequently spreads to the rest of the face. Intermittent spasms of the muscles around the eyes (*blepharospasm*) may occur in Parkinson's disease but may occur in older patients without any obvious cause. Regular rhythmic movements of the palate causing the uvula to bob up and down, and speech to become tremulous (palatal myoclonus) is a rare disorder associated with facial and tongue twitching. Sustained or intermittent spasms of the sternomastoid usually occur in infants, but in adults may be due to drug therapy, often phenothiazines.

Neuroleptic drugs, beta-adrenergic agonists and phenothiazines are some of the drugs that may cause abnormal movements and episodes of persistent spasm of muscles (dystonia), particularly in the neck.

Multiple sclerosis

Multiple sclerosis (MS) is another chronic neurological disorder. The disease, classically, pursues a relapsing and remitting course but may also be slowly progressive and is due to focal areas of demyelination in the brain and spinal cord. It has an unusual geographical distribution being of low incidence in tropical and sub-tropical zones. Its cause is unknown, although there is the possibility that it may be either a slow-virus infection of the CNS, similar to laboratory models that can be produced by the virus of chickenpox, or an immunological disorder.

The clinical features of MS are varied. The symptoms, which are usually rapid in onset, are those of brainstem disorder with diplopia, facial paraesthesia and weakness, with UMN weakness of the arms and legs. There may be inco-ordination of the limbs and trunk due to cerebellar involvement; paraesthesia in the limbs as well as the face; and visual disturbances which are usually early and transient. Less frequent symptoms are: seizures; vertigo due to damage in the vestibular tracts and cerebellum; and urinary incontinence. Facial pain may be a symptom of MS and resembles that of neuralgia, except that the subject is often young (less than 40 years of age).

Relapses may last from 2 weeks to more than a month, followed by incomplete recovery to a degree of disability that is greater than previous to the exacerbation. Treatment of relapses is usually symptomatic and by physiotherapy. Steroid therapy (prednisolone or ACTH) is sometimes given since it seems to limit the duration of exacerbations, but not the resultant disability. Long-term treatment with ACTH or prednisolone is not of benefit, even in the slowly progressive form of the disease.

The life expectancy varies considerably from less than a year to 50 years, on average 14-25. Death is usually the result of respiratory infections, accompanying bulbar nerve involvement and the consequent difficulties with swallowing, or urinary tract infection, when there is bladder denervation complicated by retention of urine with incontinence.

Facial pain and paraesthesia in the distribution of the trigeminal nerve in a patient under the age of 40 is usually due to multiple sclerosis

Motor Neurone Disease

Motor neurone disease is a progressive degenerative disorder of the motor neurones, upper and lower, principally the latter, in the brainstem and spinal cord. There are several forms of the disease with weakness affecting different parts of the body and a variable rate of evolution of the signs and symptoms.

The most prolonged form of the disease is *progressive muscular atrophy*, in which there are weakness, atrophy and fasciculation of muscles in the arms, usually proximal and initially unilateral. This form may progress to involve the bulbar motor nerves, causing features of *bulbar palsy*, which can be the initial presentation of the disorder. In patients with progressive bulbar palsy there is weakness of the tongue and pharynx, with impairment of swallowing and episodes of inhalation pneumonia. Later, jaw and facial movements are affected, and there may be nasal regurgitation of liquids due to palatal weakness. The disease may also present with progressive weakness of the limbs, initially the legs, with terminal involvement of the bulbar nerves after an interval of 2–3 years.

There is no treatment for motor neurone disease. Weakness of respiratory muscles and bulbar involvement predispose to respiratory infections and ventilatory failure, which are the usual causes of death.

◄ Difficulty with swallowing, coughing during eating, and nasal regurgitation of fluids are important symptoms of bulbar nerve involvement by disorders such as motor neurone disease, multiple sclerosis and brainstem vascular disease

Epilepsy

An epileptic seizure is the result of an abnormal paroxysmal discharge of cerebral neurones. The term 'epilepsy' is used to mean a continuing tendency to seizures, although the interval may be 30 years or more between episodes or there may be many over a brief period during adolescence but none thereafter. The variation in frequency between individuals, and sometimes between different periods of a person's life, can be explained by the seizure threshold, beyond which stimuli such as fever, alcohol, exercise, menstruation and emotion may trigger an episode.

The incidence of epilepsy declines with age up to 60 years, whereafter there is an increase. In children the frequency is 100/100,000/year falling to 30-40/100,000/year in middle age.

Seizures are classified according to the clinical manifestation, the anatomical basis, presumed cause and the electroencephalographic (EEG) changes in and between attacks. Seizures are classified as generalized, including *grand mal* convulsions; *petit mal* absences; partial seizures including Jacksonian attacks due to a 'focus' of local cerebral damage; and complex partial seizures (psychomotor epilepsy), in which disturbance of consciousness is accompanied by co-ordinated motor activity or stereotyped repetitive movements, involving the jaw and facial muscles.

The cause of and the factors which predispose to epilepsy are both intrinsic (genetic) and extrinsic. Almost half the siblings of a patient with generalized seizures may show EEG abnormalities during provocation (over-breathing and flashing lights), even though they have never had an overt attack. Among the possible structural or extrinsic causes are trauma, tumours and vascular disease, such as previous stroke. Infections of the CNS such as brain abscess and encephalitis may cause seizure discharge. Metabolic abnormalities, such as hypoglycaemia and hypocalcaemia, and drugs, such as antidepressants and alcohol, can precipitate seizures, particularly in the individual with genetic factors.

Some patients know the trigger for their seizures, by far the most common being rhythmic photic stimulation by, for example, flashing lights in a discotheque or watching TV. This form is termed 'reflex epilepsy' and may sometimes be triggered by reading, by certain musical noises, or by touching of one part of the body.

Investigation of the patient who has seizures is concerned with exclusion of structural damage and involves EEG and isotope or computerized scanning of the brain. The incidence of structural damage as a cause of seizures is greater in the older patient, about 1 in 10 of middle-aged onset epilepsy being due to tumours.

The object of medical management is to abolish seizures; but sometimes only partial control can be achieved without heavy dosage of anticonvulsants and unpleasant side effects. It is preferable to treat the patient with one drug alone in the optimum dose without causing side effects. Unfortunately most patients require two, and occasionally three drugs which may interact and produce a wide range of side effects. Other factors such as menstruation, contraception with steroid hormones, and pregnancy may disturb control of the seizure. Any seizure may, rarely, continue serially and is called *status epilepticus*. *Grand mal* is the most serious, the patient never regaining consciousness before the next seizure occurs, and death can occur from cardiorespiratory failure or brain damage. Control can usually be achieved by diazepam.

During a *grand mal* fit it is important that nothing should be put in the mouth, because of resulting damage to teeth. The tongue is bitten in the first stage of the seizure and this cannot be prevented by attempts to put an object between the teeth. All that is required , should the patient have an attack in the dental chair, is to prevent injury from falling to the floor. The patient should be turned to a semi-prone position with the head slightly lower than the shoulders, so that secretions drain out of the mouth and are not inhaled into the airways.

◄ It is wrong to place anything in the mouth during a fit since the tongue is bitten during the first stage of a seizure

Migraine and facial pain

Migraine is a periodic disorder of function of the cranial blood vessels resulting in headache of varying severity, often preceded by visual or sensory symptoms with nausea and vomiting. The occurrence is usually unpredictable but may occur at times of relaxation, after periods of stress. There are many predisposing factors, particularly dietary and psychic. An attack comprises prodromal symptoms, a variable feature occurring in classic but not in common migraine, followed by headache which is typically one-sided, but not consistent between episodes. The warning symptoms are due to cerebral ischaemia and comprise: visual loss if the retina is affected; hemiparesis or sensory disturbance if there is spasm of the middle cerebral artery; ataxia, vertigo, diplopia and paraesthesia in all four limbs with basilar artery involvement.

The headache may be generalized rather than hemi-cranial, building up rapidly from a dull ache to a throbbing intensity with vomiting and photophobia, the whole episode lasting up to 48 hours. During the headache the patient appears pale and the superficial temporal artery may be markedly pulsatile. There may be transient loss of consciousness, resembling a simple faint, associated with the headache, in the basilar artery variant.

The headache may be followed by transient neurological signs such as hemiparesis, paralysis of movements of one eye (ophthalmoplegic migraine) and facial paralysis, sometimes of LMN type. Uncommonly migraine may occur without headache, the features resembling a stroke, investigations being needed to exclude structural lesions.

There is a higher incidence of epilepsy in migraine sufferers. The development of a seizure during severe migraine is not uncommon.

Prevention of migraine is highly individual and, from experience, patients learn to avoid such foods as chocolate and fried meals. Drug therapy has largely proved ineffective in prevention but prompt administration of ergotamine, by injection or sublingually, may abort the attack in the patient who has a long aura. Oral contraceptives may influence the frequency of migraine, and the appearance of focal features requires immediate cessation of treatment.

Facial pain

Trigeminal neuralgia is one of the more important causes of facial pain of non-dental origin. It occurs in bouts that are self-limiting but which may persist many months, consisting of multiple severe, electric-shock-like pain of such intensity that the patient's face is contorted. Although the pain is described as 'continuous', careful history-taking reveals that there are many episodes lasting a few seconds limited to one division of the trigeminal nerve, usually starting in the maxillary but often spreading to the mandibular areas. There are characteristic trigger zones around the nose, the lower corner of the mouth, tongue and upper and lower gums which, when stimulated by touching, chewing, hot or cold drinks and sometimes even talking, immediately provoke an attack.

Simple analgesics are not effective in controlling the pain. Bouts often subside spontaneously, and attacks may be prevented by the anticonvulsants phenytoin and carbamazepine. If drugs are ineffective surgical treatment may be necessary. The trigeminal ganglion may either be injected with alcohol or the nerve root may be

◀ Trigger zones for trigeminal neuralgia may be in the upper or lower gums and can be stimulated by chewing, talking and hot or cold drinks

sectioned during craniotomy. Both methods result in loss of facial sensation and sometimes corneal anaesthesia with risk of ulceration.

It is more common to call other conditions 'trigeminal neuralgia', rather than to fail to recognize the disorder. Dental pain does not have the same distribution or trigger zones and atypical facial pain has none of the sharp episodes, nor the anatomical distribution.

Atypical facial pain is almost invariably in the second division of the Vth nerve, but is not strictly confined to the anatomical area and may pass over to the other side. The pain is usually described as 'burning' and persists for months or years, often related to an event such as dental procedure. The patient is invariably female and often goes from doctor to doctor or from dentist to dentist with the same complaint, although never appearing to be in severe pain.

Carbamazepine may sometimes be equally successful in atypical facial pain as in trigeminal neuralgia. Antidepressants may also be helpful in the absence of clear depressive illness.

Pain may follow *herpes zoster* of the trigeminal nerve. The first or ophthalmic division is most frequently affected but involvement of the maxillary and mandibular areas occurs. The history of the preceding vesicular rash, often with oral ulcers and herpetic scarring, are clues to the diagnosis of the pain, which is described as 'burning', 'continuous' and 'intolerable'. As in atypical facial pain, the patient does not seem to be in great pain and there may be depressive features. It is, however, a real and severe pain occurring in the older patient (over the age of 60) for which there is no universally successful treatment, including denervation.

Raeder's neuralgia is a severe pain around one eye accompanied by Horner's syndrome (small pupil and sunken eyeball) on the affected side. The pain may sometimes be confused with a migraine variant, migrainous trigeminal neuralgia, but is continuous and does not show the nocturnal clustering of attacks. The usual cause is malignancy, most often secondary deposits, in the base of the skull involving the paratrigeminal region.

Costen's syndrome consists of pain shooting down the

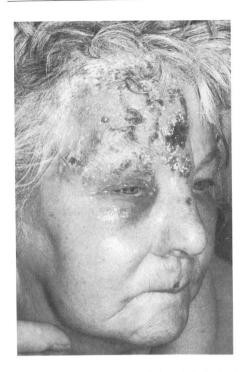

Fig. 11.6. Herpes zoster of R. ophthalmic division of trigeminal nerve. Note the clear demarcation of the rash, which does not extend beyond the midline.

mandibular area and up into the temple, accompanied by pain in the external auditory meatus. The pain is triggered by the patient chewing or perhaps by talking. The condition, which is diagnosed more often than is justified, is thought to be caused by dental malocclusion, being relieved by orthodontic procedures.

Muscle disorders

Primary muscle disorders alter the structure and function of striated muscle by changes in the muscle cell. The term 'myopathy' embraces all muscle disorders whether the defect is structural or involves the transmission of the electrical impulse, or is due to a biochemical abnormality of the metabolic pathways involved in muscle contraction. *Muscular dystrophy* is used to describe the group of genetically determined myopathies in which there is progressive destruction of muscle fibres with phagocyte invasion and fibrosis.

The symptoms and signs of muscle disorders are similar but vary in degree and distribution of the muscles affected. Weakness involves the shoulder and pelvic girdles so that the initial complaints are of difficulty in running, climbing stairs, difficulty with lifting, throwing and combing the hair. Muscle pain is uncommon except in rare disorders such as acute polymyositis, the myopathy associated with vitamin D deficiency and alcohol-induced muscle disorders. The distribution of wasting and weakness is of importance in distinguishing the various types of myopathy. Muscular hypertrophy occurs in the Duchenne type of muscular dystrophy, initially with normal power but later with profound weakness, when the enlarged muscles feel rubbery. Delayed muscle relaxation following cessation of forceful voluntary contraction (myotonia) occurs with some myopathies affecting particularly the tongue, the flexors of the fingers and the muscles of the thenar eminence.

Some muscle disorders may be associated with other, non-muscular abnormalities, such as signs of thyroid disorder. Associated bone pain and fracture suggest vitamin D deficiency, skin rashes and Raynaud's phenomenon may occur with dermatomyositis (often mistaken for scleroderma), and there may be features of Cushing's syndrome (*see* Chapter 9). Many muscle dystrophies may have associated cardiac muscle disorder presenting as heart failure, frequent dysrhythmias and sudden death.

◀ The tongue, muscles of the face and of mastication may all be affected by muscle disorders. Wasting, fasciculation, hypertrophy and fatiguability may be the clinical features

Muscular dystrophies

These disorders are usually classified on the basis of their pattern of inheritance, the age of onset, rate of progression and the distribution of muscle involvement.

The *X-linked dystrophies* occur in 20-30/100,000 live-born males, transmission occurring through the heterozygote female carrier, the affected male dying before reproducing. There are two forms: the *Duchenne* (severe) form, which begins on average by the third birthday, makes the child chairbound by the age of 9 years and causes death by the age of 22 years; and the *Becher* (more benign) form with later onset, chairbound age, and longer life expectancy. The earliest feature is a waddling gait, a tendency to fall and the characteristic sign of the child trying to get up by climbing up his own legs. Muscles that show enlargement include, calves, those of the shoulder girdle, and the masseters. Death occurs because of either heart failure or intercurrent respiratory infection.

Limb girdle dystrophies are rare. Some, the *scapulohumeral* form, are autosomal recessive disorders with varying disability which begins in the late teens or early twenties. The early symptoms affect lifting, throwing, and combing the hair. In other forms of the limb girdle group of dystrophies there may be difficulty in walking, running and climbing stairs.

Facioscapulohumeral dystrophy is a dominantly inherited disorder that varies widely in onset, from infancy to late teens, early onset being associated with a poor prognosis. Facial weakness manifests a pouting appearance of the lips and a transverse smile. There is progressive weakness of the upper limb, beginning proximally, and later leg weakness so that the patient may become wheelchair bound in the fourth or fifth decade of life.

Myasthenia gravis

Myasthenia gravis is a disorder of the neuromuscular junction which leads to fatiguability and sometimes paralysis. It is an immunological disorder in which there is a circulating antibody to the acetylcholine receptor in the junction.

The typical symptoms and signs are weakness with increasing fatigue as the day wears on. The extraocular muscles are most commonly affected with bulbar muscles, neck muscles, shoulder girdle and hip flexors next in frequency of involvement. Undue fatiguability can be demonstrated by repeated movements of the affected groups, in the case of the eyes by prolonged upward gaze, and in the case of palate movements by changes in voice during continuous counting or reading aloud. Wasting may occur after the illness has been present for some years, particularly of tongue and shoulder girdle muscles.

Anticholinesterases (prostigmine and pyridostigmine) help to restore the strength of weakened muscles, but care must be taken with adjusting the dose since intoxication may result in respiratory and bulbar muscle paralysis. Excision of the thymus gland may benefit some patients, but which is difficult to assess, although the earlier the operation the better the results. Steroids, immunosuppressive drugs, and plasma exchange, with the hope of removing circulating antibody, have all been tried with varying success.

Myasthenia may sometimes be secondary to hyperthyroidism, rheumatoid arthritis and systemic lupus erythematosus which may be masked by the muscular features. Treatment of the thyroid problem may be associated with increasing muscle power.

Some patients have long remissions but rapid onset of symptoms usually has a poor prognosis. Patients with purely ocular problems do better than others. Death occurs as the result of respiratory infections. Care must be taken in prescribing antibiotics for respiratory and other infections since tetracyclines may have harmful effects on neuromuscular transmission, as do several drugs used during general anaesthesia.

◄ Tetracyclines should not be prescribed for patients with myasthenia because of the risks of worsening of muscle weakness

Metabolic myopathies

A large number of disorders may produce a nonspecific muscular weakness and wasting, often of proximal distribution. Some of these result from specific biochemical defects in the pathways which provide energy for muscular contraction, causing either progressive limb girdle weakness and wasting, or pain and stiffness, induced by exercise and relieved by rest.

Many endocrine disorders present with weakness due to myopathy, in particular acromegaly, hyperthyroidism and Cushing's syndrome or therapeutic, steroid-induced hyperadrenalism. Myopathy occurs with vitamin D deficiency, hyperparathyroidism and with chronic renal failure, in which instances the muscles are often tender and movements are painful.

Alcohol and drugs (chloroquine and emetine as well as steroids) may cause myopathy, which is usually reversible and, in the case of alcohol, associated with pain and tenderness (*see* Chapter 7).

Myotonia

Myotonia, or slow relaxation of voluntary muscle contraction, is usually familial and occurs in two forms — one in which there is no muscle wasting (sometimes muscular hypertrophy) and the other associated with wasting of neck and facial muscles.

Myotonia congenita, in which diffuse muscle hypertrophy may occur, causes symptoms that are accentuated by rest and by cold. The condition has two forms: one autosomal dominant, the other recessive. Sometimes there is improvement with procainamide or phenytoin.

Myotonic dystrophy presents the same clinical features, but is associated with muscle wasting, as well as lens cataracts, testicular atrophy and frontal baldness. Cardiac changes occur and death is often due to cardiac failure. There is no effective treatment but myotonia sometimes responds to procainamide.

Neuropathy

Damage to peripheral nerves may cause motor, sensory or autonomic (sympathetic) symptoms and signs. Motor symptoms consist of wasting and weakness, mainly of distal muscles; sensory symptoms consist of numbness, and pins-and-needles in the limbs and sometimes the face. The symptoms of autonomic neuropathy consist of dryness of the skin, and unusual sweating responses such as on the face associated with eating, which occurs in diabetes. Diarrhoea, impotence and postural hypotension may also be features of autonomic neuropathy

Since nerves receive their blood supply from small

Table 11.11. Types and causes of peripheral neuropathy

Mononeuropathy and multiple mononeuropathies
    (including the cranial nerves)
  diabetes
  rheumatoid arthritis and systemic lupus erythematosus
  sarcoidosis
  amyloidosis
  infiltration by malignancy
  trauma
Polyneuropathy (predominantly motor)
  Guillain-Barré
  porphyria
  lead
Polyneuropathy (predominantly sensory)
  diabetes
  malignancy
  vitamin B_1 and B_{12} deficiency
  amyloidosis
Autonomic neuropathy (diarrhoea, dysphagia, hypotension,
    denervation of heart with risk of 'collapse' during GA)
  diabetes

nutrient arteries, occlusion of these vessels results in infarction of the nerve trunk with signs and symptoms involving several isolated nerves, called 'mononeuritis multiplex' (*see Table* 11.11). Mononeuritis may also follow trauma, may be due to inflammatory disorders such as sarcoidosis and to infiltration by malignant disease and amyloidosis. The cranial nerves, often the facial and hypoglossal, may be involved by the same systemic diseases that cause mononeuritis muliplex.

The peripheral nerve fibre consists of a central fibre which is an extension of the cell body, the axon, surrounded by a myelin sheath. Diseases of the peripheral nerves may be due either to axonal degeneration or to affection of the myelin sheath, segmental demyelination (*see Table* 11.11). Axonal degeneration may be due to alcohol, vitamin deficiencies, toxins, malignancies and renal failure. Demyelination occurs in diabetes (in addition to mononeuritis), leprosy and the Guillain-Barré syndrome, or acute idiopathic polyneuritis.

The clinical types of neuropathy can be classified as 'acute' or 'chronic' according to onset, and 'sensory' or 'motor' according to symptoms. Guillain-Barré syndrome, malignancy and metabolic disorders such as porphyria cause acute symptoms. A mainly motor neuropathy occurs with porphyria, Guillain-Barré syndrome and toxins such as lead. Predominantly sensory neuropathy occurs with diabetes, vitamin B_{12} and B_1 deficiencies, malignancy and amyloid.

Intracranial tumours (*Table* 11.12)

The clinical features of intracranial tumours vary widely according to site and pathological type. The onset may be abrupt and rapidly progressive but in some patients symptoms, such as generalized seizures, may be present for as long as twenty years before the appearance of other signs. Tumours present as non-localizing symptoms, or localizing symptoms and signs or the features of raised intracranial pressure, or combinations of all three.

Non-localizing symptoms consist of headache, which is usually generalized, occasionally unilateral although not always on the same side as the lesion. Pain may sometimes occur in the face and throat with posterior fossa tumours. Seizures are usually generalized but may be partial, and there may be psychological disturbances such as dementia.

The localizing symptoms of frontal lobe tumours are often vague and mild but include abnormalities of mood, urinary incontinence and dementia. Temporal lobe tumours may remain silent for a long time or

Table 11.12. Common intracranial tumours

Metastases (secondary to primary tumours of bronchus, breast, gut)
Glioma — most common primary tumour
Meningioma
Acoustic neuroma
Pituitary tumour
Vascular tumours

present as complex seizures, with an unusual aura such as olfactory and visual hallucinations. Progressive hemianopia may be the presenting feature of temporal lobe tumours and, in the case of dominant hemisphere lesions, dysphasia. Parietal and occipital lobe lesions may present as seizures with motor or sensory features. Tumours in the region of the pituitary fossa produce loss of vision in the temporal halves of the fields of vision in both eyes, often with endocrine disturbance (hypopituitarism) and lesions of the oculomotor and trigeminal nerves. Posterior fossa tumours present with raised intracranial pressure at an early stage, in combination with ataxia, nystagmus and cranial nerve palsies.

Having localized the tumour by CAT scanning, arteriography and isotope scanning, treatment is aimed at eradicating the tumour completely, which requires biopsy to make certain of the exact pathological identity. However, total removal may sometimes only be achieved by causing increased disability, and risk to life, so that partial resection is performed and/or radiotherapy given. Palliative procedures may be performed for extensive glioma or multiple metastases. Chemotherapy may be given and surgical procedures performed to drain the CSF from the lateral ventricle of one hemisphere into either a point further down the CSF pathway, by-passing the obstruction, or into the right atrium, with a tube that incorporates a one-way valve.

Joint and bone disease 12

Diseases of joint and bone are of importance to the dentist because they may involve the temporomandibular joint and the mandible, and also because of oral manifestations of the disease or because of the effects of drug therapy for the disorder.

Rheumatoid arthritis

Rheumatoid arthritis (RA) is a systemic disorder of connective tissue which predominantly affects the synovial joints. It may develop at any age, but is common between 25 and 55 years, particularly in women.

The cause of the disease is unknown but it is thought that there is a genetic predisposition in some patients and that it is this together with an environmental trigger, possibly a virus, which stimulates the production of auto-antibodies against the patient's own immunoglobulins, with tissue damage resulting from immune complex disposition in the synovium and blood vessel walls (*see* Chapter 17).

The important diagnostic features of RA are symmetrical joint involvement, with joint stiffness after periods of rest such as in the morning on waking; the involvement being mainly peripheral, in hands and feet rather than shoulders and hips. Tendons that are surrounded by a sheath of synovium may also be involved, such as those in the palm of the hands, resulting in restricted movement due to inflammation and fibrosis. Most patients have systemic symptoms such as fatigue, weight loss and low grade fever; anaemia and damage to small blood vessels occur in a few patients.

◄ RA is a symmetrical arthritis affecting the metacarpophalangeal, wrist, metatarsophalangeal and knee joints

235

In the early stages of the disease the joints are warm, swollen, tender and painful on movement. Weakening of the joint capsule and ligament damage lead to joint instability, with partial or complete dislocations (subluxation) that produce the characteristic deformities. Eventually severe joint damage may lead to fibrosis and bony ankylosis which may affect the temporo-mandibular joint, leading in the juvenile to mandibular growth disturbance.

The characteristic changes in the hands are 'spindling' of the fingers, due to swelling of the proximal interphalangeal joints, and subluxation of the proximal phalanges on the metacarpals with palmar and ulnar deviation. Similar changes occur in the feet. Involvement of the knee may result in deformities, sometimes with instability, and synovial lined cysts (bursae) which may occur at other sites such as the elbow and ankle joints. Nodules occur in relation to bony prominences, especially around the elbow and knee, and are due to pressure or friction. Nodules show similar histological features to those found in the synovium; they occasionally ulcerate with secondary infection, and may also occur in tendon sheaths, lung, heart and the sclera of the eye.

Rheumatoid changes may affect the synovial-lined apophysial joints of the spine as well as the joints in the lateral margins of the intervertebral disc and the bursa between the odontoid peg and transverse ligament. The latter changes lead to subluxation at the atlanto-axial junction with the risk that flexion of the cervical spine will be associated with excessive posterior displacement of the odontoid peg and cord compression. This instability, which can be demonstrated by radiography, is of importance if the patient is to have GA; head and neck handling that may occur during dental surgery with GA could cause damage with resulting weakness or paralysis in all four limbs.

There are many non-articular manifestations of RA involving several systems. The cardiovascular system may be involved both as an inflammatory disorder affecting the heart, the pericardium and, less frequently, the myocardium and the aortic valve, and a vasculitis, usually in the hands, causing small areas of gangrene in the nail fold and nail edge. Normochromic, normocytic anaemia is the commonest blood disorder

◄ Juvenile forms of RA (Still's disease) may involve the temporo-mandibular joint leading to disturbance of mandibular condylar growth, and in the adult to limited mouth opening or ankylosis

◄ Flexion of the cervical spine in patients with RA may, when the bursa between the transverse ligament and odontoid peg is affected, be associated with excessive posterior displacement of the peg and damage to the spinal cord

◄ RA is a systemic disorder with important non-articular features including malaise, subcutaneous nodules, and normochromic, normocytic anaemia

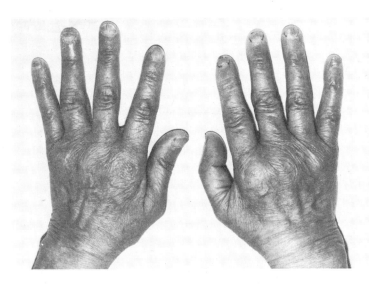

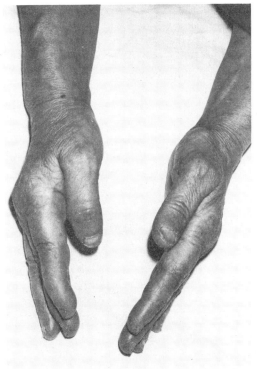

Fig. 12.1. Rheumatoid arthritis of hands. Note swelling of metacarpo-phalangeal joints and wrist. 'Swan neck' deformity of index finger of R. hand.

but some patients may have leucopenia and thrombocytopenia caused by excessive activity of the spleen, either as part of the disease process or drug-induced. Respiratory system involvement is more common in men, usually as pleurisy and pleural effusion. Rheumatoid nodules may occur in the lung and a small number of patients develop fibrosing alveolitis (*see* Chapter 5).

Peripheral nerves can be damaged by RA either by entrapment in proliferating synovium, for example, at the wrist in the carpal tunnel, or as a 'glove-and-stocking' sensory type of peripheral neuropathy (*see* Chapter 11). Renal involvement is rare except as a result of analgesic interstitial nephritis or due to secondary amyloidosis in long-standing RA.

Sjögren's syndrome is a triad of dry mouth (xerostomia), dry eyes (keratoconjunctivitis) and a connective tissue disease, most commonly RA. A chronic inflammatory disorder produces atrophy of the functioning elements of the lacrimal and salivary glands and, less often, the exocrine glands in the bronchi. The tongue is often depapillated and lobulated and there are changes in the oral flora with subsequent candidiasis. There is an increase in dental caries, inflammatory periodontal disease and enlargement of salivary glands, due either to inflammation (sialoadenitis) or, occasionally, tumours.

◀ Dry mouth, dry eyes and RA constitute Sjögren's syndrome, associated with which there is an increase in dental caries, inflammatory periodontal disease and salivary gland enlargement

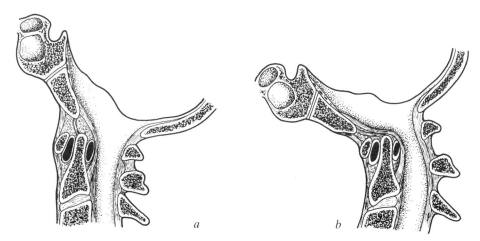

Fig. 12.2. Cervical spine (C1,C2,C3) showing posterior displacement of odontoid peg with neck flexion (*b*), causing narrowing of spinal canal.

Table 12.1. Diagnosis of inflammatory joint disease (polyarthritis)

Joint pain, swelling and stiffness

Symmetrical

Nodules
(RA definite)

No nodules

Other systems
involved
(SLE likely)

Joint disease
alone
(RA likely)

Asymmetrical

Hands, feet

Nail
changes
(psoriasis)

Urethritis
(Reiter's)

Lumbo-sacral pain

Bowel symptoms
(colitis)

No bowel
symptoms
(ankylosing
spondylitis)

Other inflammatory joint disease

The presence of macroglobulins in the serum of patients with RA, which can be detected by screening tests (RA latex test), helps to distinguish these subjects from others with inflammatory joint disease, usually associated with spinal arthritis, who have so-called 'sero-negative arthritis'. The diseases in this group are ankylosing spondylitis; arthritis associated with inflammatory bowel disease; psoriatic arthritis; Reiter's syndrome and Behçet's syndrome.

Ankylosing spondylitis is an inflammatory arthritis of the spine, sacro-iliac and sometimes peripheral joints with a strong family trait, predominantly affecting young men. Although these are associated with the tissue antigen HLA-B27 (*see* Chapter 17), there are, almost certainly, environmental factors, possibly bacterial antigens, which are additional prerequisites for development of the disease.

The clinical features include low back pain, worse on wakening and better with exercise; pain with and limitation of chest expansion; and a grating sensation in the neck when the cervical spine becomes involved. The peripheral arthritis is often asymmetrical, usually affecting the hips, knees and ankles and rarely the wrists and shoulders. Severe exacerbations may be associated with weight loss and fever.

Severe thoracic kyphosis develops after some years of active disease and is compensated by extension of the cervical spine, so producing the typical spondylitic picture. The disease may halt at any level and is sometimes limited to the lumbar spine and sacro-iliac joints.

A non-specific inflammation of the aorta occurs in nearly 50% of the patients with long-standing disease and causing aortic regurgitation and, rarely, cardiac conduction defects. Heart failure may occur, but Stokes–Adams attacks are unusual. Infective endocarditis is a risk when the aortic valve is damaged.

◄ Ankylosing spondylitis may be associated with aortic valve regurgitation with a risk of infective endocarditis following bacteraemia

Neurological complications may occur at cervical or sacral level, because of either nerve root irritation and entrapment or spinal cord damage at the higher level because of rigidity of the spine. Care is needed in positioning of the neck during general anaesthesia.

Rigidity of the thoracic cage, due to costo-vertebral arthritis, causes very little restriction of pulmonary function, because of compensation by increased dia-phragmatic excursion. Fibrosis occasionally occurs in the lung apices, and secondary fungal infections may occur.

Approximately 10% of patients with *psoriasis* suffer from an inflammatory arthritis, sometimes affecting the spine, producing a clinical picture indistinguishable from ankylosing spondylitis. Most patients present with an asymmetrical arthritis affecting two or three, occasionally only one joint, most often the knee. But a severe and extensive mutilating arthritis may also occur as well as a full-blown spinal arthritis. It is sometimes impossible to distinguish the disease from RA and, in a few patients, it is no more troublesome than an arthritis of the distal interphalangeal joints in the hands, associated with pitting of the nails. Aortitis, similar to that seen with ankylosing spondylitis, may occur with a risk of infective endocarditis.

◄ The arthritis of psoriasis usually affects only one or two joints, together with nail changes, but sometimes the condition cannot be distinguished from RA

The arthritis associated with *ulcerative colitis* and *Crohn's disease* frequently presents as single joint involvement, most often the knee, and in 1 patient in 20 with a picture of ankylosing spondylitis, which follows a course independent of the bowel problem, and is not influenced by resection of the diseased colon. The peripheral arthritis, however, which is normally self-limiting, improves with treatment of the bowel disease.

Reiter's syndrome comprises polyarthritis, conjunctivitis and non-specific urethritis which may follow sexual exposure and occurs in males, very rarely females, between 16 and 35 years of age. Any synovial joint can be involved, and the pattern is usually asymmetrical. The knee is most often affected but the spine is also involved in 20% of patients. A scaly rash on the palms and soles may occur in severe cases and the patient may suffer from buccal and lingual ulcers as well as pharyngitis. Aortitis occurs in some patients.

◄ Reiter's syndrome presents with acute arthritis, conjunctivitis, urethritis, erythematous lesions of the oral mucosa, with buccal and lingual ulcers, usually in a young male 4–6 months after sexual exposure or an attack of dysentery

Behçet's syndrome may be associated with a non-deforming arthritis. The other features of the syndrome, particularly oral and genital ulcers, are more constant.

Treatment of inflammatory joint diseases
Over recent years many non-steroidal inflammatory

drugs (NSAIDs) have been introduced and are helpful in relieving the pain and stiffness associated with all forms of arthritis, even though they do not alter the progress of these diseases. Most of them cause side effects, usually dyspepsia and gastro-intestinal symptoms, and some cause oral ulceration and lichen-planus-like reactions, as well as skin rashes that have an oral component (Stevens–Johnson syndrome) (*see* Chapter 15). Thrombocytopenia and leucopenia are rare complications of the use of NSAIDs, which may present with oral problems such as easy bleeding and gingivo-oral infections.

Corticosteroids are used in RA and other inflammatory joint disease because of their anti-inflammatory effects but, although very effective in causing suppression of symptoms, they do not appear to alter the course of the disease. In doses sufficient to control the symptoms of RA Cushing's syndrome is inevitable and the problems which this causes seem to be greater in patients with RA than in any other disease. Thin, fragile skin and mucosal surfaces which tear easily and heal poorly, weight gain, osteoporosis, infections of all kinds (including parodontal), raised blood pressure and diabetes mellitus occur frequently in patients treated with any corticosteroid. In children there is the additional problem of growth suppression.

◀ Corticosteroids exaggerate the problem of thin atrophic skin and mucosal surfaces with delayed healing in patients with RA

Drugs such as penicillamine, gold, immunosuppressive drugs and chloroquine seem to have some fundamental action on the disease's process, including the non-articular manifestations, and may enable a reduction in excessive requirement for corticosteroids. Penicillamine causes more side effects than the others, but is probably most effective in patients with RA, although it gives no benefit to the patient with either ankylosing spondylitis or psoriatic arthropathy. Loss of taste, mouth ulcers, thrombocytopenia and proteinuria develop in 10–20% of patients on penicillamine therapy.

Gold injections have been used in the treatment for RA for many years, the action being similar to penicillamine although with fewer side effects. Rash, thrombocytopenia, proteinuria and oral ulceration as well as lichenoid reactions may occur with gold therapy.

◀ Penicillamine and gold salts may cause lichenoid reactions and oral ulceration in patients with RA

Surgical management of RA of the wrist and hands is indicated where nerve and tendon compression occurs and is often advised where there is serious deformity. Arthroplasty, involving limited resection of the carpus with the insertion of a prosthesis, is the preferred procedure for RA of the wrist. Surgery of the hand is advised where there is nerve and tendon damage but established deformities can be dealt with by joint replacement and by transplantation or reimplantation of tendons.

Surgery of the major joints (hips and knees) is performed for osteoarthritis as well as rheumatoid disease and is recommended for pain, loss of function, instability, loss of mobility and radiographic evidence of joint destruction. The commonly used operations for arthritis are osteotomy, arthrodesis and total joint replacement. Osteotomy — cutting of bone in order to realign weight bearing — is particularly useful in relieving pain and is most commonly used on the hip and on the knee, when there is deformity. Arthrodesis is performed to stabilize a joint, particularly the ankle or wrist but occasionally the hip, when a stiff but painless joint is acceptable to the patient. Total joint replacement procedures are performed to increase mobility and produce excellent pain relief with, at best, near normal function. These procedures are ideal for the hip, less so for the knee, and have not been tested for the shoulder, elbow and ankle.

◄ Nerve and tendon compression associated with joint disease requires urgent surgery, preventing or relieving severe disability

◄ Surgery of the major joints in arthritis is performed for pain, loss of function, instability and loss of mobility

Osteoarthritis

The primary event in osteoarthritis is probably in articular cartilage, with biochemical changes below its surface causing disruption and alteration in the thickness of parallel collagen fibres, leading to disintegration of the surface and the development of deep clefts allowing enzymes from the synovial fluid to enter and digest the cartilage. The condition is more common in the elderly, but there are many other possible factors concerned including trauma, genetics and obesity.

The commonly affected joints are the distal interphalangeal joints of the fingers, the carpometacarpal joints of the thumb, the cervical and lumbar spine, hip, knee and foot (the big toe joint). Pain is made worse by use of the affected joint, is dull and aching in character, being worse at the end of the day. The stiffness experienced is less severe than with RA, but may occur after rest, being quickly relieved by mild exertion. Joints affected are usually swollen due to soft tissue or bony overgrowth but there is only a mild inflammatory synovitis. Heberden's nodes are bony outgrowths (osteophytes) at the base of the distal phalanx in the hand, which are initially made up of fibro-adipose tissue which later ossifies. Cartilage and bony destruction lead to generalized joint deformity, which is not correlated with pain or stiffness; the subsequent loss of function is caused by pain and muscle wasting.

Treatment involves physiotherapy, changes in the patient's life style so as to protect the affected joints, drug therapy with anti-inflammatory and analgesic preparations and surgery, usually performed to relieve pain but occasionally to restore function.

◄ The pain of osteoarthritis is made worse by use of the affected joint, the stiffness being mild and relieved with exercise

Gout

Gout is caused by the deposition of crystals of uric acid or urates into joints and other tissues, associated with

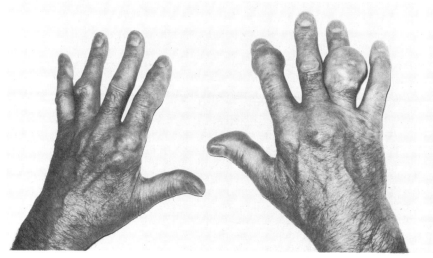

Fig. 12.3. Gouty arthritis. Note tophi related to proximal interphalangeal joint R. hand.

Table 12.2. Provocation of acute gouty arthritis

Trauma
Surgery
Severe systemic illness
Severe dieting and dietary excess
Alcohol
Drugs — diuretics and following drug allergy

an increase in these substances in the blood and other body fluids. The clinical features are usually those of an acute arthritis, sometimes with tenosynovitis (inflammation of tendon sheaths) and bursitis. Renal disease and stone formation may also occur and urates are deposited in particular tissues, notably the cartilage of the ear and tendon sheaths (tophi).

Gouty arthritis may present in a chronic form characterized by asymmetrical joint swelling after repeated episodes of acute arthropathy. Acute attacks may be precipitated by trauma, undue physical activity, surgery of any kind, severe systemic illness, severe dieting, drugs (such as diuretics) as well as excess alcohol. In 70% of patients the first joint to be affected is the metatarsophalangeal joint of the big toe: thereafter in decreasing order of frequency the ankle, knee, small joints of the feet, wrist and elbow. The axial joints are rarely affected.

Acute attacks are very sudden in onset, may wake the patient from sleep and are characterized by hot, red, swollen joints with shiny, overlying skin, plus systemic upset such as fever and anorexia. An untreated attack may last days or months and repeated episodes merge to cause chronic disability.

Uric acid stones in the kidney may occur with episodes of colicky pain due to passage of the calculus down the ureter, often associated with haematuria. A rare consequence of gout is chronic renal disease due to tubular obstruction, glomerular damage and hypertension.

Treatment of the acute attack is usually with a NSAID such as indomethacin or phenylbutazone. If there are recurrent attacks, or tophi, life-long drug therapy is given with allopurinol, an enzyme inhibitor that reduces uric acid production.

Increased production of uric acid with episodes of acute gout may occur in malignant diseases such as Hodgkin's lymphoma and leukaemia, as well as with benign disorders such as polycythaemia (*see* Chapter 8).

Connective tissue disease

Apart from RA other diseases of connective tissue have some interest for the dentist, including systemic lupus erythematosus (SLE) and scleroderma.

SLE is a relapsing and remitting disease affecting many organs and associated with circulating antibodies against both autologous and exogenous antigens. Activity of the disease is associated with fever and malaise, skin, joint, lung, renal, blood and neurological features. The classic rash of SLE is blotchy, red and light-sensitive in the malar areas and on the bridge of the nose. Another common feature is involvement of the small blood vessels of the skin, causing red, flat spots on the hands and feet, knees, elbows and scalp, the latter causing alopecia (hair loss). Symmetrical polyarthritis is common but deformity is unusual except when there are tendon contractures. Renal disease occurs in almost half the patients which may progress to chronic renal failure. Haemolytic anaemia associated with red cell antibodies, thrombocytopenia and agranulocytosis occur both during activity of the disease in other organs and, sometimes, as the sole manifestation of the disease.

◄ Oral lesions may occur with SLE, particularly on the lips, consisting of red patches with white central striae and telangiectasia

Table 12.3. Comparison of connective tissue diseases

	SLE	*Scleroderma*	*PAN*
Raynaud's phenomenon	+	+ + + +	0
Arthritis	+ + +	+	0
Swollen hands	+	+ + + +	0
Oesophageal involvement	0	+ + + +	0
Renal disease	+ + +	+	+ + + +
CNS disease	+ + +	0	+ + +
GIT bleeding	+	0	+ + +

Involvement of CNS occurs at some stage in most patients with SLE and the features are varied according to the region involved. There may be minor personality changes, with depression and psychosis as well as seizures, cranial nerve palsy, meningitis, hemiparesis and chorea. The features of pulmonary involvement are usually pleurisy and, less often, interstitial lung disease.

Treatment consists of corticosteroids combined with either chloroquine, particularly for skin and joint disease, and immunosuppressants. The outcome is difficult to predict but is best in those patients in whom the disease has been caused by drugs that induce antinuclear antibodies such as hydrallazine (used in hypertension), isoniazid (an antitubercular drug) and procainamide (used to treat cardiac dysrhythmias).

Scleroderma presents with both cutaneous and internal organ involvement, the prognosis being determined by the latter. The early phase of the disease is characterized by puffiness of the fingers, due to oedema, and episodes of pain with whiteness of the digits which subsequently become blue (Raynaud's phenomenon). The classic fibrotic stage occurs later, the skin becoming thickened and tethered with resultant loss of joint mobility, diminution in mouth size and difficulty inserting dentures, loss of skin creases and reduced elasticity over the nose and below the eyes.

◄ The earliest feature of progressive scleroderma is loss of elasticity of the skin over the nose and below the eyes, with telangiectasia on the lips, and widening of the periodontal ligament seen on X-ray

Arthritis, muscle inflammation (myositis) and tendon involvement may occur in scleroderma. Involvement of the gut causes reduced motility, most common at the lower end of the oesophagus, producing heartburn and reflux of food in the stomach. The lungs may be affected by interstitial fibrosis and the heart may be affected either directly or as a consequence of increased blood pressure, secondary to renal involvement.

A mild form of the disease can be recognized — the CRST syndrome, occurring in middle aged to elderly females. CRST is an acronym for calcification in the soft tissue of the fingers, Raynaud's phenomenon, sclerodactyly (thickening of the skin over the digits) and telangiectasia.

There is no convincing evidence that any drug retards the progression of the disease, but many patients are treated with corticosteroids and penicillamine, both of which produce some symptomatic relief. Careful attention to skin care in the areas involved is important.

Periarteritis nodosa (PAN)

PAN is a widespread arteritis involving medium-sized vessels causing multisystem symptoms due to ischaemia or infarction of tissues supplied by the affected artery. Hepatitis B surface antigen has been demonstrated in the wall of damaged vessels in a variable number of patients and the disease may be associated with drug addiction.

◄ Hepatitis B surface antigen is carried by 5–40% of patients with periarteritis nodosa

Apart from non-specific symptoms such as fever, malaise and weight loss, the commonest features are abdominal pain and raised blood pressure, the former due to infarction of bowel, liver and gallbladder and the latter to renal damage. Cutaneous features include digital gangrene or ulcers and there may be mono-neuritis, often involving the cranial nerves, due to vasculitis (*see* Chapter 11). The coronary arteries may be affected causing angina and myocardial infarction.

Diagnosis is established by biopsy of muscle or an affected organ, such as the kidney, and by arteriography of the abdominal vessels where the vascular lesions are most frequent. Treatment consists of prednisolone with an immunosuppressant drug, such as azathioprine or cyclophosphamide. Remissions may occur with such treatment but the outcome depends on the residual problems of hypertension and renal failure.

Soft tissue lesions

Soft tissue lesions are common problems being caused, in most instances, by local trauma and/or over-use — often named after sporting or occupational associations, such as 'tennis elbow', or 'golfer's elbow'. Occasionally such local lesions may be part of generalized disorder such as rheumatoid arthritis, SLE and polymyositis. Similarly, generalized soft tissue pain may occur with osteoarthritis affecting many joints, as well as

Paget's disease of bone, osteomalacia, malignancy and Parkinsonism.

Soft tissue symptoms may be due to tendon rupture, damage to the insertions or inflammation of the sheath. Rupture may occur with vigorous sporting activity, but sometimes spontaneously (particularly the Achilles tendon) with steroid therapy. Inflammatory lesions of the tendons occur with disorders such as RA, usually associated with involvement of the sheath; or may be due to over-use, such as tennis elbow.

Inflammation of bursae can sometimes be the cause of localized soft tissue pain. There are many of these synovium-lined cavities throughout the body but those which become chronically inflamed due to over-use and trauma with sport or associated with occupations are those in relation to the elbow (miner's or student's elbow), the knee (prepatellar bursitis or housemaid's knee) and the heel (posterior to the Achilles tendon).

Inflammatory lesions of the capsule may follow tears and major ligamentous damage. The shoulder is the most commonly affected joint, beginning with minor tears of the supraspinatus tendon with resulting inflammatory change which spreads to local bursae and further restricts the movement of the joint by pain and stiffness. The condition is sometimes known as 'frozen shoulder'.

Treatment of these soft tissue lesions usually involves physiotherapy, ultrasound and local heat, and local injection of corticosteroids or anaesthetics.

Bone disorders

Diseases that affect bone may involve not only the mineral component but also the collagen element on which the calcium is deposited. The metabolism of calcium is carefully controlled to adapt to changing circumstances such as pregnancy and ageing. Where there is failure to adapt to such stress bone disease occurs.

Ninety-nine per cent of the calcium in the body is in the bones and is continually being exchanged with that in the plasma. The plasma–calcium level is controlled within narrow limits by parathormone (PTH), calcitonin and vitamin D. Parathormone increases calcium absorption from the gut, resorption in the renal tubules and resorption from bone. The action of PTH is blocked by calcitonin and this tends to reduce calcium level. Vitamin D, which is normally obtained from the action of sunlight on the skin and from a limited number of foods, is converted in the liver and in the kidney to a hormone which acts on the gut to increase calcium absorption; its production is promoted by PTH, which therefore has an indirect action on the bowel mediated by this hormone (1,25-dihydroxy-vitamin D).

The clinical manifestations of most bone disorders are those of bone pain, particularly with physical stress, sometimes associated with tenderness; spontaneous fracture; and gradual development of skeletal deformity which may affect any bone, especially the weight-bearing ones but occasionally the skull and mandible. Bone deformity is more common in the younger patient in whom growth failure usually occurs.

Osteomalacia

The term 'osteomalacia' means softening of bone and results from vitamin D deficiency in any form. Vitamin D deficiency may occur because of deficient dietary sources and lack of exposure to sunlight, which facilitates synthesis in the skin. In Britain the people

Table 12.4.   Causes of osteomalacia and rickets

Deficient synthesis and supply of vitamin D
  infants, elderly housebound, Asian immigrants to U.K.
Impaired absorption of vitamin D
  malabsorption
Impaired hydroxylation of vitamin D
  chronic liver disease
  chronic renal disease
Osteomalacia in spite of normal levels of hydroxylated
    vitamin D
  familial hypophosphataemic rickets
Other renal diseases such as renal tubular acidosis

most commonly affected are Asian immigrants of all ages and the elderly, confined to their homes, who do not have adequate sunlight exposure and a diet poor in oily fish, margarine, milk concentrates and eggs.

Osteomalacia may also occur in liver and renal disease because of failure of hydroxylation of vitamin D_3 and in the rarer tubular defects with altered sensitivity to the action of the activated form and loss of phosphate in the urine (*see* Chapter 10). Failure of absorption of vitamin D due to small bowel disorder, such as coeliac disease and other causes of malabsorption, may also be associated with osteomalacia (*see* Chapter 6).

◀ Babies fed by bottle with non-vitamin supplemented feeds and little exposure to sunlight are at risk of developing rickets

The changes in the bone are softening and deformity with spontaneous fractures in some. These effects are the result of the histological changes in the bone consisting of excess uncalcified osteoid tissue within normal-sized trabeculae.

The clinical features depend on the age of presentation. In childhood the condition, termed 'rickets', normally occurs in bottle-fed babies with little sunlight exposure or breast-fed by a mother with marginal vitamin D stores. Rapidly growing bones are most markedly affected by rickets, with frontal bone prominence ('bossing'), bowing and deformity of long bones and expanded epiphyses, usually at the wrist.

Osteomalacia presents with bone pain, often mistaken for arthritis, spontaneous fractures and weakness of proximal muscles producing a waddling gait. The condition may sometimes be recognized on bone radiographs which show generalized decrease in bone density, which may be incorrectly · interpreted as osteoporosis. The pulp chambers of teeth may be extremely large.

◀ Bone pain, spontaneous fracture and proximal myopathy may be the presenting features of osteomalacia and in children there may be wide pulp chambers of the teeth seen on X-ray

Diagnosis depends on bone biopsy and the finding of either a low serum calcium or low phosphate and a raised alkaline phosphatase, a not invariable feature.

Treatment consists of vitamin D_2 (calciferol) in appropriate dose, 1000–2000 IU in cases of dietary deficiency but 50 000 IU orally or by intramuscular injection twice a month in malabsorption. Renal tubular defects are treated with phosphate and large doses of vitamin D and correction of acidosis in those patients with RTA (*see* Chapter 10). The osteomalacia associated with renal disease is mainly confined to the end-stage and is treated with the synthetic form of vitamin D_3 (1-alpha-hydroxycholecalciferol) or with 1,25-dihydroxycholecalciferol, plus phosphate-binding drugs (aluminium hydroxide) and additional calcium by mouth.

Osteoporosis

Osteoporosis is a reduction in bone mass per unit volume, mineral constituent and chemical composition being normal, unlike osteomalacia in which mineral content per unit mass is diminished.

The major clinical features are spontaneous fracture, most often in the vertebral bodies causing severe localized pain in the mid-thoracic or lumbar spine. Fractures may also occur in the forearm bones and the upper end of the femur.

The commonest cause of osteoporosis is ageing. It is especially common in the two decades that follow the menopause, and may be related to fall in oestrogen levels. Osteoporosis may occur secondary to endocrine disease such as Cushing's syndrome, hyperthyroidism, hyperparathyroidism and hypogonadism; with drugs such as corticosteroids; in chronic renal failure; in myeloma and secondary carcinoma; and with immobility.

Diagnosis depends on excluding other causes of radiolucent bones such as osteomalacia and osteogenesis imperfecta. Serum calcium, phosphate and alkaline phosphatase are normal. Exclusion of

Table 12.5. Causes of osteoporosis

Primary
    commonest in postmenopausal women, elderly
Secondary
    Cushing's syndrome and corticosteroid therapy
    hyperparathyroidism
    hyperthyroidism
    chronic renal failure
    multiple myeloma and secondary carcinoma
    immobilization, e.g. after fracture or injury

secondary causes for osteoporosis requires assessment of thyroid and endocrine function and a search for myeloma and secondary carcinoma.

Having treated the remediable causes for osteo-porosis there are few measures that are effective, particularly in reducing the frequency of fracture. In the female it may be justified to give oestrogens and supplemental calcium, but other measures such as fluoride, anabolic steroids, parathormone and vitamin D have not been proved to be effective.

Osteogenesis imperfecta

In osteogenesis imperfecta collagen metabolism or structure is abnormal, producing brittle bones of vary-ing clinical severity. The most severe forms, which are recessively inherited, produce extensive intrauterine fractures and neonatal death. The more common autosomal dominant form has less severe osseous fragility, associated with blue sclerae of the eyes, impaired hearing due to involvement of the ossicles and dentinogenesis imperfecta. The less severe form is compatible with survival into adult life but with impaired growth and deformity due to repeated fractures.

The teeth may appear blue or brown and are characteristically opalescent. The junction of dentine with overlying enamel is abnormal. Radiography may show obliteration of the tooth pulp chamber, short roots which may fracture, and marked attrition of the tooth crown.

◀ Dentinogenesis imperfecta is manifest as bluish translucency of teeth with marked attrition of some which may then be brown in colour

The biochemical basis of the collagen disorder is unknown and no specific treatment is available.

Fibrous dysplasia of bone

Fibrous dysplasia of bone occurs more often in girls in association with precocious puberty plus cutaneous and mucosal pigmentation in some instances. The bone disease is asymmetrical and may be monostotic, affecting the jaws in some patients, although the femur and tibia are most frequently involved. The affected

◀ Fibrous dysplasia of the bones may be monostotic, affecting the maxilla and jaws with expansion, impeded tooth eruption and pathological fractures

bones may fracture but heal readily with callus. The cortex of affected bones is thin due to replacement by fibrous tissue and radiographs may show cystic areas.

Tooth eruption may be impeded and pathological fractures of the mandible occur. The aetiology is unknown but is not familial and there is no specific treatment.

Osteopetrosis

There are two genetically determined forms of osteopetrosis, a severe form with autosomal recessive inheritance and a mild form which is determined by an autosomal dominant. There is a generalized increase in bone density with varying clinical features — fractures and bone-marrow replacement, causing anaemia and thrombocytopenia. The mild form is sometimes an incidental radiological finding. Involvement of the skull may lead to narrowing of the foramina and cranial nerve palsies. Delayed tooth eruption and impacted teeth may occur and there is a risk of fracture and osteomyelitis with dental treatment.

Osteopetrosis may be due to deficiency of osteoclasts, but specific treatment is not available.

◄ Osteopetrosis may lead to delayed tooth eruption, impacted teeth and a predisposition to pathological fractures and osteomyelitis

Paget's disease of bone

The disease is a reflection of increased bone turnover due to excessive osteoclastic absorption and increased but disorganized bone formation. The exact incidence is not known but it is a common incidental finding with a geographical distribution, being prevalent in U.K. and U.S.A. but rare in Scandinavia, the Middle and Far East. It is seldom found in patients under the age of 50. Although the cause is not known there is some evidence that it may be due to an abnormal immunological response to a virus.

The majority of patients are asymptomatic. The most common symptom is pain in affected bones, unrelieved by rest and unaltered by movement, sometimes waking the patient at night. Affected bones may be tender, warm and deformed, the latter resulting in limb shortening with abnormal stress on hip and knee joints. Pathological fractures occur and there may be delayed union. Neurological problems can complicate involvement of the spine (cord compression and paraplegia) and skull (cranial nerve lesions due to constricted foraminae, frequently deafness). An increased blood supply to bone may cause cardiac problems, particularly in those with heart disease, and heart failure may occur. Osteosarcoma may occur in some patients and has a grave prognosis.

The maxilla may be affected and there may be expansion of the jaw resulting in pain under a denture, tilting of teeth and malocclusion. Radiography may show a cotton-wool pattern of the jaws with expansion of affected areas, thinning of the lamina dura and hypercementosis of the tooth roots. Tooth extractions can be difficult and may be complicated by osteomyelitis.

◄ Expansion of bones in Paget's disease may cause pain under a denture, tilting of teeth and malocclusion. Extractions can be difficult

Treatment is indicated where there is gross deformity in weight-bearing bones, when neurological complications occur and pain is very severe. Three drugs have been shown to be effective — a cytotoxic antibiotic mithramycin, which has a direct effect on osteoclasts; calcitonin, a peptide hormone, secreted by the thyroid, which also inhibits the osteoclast; and diphosphonates which also prevent osteoclast functioning. Surgery is sometimes needed to correct deformity or to relieve neurological damage.

Bone tumours

The primary tumours of bone may arise from bone- (or cartilage) forming cells, from the bone-marrow cells (myeloma) or from connective tissue elements. Secondary tumours in bone are, however, more common than primary neoplasms.

Tumours of the osteoblast may be benign (ivory osteoma) or malignant (osteogenic sarcoma). *Ivory osteoma* is rare and occurs mainly in the skull, causing pressure symptoms and occasionally becoming infected, causing osteomyelitis in adjacent bone. *Osteogenic sarcoma* occurs in two age groups, a younger group aged 10–25 years and an older, where

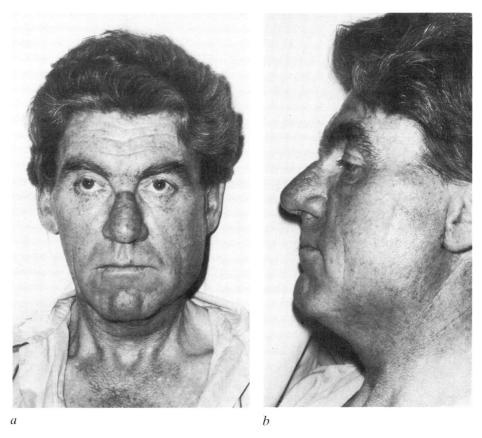

a   *b*

Fig. 12.4. Mandibular swelling due to bone tumour. Secondary carcinoma (primary bronchus) with pathological fracture.

the condition occurs in association with Paget's disease of bone. The tumour may occur in any bone, but particularly near the ends of long bones, such as the femur around the knee joint, spreading locally or via the blood to the lungs. The prognosis is very poor unless early diagnosis is made and radical treatment by amputation and radiotherapy is given.

Benign tumours of cartilage (*enchondroma*) are usually found in the centre of long bones and may be single or multiple. They can also occur in the phalanges of the fingers, causing pain and deformity. *Chondro-*

sarcoma is the most frequent primary malignant tumour of bone, occurring in the age group 30–60 years, particularly in the pelvis, long bones around the knee, but rarely in the arm. The rate of growth is slower than for osteogenic sarcoma, blood invasion occurring late. Amputation or surgical extirpation is successful in achieving a 50% 5-year survival.

Fibrous tissue lesions in bone may be benign (*fibroma*) or malignant (*fibrosarcoma*), the latter being the more common of two rare tumours and occurring at the ends of long bones, spreading by direct invasion or via the blood.

Tumours of the *osteoclast* have many histological and clinical imitators, called 'giant cell variants'. The giant cell tumour of osteoclasts occurs mainly at the ends of long bones, those around the knee joint accounting for over 50% of cases. The true giant cell tumours are locally malignant, metastasizing only late to the lungs. The impersonators of the true osteoclastoma also contain giant cells and have other similar features. One of these may involve the jaw, the *giant cell reparative granuloma*, causing destruction and osteolytic lesions. It is, however, benign.

◄ Giant cell tumours of the jaw have histological similarities with osteoclastoma but are benign

Secondary tumours of bone usually arise from primary sites in bronchus, breast, thyroid, prostate and kidney. Single or multiple deposits may occur and pathological fractures are common, particularly in the vertebrae and long bones. Deposits in the maxilla and mandible are rare, but may on occasion be the presenting feature with pain or sensory disturbance, swelling, loosening of teeth, failure of extraction sites to heal and pathological fractures.

Infections of bone

Acute infections of bone occur by haematogenous spread from infection elsewhere (skin sepsis in the case of *Staphylococcus*, from the bowel in the case of *Salmonella*), occasionally by direct spread from an adjacent infective source, such as an incorrectly treated apical abscess (*Staphylococcus* and anaerobes) or mastoiditis, and following compound fracture of bone.

◄ Osteomyelitis occurs with haematogenous spread from infection elsewhere and by spread from an adjacent focus such as incorrectly treated apical abscess

Infection may occur in any bone, but particularly at the metaphysis of long bones as well as the pelvis and vertebrae.

The infection usually begins in the medullary cavity or in subcortical bone, spreading up the medulla or bursting through the cortex to produce elevation of the periosteum. Bone destruction with pus formation follows and, in severe cases, the cortex dies due to deprivation of blood supply resulting in sequestrum formation. New subperiosteal bone is formed in progressive cases (the involucrum) with defects (cloacae) through which pus and nectrotic debris are discharged.

Septicaemia and metastatic abscess may complicate osteomyelitis, and, when infection extends into neighbouring joint space, septic arthritis. Chronic osteomyelitis may develop with osteosclerosis of surrounding bone and subperiosteal new bone formation, and in some cases chronic abscess, frequently at the upper end of the tibia.

Haematogenous spread to bone from a tuberculous focus may cause a granulomatous osteomyelitis. The vertebral bodies are the commonest site (Pott's disease of spine) but the long bones, fingers and joints may be affected. New bone formation does not occur in tuberculous osteomyelitis and pathological fracture through caseous material can occur, as well as extension through the periosteum to produce a cold abscess.

Bone involvement may occur with both congenital and acquired syphilis. Periostitis with new bone formation occurs in either form, gumma occurring in the acquired variety.

Bone pain is the most important symptom of osteomyelitis, varying from severe, when there is a subperiosteal abscess, to aching in chronic infection. Rapid diagnosis is essential, especially in children, to prevent irreversible damage. Tenderness on pressure is the most important sign. Radiological changes may take at least 10 days to develop.

◄ Radiological abnormality takes up to 10 days to develop in acute osteomyelitis.

Treatment of acute osteomyelitis consists of antibiotic therapy; if diagnosis and treatment are delayed, drainage of pus is performed. Choice of antibiotics depends on the organism identified with drainage or needle aspiration. Treatment is given for at least 6 weeks, or longer in chronic infections. Removal of the sequestrum is usually necessary in chronic osteomyelitis.

Diseases of the head and neck   **13**

Middle ear disease

Acute bacterial inflammation of the middle ear (*otitis media*) is usually due to spread of infection from the tonsils, adenoids and sinuses via the Eustachian tubes. It is frequently bilateral and particularly common in children, complicating infectious diseases such as measles, scarlatina and whooping cough. The infecting organism is usually haemolytic streptococcus, or *Streptococcus pneumococcus* or *Staphylococcus pyogenes*.

The organisms invade the mucous membrane and oedema closes the usual drainage route via the Eustachian tube. Exudate and pus formation increase pressure in the middle ear with bulging of the tympanic membrane which eventually ruptures, and discharge through the external ear (otorrhoea) continues until infection resolves.

The symptoms of acute otitis media are earache (otalgia) and deafness. There is usually a high temperature with mucoid or purulent discharge from the external meatus and tenderness over the mastoid bones.

Treatment consists of antibacterials (penicillin or erythromycin), analgesics and incision of the tympanic membrane (myringotomy) if pain persists despite treatment. Adequate early treatment causes rapid resolutions of signs and symptoms, discharge stops and hearing returns to normal. Rarely, symptoms persist with acute mastoiditis or extension of the infection to the meninges, causing extradural and intracerebral abscess or lateral sinus thrombosis.

Chronic otitis media

Infection persists in some cases of otitis media, the tympanic membrane perforation fails to heal and discharge continues. Progressive damage occurs; as does the degree of deafness. There are two main types of chronic otitis media: the mucosal type, with chronic mucoid discharge, and the bony type in which the ossicles, mastoid air cells and walls of the tympanic cavity are affected.

Mucosal infection rarely leads to serious complications although deafness can progress as the perforation gets larger. Treatment involves removal of the source of infection and repair of the tympanic membrane (tympanoplasty). Discharge is usually purulent in the *bony* type of infection and there may be acute exacerbations, with pain and fever. The disease progresses to cause increasing deafness and accumulation of epithelial debris which destroys the mastoid bone by pressure (cholesteatoma) — a precursor of intracranial complications such as meningitis and abscess formation. Failure to respond to conservative treatment (toilet of the ear and eradication of chronic infection in the oro-naso-pharynx) is an indication for mastoidectomy, in which the mastoid cells are exposed, all disease tissue removed, leaving a large cavity which can drain freely and eventually heal, but leaving the patient very deaf.

Otalgia

Although earache is associated with inflammatory diseases of the external and middle ear and mastoiditis, it may, however, be referred via the trigeminal, glossopharyngeal, vagus and 2nd cervical nerves. Dental and oral problems as well as pharyngeal, laryngeal and other diseases of the neck can present with earache. Dental abscess, caries, impacted lower molars and disease of the temporo-mandibular joint cause pain referred via the auriculo-temporal branch of the trigeminal nerve (first division).

Enlarged lymph nodes in the anterior and posterior triangles of the neck can cause otalgia, pain being referred via the great auricular nerve, a branch of the

◄ Otalgia (earache) may be referred from the oral cavity via the auriculo-temporal branch of the trigeminal nerve

Table 13.1. Earache

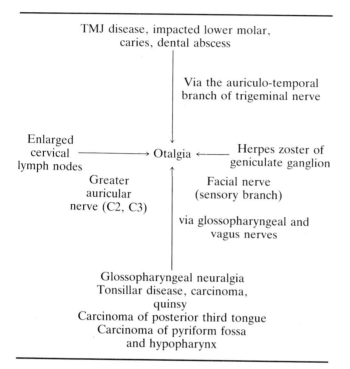

TMJ disease, impacted lower molar,
caries, dental abscess

Via the auriculo-temporal
branch of trigeminal nerve

Enlarged
cervical ————————→ Otalgia ←——— Herpes zoster of
lymph nodes   geniculate ganglion

Greater   Facial nerve
auricular   (sensory branch)
nerve (C2, C3)

via glossopharyngeal and
vagus nerves

Glossopharyngeal neuralgia
Tonsillar disease, carcinoma,
quinsy
Carcinoma of posterior third tongue
Carcinoma of pyriform fossa
and hypopharynx

2nd and 3rd cervical nerve roots. Herpes zoster of the
geniculate ganglion (Ramsay Hunt syndrome) also
causes earache via the sensory branch of the facial
nerve, in addition to facial paralysis and loss of taste on
one half of the tongue.

Referred earache also occurs with a variety of
oropharyngeal and laryngeal conditions via the glossopharyngeal and vagus nerves. Among these diseases
are glossopharyngeal neuralgia, tonsillitis, following
tonsillectomy, carcinoma and foreign bodies in the
faucial area, tumours of the posterior third of the
tongue, pyriform fossa and larynx, as well as foreign
bodies in the hypopharynx.

Since earache may radiate to the lower jaw it is
important to exclude other causes to account for the
pain — in patients without dental disease. The
combination of earache with increasing deafness is
often an indication of serious disease.

◀ The combination of
earache and increasing
difficulty with or painful
swallowing may be the
earliest signs of carci-
noma of the posterior
oropharynx

Other symptoms of middle ear disease

Tinnitus (ringing, buzzing or hissing in the ears) may be due to aural disease, conditions that cause referred otalgia and can be associated with systemic upset and neurological disorders.

Aural causes vary in seriousness from wax in the external meatus to labyrinthine disorders, such as Menière's disease, and middle ear disease. Impacted lower molars, dental caries, TMJ abnormalities (Costen's syndrome) and cervical lymph node enlargement may cause tinnitus as well as referred otalgia. Hypertension, anaemia, large doses of salicylates, drugs such as streptomycin, and high fever are some of the systemic problems that may be associated with tinnitus.

◀ Referred otalgia caused by impacted lower molars, dental caries and TMJ abnormalities may be accompanied by tinnitus

Vertigo may accompany tinnitus but is a separate condition that must be distinguished from 'dizziness'. The patient with true vertigo complains of the intermittent sensation of rotation, either subjective or objective, and not of faintness or of feeling 'lightheaded'. Vertigo can be caused by vestibular nerve lesions, disorder of the labyrinth and neurological diseases. Wax and Eustachian tube obstruction may also cause vertigo.

Attacks of vertigo are often accompanied by nausea and vomiting and occasionally the attacks are positional, often related to chronic suppurative otitis media, and provoked by head movements, such as lying back on a couch.

Table 13.2.   Vertigo

Acute vertigo
    vestibular neuronitis (often severe systemic upset)
    labyrinthitis (acute or chronic otitis media)
    vertebro-basilar artery ischaemia (usually with diplopia, dysarthria and facial paraesthesiae)
    multiple sclerosis
    positional vertigo (provoked by lying flat and turning head)
    Menière's disease
    basilar migraine (headache follows attack)
Persistent vertigo
    acoustic neuroma, drugs (streptomycin), brainstem lesions

---

Deafness may occur with middle ear disease (conductive), with VIIIth cranial nerve and inner ear damage (perceptive) or a mixture of both. Menière's disease is the association of progressive deafness, with tinnitus and episodes of vertigo, due to labyrinthine damage resulting from increased fluid formation in that organ, of unknown cause.

Nasal disorders

The sensation of *nasal obstruction* is usually bilateral and often associated with discharge (rhinorrhoea) and postnasal drip, causing persistent, unproductive, nocturnal coughing.

The common causes for nasal obstruction are fractures of the nasal bones; simple inflammatory conditions (coryza); allergic disorders, such as hay fever usually with polyp formation; and vasomotor rhinitis, a condition due to vascular change in and oedema of the mucosa. Malignant disease can also cause nasal obstruction, sometimes associated with swelling of the cheek, alveolus or palate, causing such problems as ill-fitting dentures, painful, loose teeth and facial pain. The first sign of malignant disease in the nasopharynx may, however, be an enlarged metastatic cervical lymph node.

Uncommon granulomatous conditions such as Wegener's granuloma and sarcoidosis may also cause nasal obstruction.

Epistaxis (nasal haemorrhage) can be due to nasal or systemic causes. Local factors, which are more common, include trauma and telangiectasia (sometimes part of multiple hereditary telangiectasia). Bleeding often arises from blood vessels in the area on the anterior part of the septum known as Little's area.

Systemic causes of epistaxis include hypertension; blood disorders including leukaemia, thrombocytopenia, scurvy and haemophilia; fevers, such as influenza; or drugs, such as anticoagulants.

Recurrent epistaxis requires careful examination of the source of bleeding and a search for signs of systemic disorder such as purpura. Cautery of Little's area will control spontaneous epistaxis but occasionally ligation

◄ Recurrent, heavy epistaxis may be a sign of systemic disease including haemorrhagic disorders such as thrombocytopenia and haemophilia

of the ethmoid branches of the maxillary artery (via the maxillary antrum) is needed.

Diseases of the sinuses

The maxillary sinus is related inferiorly to the hard palate, and the roots of the second pre-molar and first two molar teeth, and anteriorly to the bucco-alveolar sulcus. It is lined by ciliated columnar epithelium containing numerous mucous cells. Mucus produced is swept by ciliary action towards the ostium, which drains into the nose from the upper part of the medial wall and may be blocked by oedema of nasal mucosa.

Acute and chronic maxillary sinusitis can cause symptoms that are mistaken for dental disease. Conversely, dental disease such as apical abscess draining into the sinus may predispose to infection of the maxillary antrum. Root dislocation into the antrum and oro-antral fistula following extraction of a maxillary pre-molar or molar may also cause sinusitis.

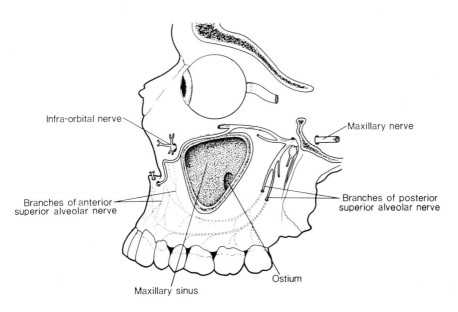

Fig. 13.1. Relationships of maxillary sinus.

Table 13.3. Oro-antral fistula

Antral disease
    carcinoma invading the alveolus
Oral disease
    following extraction maxillary molar/premolar
    fracture maxillary tuberosity
Symptoms
    maxillary infection
    discharge into oral cavity
    fluids pass from mouth to nose
    escape of air into mouth when blowing nose

The symptoms of acute sinusitis are facial pain (often resembling that of dental origin) made worse by bending, lying down and even walking, plus nasal obstruction, with scanty nasal discharge. The patient has usually had a recent upper respiratory infection, dental infection or extraction. The clinical features consist of fever, tenderness over the antrum, with puffiness over the sinus, particularly if the cause is of dental origin, or due to antral carcinoma.

◄ Acute maxillary sinusitis causes throbbing facial pain made worse by head movement, walking or stooping

Treatment consists of analgesics to reduce pain, control of infection with antibacterials, and attempts to improve drainage by reducing mucosal swelling with ephedrine nasal drops, or puncture of the antrum, through the nose, and washing out. If a cause can be identified such as deviated nasal septum, nasal polyps or root fragments, these are treated. Polyps in the antrum or grossly thickened mucosa can be removed via the Caldwell–Luc approach, an incision being made in the muco-periosteum of the canine fossa and a window made in the antrum, through which the antro-nasal wall can be removed, allowing drainage.

Acute maxillary sinusitis may be complicated by involvement of other sinuses, and by otitis media. The condition can become chronic, particularly if there is poor drainage, and when there are dental problems. Chronic sinusitis results in polyp formation, which causes persistent discomfort over the antrum, nasal stuffiness, chronic nasal or postnasal discharge, huskiness and cachosmia (an awareness by the patient of the foul smell of the discharge and breath). The principles

◄ Chronic antral infection may result from apical abscess related to a maxillary molar or premolar

of treatment of chronic sinusitis are to improve drainage by antral puncture or antrostomy, and removal of mucosal abnormalities.

Frontal sinusitis usually follows coryza or may complicate infection of the antrum and ethmoidal sinuses. The prominent symptom is supraorbital pain which is periodic, with peaks of severity at midday, subsiding during the afternoon. There may be acute tenderness over the sinus plus swelling of the upper eyelid. Although most cases improve with antibiotics and with attempts to improve drainage with ephedrine nasal drops, orbital cellulitis can occur and, rarely, osteomyelitis in the frontal bone. Meningitis with extra or subdural abscess, as well as frontal lobe cerebral abscess, are very rare complications.

Fistula between the maxillary antrum and the oral cavity may occur because of antral carcinoma eroding through the alveolus; follow fracture of the maxillary tuberosity; and complicate extraction of an upper molar or premolar, when there is only a thin layer of tissue between the roots and sinus. The symptoms, in addition to those of maxillary sinusitis, include discharge into the oral cavity; escape of air into the oral cavity during nose blowing; and the escape of liquids through the fistula and down the nose during drinking.

Larger fistulas require surgical closure after treatment of any antral infection and antrostomy to provide drainage into the nasal cavity. Small fistulas following extraction are often undetected, do not cause clinical problems and heal spontaneously.

Carcinoma of the maxillary sinus is seldom diagnosed until there has been spread to surrounding structures. The condition often occurs in the context of chronic catarrh and sinus infection producing, in its earliest stages, blood-stained nasal discharge and unilateral nasal obstruction. Late symptoms include swelling of the cheek, swelling or ulceration in the bucco-alveolar sulcus or palate, eye-watering (epiphora) due to naso-lacrimal duct obstruction, double vision, squint and prominence of the eye (proptosis). Pain occurs in the distribution of the maxillary division of the trigeminal nerve, sometimes radiating to the ear and mandible via other branches.

Apart from local spread to the cheek, bucco-alveolar sulcus, palate, orbit and nasal cavity, the usual features

◀ Swelling of the cheek, the bucco-alveolar sulcus and palate may be the first signs of maxillary antral tumour

of extension are enlargement of the sub-mandibular and deep cervical lymph nodes.

The tumour is, histologically, an undifferentiated squamous carcinoma. Treatment by wide-field mega-voltage radiation and block excision of the regional lymph nodes in the neck is largely palliative. The prognosis is poor.

Carcinoma and other malignant tumours (lymphomas) of the *naso-pharynx* present with similar symptoms to antral malignancy with the addition of conductive deafness and involvement of the Vth, VIth and bulbar cranial nerves, due to invasion of the foramen lacerum and jugular foramen. The disease is particularly common in South China and there is often evidence of Epstein–Barr virus infection. The prognosis is poor and treatment consists of radiotherapy.

◄ Malignant disease in the nasopharynx may invade the base of the skull, involving the trigeminal nerve as well as the lower cranial nerves via the jugular foramen

Tonsillar disease

Acute tonsillitis is common in children under 9 years of age, and is recurrent, resulting in hypertrophy of the lymphatic tissues in the mouth and pharynx (adenoids). The symptoms are sore throat and dysphagia, earache,

Table 13.4.   Differential diagnosis of acute tonsillitis

Vincent's angina
  acute necrotizing ulcerative gingivitis — yellowish
    membrane
  Borrelia vincentii present in large numbers
Scarlet fever
  typical rash and 'strawberry' appearance of tongue
Infectious mononucleosis
  cheesy white membrane on tonsils, palatal petechiae,
    cervical lymphadenopathy
Diphtheria
  greyish-yellow true membrane, is in one piece and
    attached with no spread beyond tonsil
Agranulocytosis
  ulceration and false membrane (exudate not attached to
    tonsils)
  extensive lesions on pharyngeal and buccal mucosa

headache and malaise. The child is usually feverish, and has halitosis. The pharynx and tonsils are hyperaemic with debris between follicles, the cervical lymph nodes, particularly that at the angle of the jaw, being enlarged and tender.

Acute otitis media is the most common complication of tonsillitis but occasionally the infection may progress to quinsy (peritonsillar abscess) and spread to lymph nodes in the parapharyngeal space. The patient with *quinsy* is more ill than with acute tonsillitis, having very high fever and dysphagia. The typical features are distortion of the oro-pharyngeal isthmus with downward deviation of the related tonsil and oedema of the uvula. With early antibiotic therapy quinsy is uncommon, requiring incision through the mouth, if spontaneous rupture does not occur. *Parapharyngeal abscess* presents as swelling to one side of the midline of the posterior wall of the oro-pharynx. Incision may also be required.

Sore throat may be caused by other conditions including pharyngitis (often with postnasal discharge); pharyngeal ulceration of whatever type; trauma by foreign body (fish or chicken bone); with gastro-oesophageal reflux and with glossopharyngeal neuralgia. Sore throat may also be related to systemic disorders such as iron-deficiency anaemia, agranulocytosis and leukaemia, as well as diffuse local infection with *Candida* and Vincent's angina.

Enlargement of the adenoids usually occurs in combination with tonsillitis but occasionally malignant tumours in the postnasal space mimic symptoms of inflammatory adenoidal hypertrophy. The clinical features of adenoidal enlargement are mouth-breathing and snoring due to nasal obstruction; recurrent otitis media due to Eustachian tube obstruction; and postnasal discharge and cough. Adenoidectomy relieves these symptoms.

Squamous carcinoma may present as an indurated ulcer on fauces, tonsil or pharyngeal wall associated with earache and slight headache. Unilateral and progressive enlargement of the tonsil requires biopsy to establish the cause. Lymphomas can also present with enlargement of the tonsils, usually bilateral and, rarely, ulcerating.

◀ Progressive unilateral tonsillar enlargement should be biopsied

Table 13.5. Hoarseness

Laryngeal causes
    Acute laryngitis — painful (dysphonia)
    Chronic laryngitis — vocal fatigue, smokers,
      actors, alcohol excess
    Tumours — persistent hoarseness
    Neurological — cord paralysis (recurrent laryngeal
      N.palsy), myasthenia gravis
Pharyngeal causes
    Malignant disease oropharynx
General causes
    Hypothyroidism, RA involving cricoarytenoid joints
Functional dysphonia

Laryngeal disorders

Most laryngeal disorders present with change in the voice, varying from aphonia (loss of voice) to pain with phonation (dysphonia) and changes in the pitch, any of which symptoms being termed 'hoarseness' by the patient.

Hoarseness may be caused by laryngeal conditions — tumour, inflammation, paralysis of the vocal cords by neurological lesions — and by pharyngeal disorders, usually malignant disease or pharyngeal pouches.

Acute laryngitis is usually associated with upper respiratory infections, often in the context of over-use of the voice and heavy smoking. There may be loss of voice or dysphonia and, sometimes, pain and tenderness of the larynx.

Chronic laryngitis presents as hoarseness, vocal fatigue, cough and a constant tendency to clear the throat. It usually occurs in those who over-use their voices (teachers, actors, soldiers) and with over-indulgence in alcohol and tobacco. Chronic sinus infection and sepsis of the tonsils or lungs also cause the same symptoms. The diagnosis of chronic laryngitis is only made after other lesions have been excluded, including carcinoma of the larynx, laryngeal tuberculosis and vocal cord paralysis. Hoarseness present for more than 2–3 weeks should be investigated.

Laryngeal tuberculosis is a rare complication of pulmonary infection, causing aphonia, change in pitch of the voice and painful dysphagia. *Gummatous infiltration* of the larynx and epiglottis can occur in the tertiary stage of syphilis, causing damage to cartilage of the larynx and subsequent stenosis.

Benign laryngeal tumours (papilloma and fibroma) are rare, and cause persistent hoarseness. Removal with forceps under general anaesthetic is the only treatment needed.

Malignant tumours of the larynx are usually squamous cell carcinomas and occur either on the vocal cords (intrinsic) or on the vestibular folds and the epiglottis (extrinsic). Persistent hoarseness, often for months, is the characteristic symptom. Dysphagia, dyspnoea, earache, dry cough and haemoptysis are later symptoms. Diagnosis is made by direct laryngo-scopy and biopsy.

◀ Hoarseness that persists for more than 3 weeks must be investigated by laryngo-scopy to exclude malignancy

Carcinoma of larynx spreads both locally and via the lymphatics to the deep cervical nodes, relatively late. Tumours are treated, in the first instance, by X-irradiation. If the lesion does not regress, if it recurs, or if the disease is extensive, total laryngectomy with block dissection of cervical lymph nodes is performed. These patients have a permanent tracheostomy but, after suitable training, can converse with the use of oesophageal speech.

Paralysis of the vocal cords is usually due to lesions of the recurrent laryngeal nerve, a branch of the vagus, only the tensors of the cords being supplied by the superior laryngeal. Paralysis due to left recurrent laryngeal nerve damage is caused by lesions in the thorax, particularly carcinoma of bronchus, mediastinal lymph node enlargement and aortic aneurysm and, less often, by lesions in the neck such as carcinoma of the thyroid gland, trauma during thyroidectomy and malignant cervical lymph nodes. The right recurrent laryngeal nerve does not have an intrathoracic course and is damaged less frequently by thyroid cancer and surgery. The symptoms are change in voice pitch and cough with difficulty in expectoration of sputum.

Systemic disorders can cause hoarseness, particularly hypothyroidism, and weakness of cord movements occurs in myasthenia gravis, usually after prolonged conversation. Involvement of the cricoarytenoid joints occurs, occasionally, in rheumatoid arthritis, causing pain and tenderness over the larynx as well as hoarseness.

Mouth and tongue

The oral manifestations of systemic disease are dealt with in other chapters. This section deals with local disease of the buccal cavity, the tongue and gums.

Cysts in the mouth occur at many sites and are of nuisance value only. *Mucous retention cysts* are usually found on the inside of the lips and cheeks, having a bluish appearance and containing mucoid fluid. These lesions are often chewed by the patient which may 'ease' the problem although excision is usually required. *Ranula* is a cyst on one or other side of the floor of the mouth, arising either in the sublingual or one of the accessory salivary glands. Midline *dermoid* occupies the floor of the mouth and may project as a swelling below the chin, representing an implantation during fusion of the two mandibular processes. Both ranula and dermoid cysts are dealt with by excision.

Oral infections may be bacterial, fungal or viral. Bacterial infections are most often due to *Streptococcus pyogenes*, which may be cultured from throat swabs in patients with sore throat and tonsillitis. Infection may be followed by scarlet fever and, in some patients, after an interval of two to three weeks, by rheumatic fever and acute glomerulonephritis. *Scarlet fever* is characterized by circumoral pallor, seen in some other fevers, and an extensive erythematous rash on the limbs and trunk which desquamates. The surface of the tongue may peel as the condition progresses, leaving the papillae prominently visible — the 'strawberry' appearance.

Other streptococci, notably *viridans*, occur normally in the mouth in large numbers but rarely cause oral infection, although they may enter the bloodstream during chewing and dental manipulation. The transient bacteraemia is of importance in patients with rheumatic heart disease, congenital cardiac defects and patients with prosthetic valves (*see* Chapter 3).

Diphtheria occurs most commonly in children under the age of 14 living in crowded conditions. The disease can be transmitted by droplet infection from the patient

◀ Circumoral pallor occurs not only with scarlet fever but with other fevers that cause facial flushing

and carriers. The infection occurs anywhere in the oro-naso-pharynx presenting as nasal discharge, sore throat with a greyish-yellow membrane on the tonsils and swelling of the neck due to tender oedema and lymph node enlargement. Systemic effects occur most often in the patient with pharyngeal involvement, and are due to an exotoxin that causes cardiovascular complications, including peripheral circulatory failure and neurological complications such as palatal palsy and, in the most serious cases, paralysis of the nerves to the heart, respiratory muscles and the limbs.

Diphtheria is treated with a specific antitoxin and antibiotics (penicillin or erythromycin) which eradicate the bacilli from the throat.

Actinomycosis is another uncommon infection, although the majority of cases occur in the neck and face. The infection, which is endogenous and due to *Actinomyces israelii*, presents as a suppurative lesion of soft tissue, although bone (e.g. mandible) may be involved. Swelling occurs over the angle of the jaw and there may be pain with trismus. Treatment consists of drainage of pus and prolonged, high-dose penicillin therapy.

Candida infections occur under special circumstances such as during treatment with broad-spectrum anti-bacterials, immunosuppressive drugs and cortico-steroids, and with blood disorders such as leukaemia and agranulocytosis. The yeast normally occurs in small numbers in the mouth and proliferation under these circumstances, invading the mucosa, produces the features of oral thrush: inflammation of the mucosa with characteristic white adherent patches. Very rarely, in patients with impaired immunity,

Table 13.6. Factors predisposing to candidiasis

Drugs
    immunosuppressives
    steroids (including the oral contraceptives)
    antibiotics
    aerosol propellants (particularly steroids)
Carcinoma and leukaemia
Neutropenia
Diabetes mellitus (uncontrolled)

Candida may invade the blood causing foci of infection in the brain, heart, kidney and muscle.

Treatment of oral candidiasis is with topical antifungal agents (nystatin or amphotericin B) as lozenges, and correction of the predisposing cause, if possible.

Herpes simplex is a DNA virus that has two serotypes; type I causing skin and membrane lesions, type II causing genital and perineal infections. Type I commonly presents in childhood as an ulcerative stomatitis involving the tongue, gums, buccal mucosa and lips. Systemic infection, causing encephalitis in some patients, occurs in immunosuppressed subjects. Recurrent herpes simplex presents as the 'cold sore', the virus remaining dormant in the trigeminal ganglion following a primary infection and later producing vesicular lesions around the lips in response to sunlight, emotion, trauma and infection.

Oral vesicles, which ulcerate, may occur in *chicken pox* and *herpes zoster*, the latter caused by reactivation of the same virus which has remained dormant in a sensory ganglion. Although the first division of the trigeminal nerve is most commonly affected, the maxillary division may, sometimes, be involved.

Coxsackie A virus infections are common in children and two clinical syndromes, herpangina and hand, foot and mouth disease, occur. *Herpangina* is characterized by fever, headache, sometimes vomiting, and small vesicles on the palate and tonsils which coalesce to form shallow ulcers. *Hand, foot and mouth disease* is principally a disease that occurs in childhood, with outbreaks in schools, presenting with vesicular stomatitis and a maculopapular rash on the hands and sides of the feet, which later blisters. Both conditions are self-limiting and do not require special treatment.

Malignant disease of the mouth and pharynx. (*see also* Chapter 18)

The broad principles of the pathology, diagnosis and treatment of malignant disease in the oral cavity and pharynx can be considered together.

With the exception of the postcricoid area, tumours in this region are more common in the male. There are several known predisposing factors including chronic irritation by smoking, alcohol, gross dental caries and chewing of betel nuts in some areas of the Indian subcontinent. Chronic mucosal atrophy from iron deficiency (Plummer–Vinson syndrome), candidiasis and syphilis are other predisposing factors.

These factors cause a pre-malignant condition of the mucosa (*leucoplakia*), consisting of a white, thickened patch, which cannot be rubbed off, with cracks and fissuring. Histologically, there is hyperplasia of the squamous epithelium with hyperkeratosis. Malignant change occurs in only a few cases of leucoplakia, which can be recognized by dysplastic changes in biopsy material. Red, velvety mucosal thickening (*erythroplasia*) may also be pre-cancerous.

Macroscopically, malignant tumours present as either single or multiple lesions (in chronic mucosal atrophy) having a nodular appearance, showing ulceration and fissuring or features of a warty, papilliferous growth. The histological changes are usually those of squamous carcinoma, although transitional cell tumours occur in the posterior third of the tongue, tonsil and nasopharynx.

Although diagnosis depends on the history, clinical presentation, and histological examination of the lesion, some features are suggestive of malignancy. Progressive growth, ulceration, haemorrhage without evidence of infection, induration and fixation to deep tissues such as bone, involvement of nerves, and enlargement of the regional lymph nodes, all suggest malignancy.

◄ Oral tumours frequently present first to the dentist. Any features suspicious of malignancy require referral for specialist investigation

Having confirmed the diagnosis and identified any predisposing factors, such as syphilis or iron-deficiency anaemia, the treatment of any tumour must be considered with respect to the primary site and the regional lymph nodes. *Surgical treatment* involves local excision and block dissection of neck lymph nodes. The excision of the lesion may leave large mucosal and skin defects which cause disfiguration, swallowing and speech problems, and trismus, especially if bone is resected. Plastic surgery techniques are needed to reconstruct and reduce subsequent deformities, flaps of skin and muscle being reflected from the forehead and upper thorax.

Table 13.7.   Effects of radiotherapy

Skin — acute erythema
    pigmentation, following erythema
    desquamation — usually dry
Mucous membrane
    erythema
    fibrinous mucositis
Late changes
    atrophy skin and mucosa
    telangiectasia
    loss of hair, mucus and sweat glands
    increased incidence infection with trauma

Radiotherapy may be used before or after surgery and as the primary treatment. Large tumours of the tongue, mouth, palate, tonsil, nasopharynx and laryngopharynx are usually treated by external supervoltage therapy. Radiotherapy causes acute changes in the skin (erythema, pigmentation and desquamation) and mucous membrane (erythema and fibrinous changes) which heal within 2–4 weeks. Late damage to the subepithelial connective tissues may occur causing small blood vessel occlusion, and resulting in mucosal atrophy, telangiectasia, loss of sweat and mucus glands and hair. Areas exposed to therapeutic radiation are easily damaged by trauma leading to infection and necrosis. Irradiation of the jaw can cause necrosis, developmental and structural abnormalities of teeth and arrest of normal condylar bone growth in children.

Chemotherapy may be used in locally advanced tumours, usually in combination with radiotherapy or surgery, with the aim of controlling the rate of growth of the primary tumour before the other treatment. Drugs can be given by regional perfusion through a branch of the external carotid artery. Among the drugs used are bleomycin, methotrexate, cyclophosphamide and vincristine, usually in combination régimes, which are more effective.

Chemotherapy can cause superficial ulceration of the mucosa, often accompanied by leucopenia and thrombocytopenia, reduced salivary flow and increased susceptibility to Candida infection. It is important that good oral hygiene is maintained during this form of

◀ Chemotherapy for malignancy predisposes to ulceration of the mucosa; causes reduced salivary flow and increases susceptibility to oral infections

treatment and the dentist is often asked to deal with caries and periodontal disease. If extraction is necessary, the blood count must be checked (particularly platelets and white cells) before surgery, which should be performed after a course of therapy. There is an increased risk of septicaemia in these patients and prophylactic antibiotics should be given.

When the regional lymph nodes are obviously involved they may be treated by block dissection of the nodes on both sides of the neck, since lymphatic drainage tends to be bilateral. If the nodes are fixed and obviously irremovable, palliative radiotherapy is given.

Carcinoma of the lip commonly affects elderly men who have been exposed to a weather-beaten outdoor life. The lower lip is the most common site, presenting as a fissure, ulcer or warty growth. Upper lip and angle of the mouth lesions are less common but have a poorer

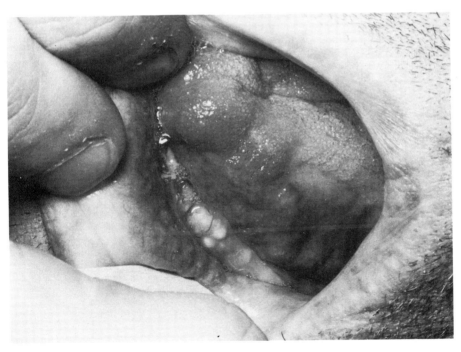

Fig. 13.2. Carcinoma of tongue. Nodular lesion on undersurface of tongue, with ulceration and bleeding.

prognosis. The lymphatic spread is initially to submental and mandibular nodes. A lip swelling may also be a simple wart, chancre, haemangioma, herpes simplex or mucous cyst. Treatment of carcinoma of lip consists of wedge resection combined with plastic surgery to resurface the defect.

Carcinoma of the tongue on the anterior two-thirds begins as a nodule, fissure or ulcer which is rarely painful unless secondarily infected or there has been invasion of deeper structures. Pain may be referred to the ear. When the tumour extends onto the floor of the mouth and the alveolus, swallowing and speech become difficult because of tongue fixation. Tumours on the posterior third are poorly differentiated, and spread to the regional lymph nodes early, presenting with bilateral enlargement.

◀ Posterior third tumours of tongue are poorly differentiated and spread to regional nodes at an early stage

Any nodule or chronic ulcer of the tongue must be regarded as malignant until proved otherwise, particularly if associated with leucoplakia. The lesion must be differentiated from benign tumours such as papilloma, haemangioma and fibroma. The nervous patient may think that a circumvallate papilla is a tumour.

Small carcinomas of the tongue are treated by excision or by implantation of an iridium wire, structured as a grid, and left in place for several days so as to give the required dose of irradiation. Posterior third and larger anterior lesions are treated by irradiation of the tumour and excision of the draining lymph nodes.

Palatal tumours are often warty and must be differentiated from antral lesions spreading downwards and from mixed salivary tumours, which can arise in accessory glands scattered over the hard palate. Treatment consists of excision and/or a radioactive mould, fashioned as an upper dental plate containing iridium wire. Larger lesions are treated by external beam irradiation.

Tumours of the tonsil are usually squamous carcinoma but may be lymphoma. Carcinoma usually presents with metastatic lymph node enlargement and otalgia. Treatment consists of external irradiation including the draining nodes. Lesions of the floor of the mouth, alveolus and cheek also spread early to lymph nodes as well as to the root of the tongue; they must be

◀ Tumours of the tonsil are usually squamous carcinoma but may also be lymphoma

Table 13.8.   Tumours of jaw

Of bone itself
 osteoma and osteogenic sarcoma
 chondroma and chondrosarcoma
 osteoclastoma
 haemangioma and fibrosarcoma from periosteum
 myeloma
 secondary deposits (lung, breast, prostate, kidney)
Surface tumours invading bone
 carcinoma and mixed salivary tumour
 melanoma
Invasion from carcinoma of the maxillary antrum

differentiated from tumours, including adenocarcinoma, of the salivary glands. Lesions are excised, where possible, or treated by external irradiation.

Malignant tumours of the gums are rare (fibrosarcoma or osteoclastoma) and must be differentiated from other forms of epulis. Localized swelling of the gums may be: a nodule of vascular fibrous tissue arising from the periosteum; a benign giant-cell lesion, which mimics an osteoclastoma, and is found frequently in association with primary hyperparathyroidism; or an angioma.

Tumours of the jaw may arise from the bone itself, by invasion from overlying tissues or extension from the maxilla. Bone neoplasms originate in cartilage (chondrosarcoma), the osteoid (osteoma, osteogenic sarcoma, osteoclastoma), the medulla (myeloma) and the periosteum (fibrosarcoma). The jaw is also an occasional site for secondary deposits, the primary lesion being in bronchus, breast, prostate, thyroid or kidney.

Benign tumours of bone are treated by excision, which in the case of the mandible requires bone graft. Malignant tumours are treated by either hemimandibulectomy or radiotherapy, the latter causing radionecrosis and the risk of osteomyelitis following tooth extraction, even many years after treatment, and thus requiring prophylactic antibiotic therapy.

Development abnormalities of lip and palate

In half the cases cleft lip and palate coexist and in a quarter the palatal defect occurs alone. As in all congenital anomalies, it is important to search for other developmental defects, which occur in up to 10% of patients with clefts.

Cleft lip is rarely in the midline. It may be bilateral, and vary from a small defect to a large anomaly that extends into the nostril, or as far as the orbit, and splits the alveolus. Rarely, there may be associated cleft of the tongue and of the mandible.

Cleft lip alone presents no feeding or nursing problem. Early repair, usually between the third and six month, permits normal moulding of the facial bones during growth. Optimum management for lip and palatal clefts requires co-ordinated treatment by orthodontist, plastic surgeon, ENT and dental surgeon with a speech therapist.

Palatal clefts may be partial, involving the soft palate alone, or complete. Complete clefts may be unilateral, running the full length of the maxilla, or bilateral in which there is an anterior V separating the premaxilla completely, which can move about, causing gross deformity.

Cleft palate interferes with the sucking mechanism in infants and to aid feeding a plate may be used, or a spoon rather than a bottle. The defects are repaired at about 12 months of age in order to allow normal speech to develop. Where hair-lip coexists, this is repaired at about 8 weeks and the palate repaired as a second stage at 1 year.

Secondary surgical procedures may be needed to correct persistent problems after primary repair, including nasal escape of air during speech. Correction of nasal defects, and facial bone surgery to correct deformity resulting from maxillary hypoplasia are also sometimes needed.

Salivary glands (*see* Chapter 2)

Stone formation is common in the submandibular gland and its duct, but is rare in the parotid and unrecorded in the sublingual. The cause of stone formation is

Table 13.9. Symptoms of salivary gland disease

Swelling
    single gland (mixed tumour) or several (sarcoid)
    painful (parotitis or carcinoma or mumps)
    varies in size (calculus)
Xerostomia
    calculus
    Sjögren's syndrome (plus dry eyes)
Excess saliva
    drugs
    psychiatric disorders and Parkinsonism
Abnormal taste
    calculus or sialadenitis
    others include ENT disease, gastro-oesophageal reflux,
        drugs

---

unknown. They are composed of calcium, phosphate and carbonate and hence are radio-opaque.

The clinical features are painful swelling of the affected gland, aggravated by food, abnormal taste due to purulent discharge and dry mouth (xerostomia). On examination the gland is swollen and tender; the duct opening may be reddened with a discharge. The calculus is usually palpable.

A single stone in the duct can be removed through the mouth but if there are more, or if one is impacted, the gland is excised.

Salivary gland inflammation may occur with *mumps*, a viral disease; the swelling is usually bilateral, affecting the parotid more often than the submandibular or sublingual. Other organs may be involved by mumps including the testes, pancreas, thyroid and ovary.

Ascending infection of the parotid, via its duct, may occur in association with dental sepsis, dehydration, poor oral hygiene after operation and the prolonged use of a naso-gastric tube. The disease may be unilateral and associated with intense pain in and firm enlargement of the gland, with purulent discharge from the duct. Prevention is important, but in the established case the patient is fully hydrated and antibiotics are given; drainage procedures are rarely necessary.

Recurrent parotitis, usually affecting one gland in children, is associated with dilatation of the duct system (sialectasia), demonstrated by a sialogram, and is due to stone or stricture.

Sarcoidosis, lymphomas and, rarely, *tuberculosis* may also cause parotid and submandibular gland enlargement which is usually painless and not associated with xerostomia or taste problems. Sarcoidosis involving the parotid is often accompanied by acute iritis and sometimes by facial paralysis (*see* Chapter 5).

Neoplasms of the salivary glands may be nodular or diffuse and commonly affect the parotid. Diffuse tumours are always *malignant*, are often painful and grow rapidly, involving the facial nerve and regional lymph nodes. Eventually surrounding tissues are infiltrated and skin or mucosal ulceration may occur. If carcinoma is confined to the parotid, radical parotidectomy is performed, sacrificing the facial nerve, combined with block dissection of the regional lymph nodes and external irradiation. The prognosis for salivary gland carcinoma is poor, particularly when it originates in the submandibular gland.

Nodular salivary tumours are usually benign, although adenocystic carcinoma, a slowly growing, malignant lesion, can resemble the pleomorphic adenoma (mixed parotid tumour) and adenolymphoma. *Mixed parotid tumours* usually begin in the lower pole of the gland, around the angle of the jaw. Although superficial there may be deep prolongation with projection into the pharynx. The facial nerve is never involved except when there is malignant transformation.

◀ Paralysis of the facial nerve with parotid tumour only occurs with carcinoma and malignant transformation in mixed salivary tumours

The microscopic features of the pleomorphic adenoma range from typical adenoma to frank carcinoma, with an appearance of the stroma that resembles cartilage, hence the term 'mixed tumour'. Enucleation of the tumour is a satisfactory treatment, but recurrence is not uncommon because the capsule is often incomplete and penetration occurs. Implantation of tumour cells in the wound can occur. Care is taken during partial parotidectomy to preserve the facial nerve and provided that a wide excision is performed the prognosis is excellent.

Adenolymphoma occurs in the parotid and may be bilateral, the tumour being soft and cystic. It probably arises from salivary duct epithelium and shows lymphoid stroma on microscopy. Prognosis is excellent after local removal.

The salivary glands may be enlarged in *Sjögren's syndrome* but are, more often, smaller than normal (*see* Chapter 12). The lacrimal, as well as salivary, glands are infiltrated by chronic inflammatory cells, with acinar atrophy and fibrosis and reduction in secretions. Other salivary glands, apart from the parotid and submandibular, can be involved and the diagnosis may be confirmed by lip biopsy.

There may be association between Sjögren's syndrome and other autoimmune disorders. Patients with Sjögren's syndrome and rheumatoid arthritis seem to have an increased incidence of malignant lymphoma.

Bilateral parotid swelling occurs with alcoholism and alcohol-induced liver disease (*see* Chapter 7). The cause is not known.

Swellings in the neck

The differential diagnosis of swellings in the neck is considered in Chapter 2. They may arise from any of the anatomical structures in the neck — lymph nodes, lymphatics, arteries, salivary glands, pharynx, branchial arch remnant as well as from the skin and superficial fascia.

Branchial cysts arise from the cervical sinuses created in the embryo by growth of the 2nd branchial arch over the 3rd and 4th arches. This sinus usually disappears but may persist, presenting in early adult life as a soft swelling which bulges from beneath the anterior border of the sternomastoid. The cyst fluid contains cholesterol crystals and is usually sterile. Treatment is by surgical excision.

Branchial sinus presents as a small discharging orifice, opening over the anterior border of the sternomastoid, low in the neck, the tract extending upwards between internal and external carotid arteries to the side wall of pharynx or tonsillar fossa. Although usually present at birth, a secondary sinus may form if an infected branchial cyst ruptures.

Enlarged cervical lymph nodes may be due to infection or neoplasm. Enlargement of nodes due to infection may be secondary to lesions in the mouth, nose, ear, scalp, sinuses or pharynx. The nodes are usually tender and the overlying skin may become reddened, and an abscess forms which requires drainage. Systemic antibiotics are prescribed to treat the primary source and nodes with the site of recurrent infection, such as an enlarged tonsil, removed.

Infectious mononucleosis and *syphilis* may cause bilateral infective cervical lymphadenopathy. Recognition depends on specific serological tests, the Paul–Bunnell test for heterophil antibodies in the case of glandular fever, and the VDRL test for syphilis.

Tuberculous lymphadenopathy is now uncommon. The nodes are, at first, small and discrete, becoming matted together as they enlarge and undergo the typical caseation. The abscess formed bursts through the deep fascia to produce a 'collar-stud' lesion, which discharges onto the skin resulting in a chronic sinus. Diagnosis depends on demonstrating tubercle bacilli in the abscess or discharging fluid. Treatment consists of antituberculous drug therapy for at least 6 months and removal of the node in a collar-stud abscess. It is not necessary to deal with the primary focus, which may be in the tonsillar region, the adenoids and even the dental roots.

All cervical lymph nodes can be involved with *metastatic carcinoma* from the postnasal space, oral cavity, tonsil, larynx and thyroid. Enlargement may also be due to carcinoma in distant sites such as bronchus, oesophagus and stomach. Although some lymph node groups are more likely to be enlarged with certain tumours (submental nodes with carcinoma of lip) the pattern is not constant, the carcinoma apparently missing some groups in direct line of drainage. Treatment depends on the primary site, but block dissection or irradiation of nodes with treatment of the tumour itself is effective for most head and neck lesions. Where the primary site is more distant the prognosis is poor and cervical lymphadenopathy is not treated, except when there are pressure symptoms, such as superior mediastinal obstruction.

Hodgkin's disease, non-Hodgkin's lymphoma and *chronic lymphatic leukaemia* present with bilateral firm, discrete enlargement of nodes. Diagnosis depends on biopsy and/or the blood film. Treatment depends on cause but combined chemotherapy and/or irradiation produce good 5-year survival figures (*see* Chapter 8).

Tumours of the *carotid body* are rare and, although occasionally malignant, spreading via the lymphatics, are slowly growing. They must be differentiated from aneurysms of the carotid artery. Treatment is by dissection away from the vessels and excision.

Cystic hygroma arises from embryonic lymph channels in the neck and usually presents in infancy or childhood, being recognized by the characteristic transilluminability with a pencil torch. Excision may be difficult because of ramifications throughout the structures in the neck. Other congenital lymphatic swellings (lymphangiomas) may occur on the lips, tongue, cheek and in the tongue.

Fistulas and cysts may form in the embryological line of descent of the thyroid gland from the foramen caecum to its normal site in the neck. Rarely the thyroid may fail to descend and presents as a lump in the tongue or midline of the neck. Sometimes the gland may descend below its usual position into the superior mediastinal region causing stridor and other features, due to obstruction of the great veins.

Swellings of the thyroid move with swallowing, those from the thyroglossal tract with projection of the tongue. Thyroglossal cysts are usually excised but it is important to exclude the possibility that the swelling is composed of functioning thyroid tissue by radioisotope scanning of the neck and upper mediastinum. Midline swellings of thyroid origin may, rarely, be the only functioning tissue and should not be excised.

Psychological disorders, behavioural problems and mental illness

14

Psychological disorders, problems of behaviour and mental illness are commonly encountered in all forms of clinical practice, either on their own or accompanying, although not always related to, organic illness.

The symptoms of psychological disorder can be mistaken for those of organic illness although, usually, the diagnosis is made without need for extensive investigation. Alternatively, a mistaken diagnosis of psychological disorder can be made if there is no obvious physical explanation for the patient's symptoms — an incorrect diagnosis of depression or hysterical conversion delaying recognition of a serious illness.

Disorders of mood are common, ranging from acute anxiety to severe depression, and are more frequently encountered in clinical practice than thought and ideational abnormalities or disorders of perception. Most psychological problems and behaviour disorders are not associated with organic disease but the possibility of endocrine disturbance, vitamin or electrolyte deficiency, and organic brain syndromes has always to be considered, particularly with acute problems, because the underlying cause might be reversed by treatment.

◀ Acute changes in mood, thought and perception may be associated with reversible causes such as endocrine or dietary deficiencies

Symptoms of *anxiety* may be chronic (over a period of months and years) or acute. Many anxious patients experience associated symptoms due to increased autonomic activity — palpitations, sweating, dryness of the mouth, diarrhoea and other gastrointestinal symptoms. Anxious patients often have a heightened

◀ Anxious patients may require large amounts of analgesics and local anaesthic agents because of increased awareness of pain

286

awareness of pain, requiring large amounts of analgesics and local anaesthetic agents. Anxiety is a physiological phenomenon and cannot be regarded as abnormal, unless the degree is greater than cause would justify, unduly prolonged or if it occurs without cause.

◄ Anxiety is pathological only if greater than events would merit, unduly prolonged or without cause

The clinical distinction between chronic anxiety and hyperthyroidism can be difficult, requiring measurements of serum thyroxine. The presence of goitre, cardiovascular abnormalities and, in the case of Graves' disease, ocular signs are of help in the differentiation (*see* Chapter 9).

◄ Clinical distinction between chronic anxiety and hyperthyroidism is often difficult

Pathological anxiety may be manifest as a phobia for particular objects or certain situations and can occur acutely with drug intoxication or infections (toxic confusional states).

Drugs of the benzodiazepine group are widely used to treat anxiety and are only helpful in the short term situation. They are of little value in long-term use and can be addictive. Large doses of intravenous diazepam may be needed to control the anxiety which can be a feature of alcoholism.

◄ Long-term use of benzodiazepines is not helpful in the treatment of chronic anxiety states and may lead to addiction

Psychotherapy, hypnosis and other relaxation techniques; behaviour therapy for specific phobic anxiety states; and attempts to explain the psychogenic nature of the physical symptoms are helpful in some patients.

Feelings of sadness, failure and despair are the features of the *depressive mood* which can become so severe that suicide is considered. There may be associated symptoms such as anorexia, sleep disturbance (early waking) and an inability to concentrate. These 'vegetative' features occur with equal frequency in depression provoked by grief or some other family/social problem, as in the endogenous form. Reactive depression is excessive to the underlying cause. There is no obvious cause for endogenous depression, which may be accompanied by agitation, hypochondriacal complaints and both mental and physical slowing. Some patients present a mixed picture.

◄ Endogenous depression may be accompanied by agitation and hypochondriacal complaints

Drug therapy for depression may be successful. Severe endogenous depression with strong vegetative features often requires ECT, modified by muscle relaxants to prevent muscular contractions associated with the 'shock', which can cause dental and bone injuries. Psychotherapy may be effective in reactive depression.

In a few patients with depression there may be alternating periods of overactivity (physical and mental), feelings of great optimism and irritability which may become so severe as to be socially harmful to the patient and others. Lesser disorders of this kind (mania) may occur in other depressive patients, who have insight into their illness, and attempt to overcome their mood.

Abnormal thoughts and ideas may take the form of *obsessive* and *compulsive reactions*, which are usually recognized by the patient as irrational or out of proportion. The reaction may be one of repetitive thoughts or actions. Obsessions about dirtiness or contamination of self or objects occur, with excessive attempts at cleanliness. Concern about the state of a part of the body (sometimes the mouth and teeth) can lead to demands for surgical treatment. Some depressive patients have obsessive features which disappear once the mood has lifted. These disordered thoughts may, rarely, become severely disabling, leading to total preoccupation: this can be a feature in patients with schizophrenia.

◄ Obsessive reactions may be concerned with the state of health of parts of the body, including the mouth

Tranquillizers and antidepressants can be helpful for some of these patients although behaviour therapy, to enforce resistance to the thoughts, is probably a more logical approach.

Delusions are false beliefs held by the patient despite contrary evidence and which, in spite of assurances, are not doubted; they may be associated with schizophrenia or with depression. Thoughts can take the form of hypochondriacal belief that a part of the body (teeth included) is diseased, or can induce feelings of persecution, overestimation of personal abilities, and belief that some external force influences self.

◄ Delusions may take the form of belief that a part of the body, teeth included, is diseased

Illusions and *hallucinations* are disorders of perception, or awareness of objects and sensations following stimulation of sensory organs. *Illusions* are perceptual misinterpretations of real sensory experiences, usually accompanied by anxiety which heightens the distortion. *Hallucinations* are disorders of perception of external objects without sensory stimulation; commonly the patient sees or hears 'things'. Both illusions and

◄ Illusions and hallucinations may occur during recovery from general anaesthesia and during intravenous administration of benzodiazepines in apparently normal subjects hallucinations can be a feature of schizophrenia, organic brain disease, toxic confusional state and drug abuse; they may also occur on recovery from general anaesthesia or during sedation with intravenous benzodiazepines.

Schizophrenia is the name given to a group of disorders in which there is progressive disintegration of emotional stability and judgement, and loss of contact with and appreciation of reality. There may be secondary impairment of intellectual function. The condition may begin at any age, even in those over 70, and can be acute or insidious in onset, occurring in between 0·5 and 1% of the population. There appear to be genetic factors involved in the cause of the condition but environmental factors can influence the onset.

The characteristic features of schizophrenia are abnormalities of thought and belief, so that the boundaries between self and the external world become blurred. There is emotional impairment, the patient appearing 'flat', without variation in response to stimuli. Delusions (usually paranoid) and hallucinations (often auditory — 'someone speaking to me') occur; as does depression, often complicated by suicide attempts.

Loss of drive and disturbances of posture (catatonia — in which bizarre poses or wild activities occur) may be accompanied by self-neglect and deterioration in the patient's physical health.

The phenothiazines and butyrophenones (e.g. haloperidol) have improved the outlook for sufferers from schizophrenia by control of symptoms, although they have side effects including cholestatic jaundice and Parkinsonian features. Oral dyskinesia including champing may cause problems in patients with dentures.

◄ The phenothiazines and butyrophenones given to schizophrenic patients may cause oral dyskinesia — champing movements that may cause denture problems

Attempts to care for schizophrenic patients in non-hospital accommodation have been successful. One-quarter of patients recover completely; another quarter have only mild disability and do not require treatment, other than rehabilitation and occupational therapy; one-quarter require long-term drug therapy and sheltered accommodation; and one-quarter require long-term institutional care.

Paranoia may be a feature of schizophrenia but may occur transiently in normal but shy people. Persistent ideas of reference and persecution also occur with acute confusional states, brain damage, drugs (amphetamines, LSD and other hallucinogens) and those with physical and social disabilities.

Hysterical reactions are attempts, never fully conscious and frequently unconscious, by the patient to obtain relief from intolerable stress. These attempts may consist of conversion symptoms (symptoms without apparent organic basis) such as paralysis, loss of voice and other neurological complaints. The patient is either calm or shows a histrionic reaction. Some patients have amnesia, selective for the upsetting event, dissociating themselves from these happenings.

Dementia is the deterioration of previously normal mental function affecting all three aspects of personality: intelligence and memory, emotional integration (mood disturbance — often excessive anxiety) and behaviour. The clinical picture is varied.

Dementia may be primary or secondary to physical injury such as alcohol, vitamin deficiencies (B_1), endocrine disturbances (thyroid and adrenal disorders) and infection (syphilis and viral encephalitis). *Acute toxic confusional states* are usually secondary to drug or alcohol intoxication, and other organic causes of secondary dementia. *Chronic dementia* can occur in middle age and becomes increasingly common with advancing years. The onset is so insidious that close relations may be unaware of the patient's deteriorating intellectual function. Organic dementia (chronic brain syndrome) may be primarily due to diffuse atrophy of cerebral neurones or secondary to arterial disease, brain injury and severe vitamin (B_1) deficiency.

The management of dementia depends on identifying potentially reversible causes and control of excessive anxiety or hyperactivity with phenothiazines and butyrophenones (haloperidol).

The *mentally handicapped* patient has suffered an arrest in mental development either from birth or in infancy, due to genetic causes or intrauterine damage to the fetal nervous system. The degree of subnormality varies considerably, from the lower end of the range of normal ability to such severe handicap that institutional care is needed.

There may be oral manifestations of mental subnormality, in particular a predisposition to inflammatory periodontal disease and poor dental health. Enamel hypoplasia occurs in congenital rubella syndrome together with lens cataracts, deafness, cardiac defects and mental handicap. Self-mutilation can also occur with chronic traumatic ulcers of the lips and tongue. In many of these patients there appears to be hypersalivation due to poor muscle co-ordination. *Down's syndrome* (mongolism) has some characteristic oral features including a large, deeply fissured (scrotal) tongue, maxillary hypoplasia with palatal abnormalities, partial adontia and malocclusions. *Cerebral palsy* may be associated with dental attrition due to bruxism.

◀ Periodontal disease and poor dental health are common with mental subnormality

These patients require careful management during dental treatment, excessive anxiety being a feature that requires support from relatives and nurses and control by drugs, including benzodiazepines. Many have sensory defects, including deafness, which can make management difficult. The general principles of management of mental handicap are provision of appropriate level of support, supervision, education (as far as is possible) and training for a useful role.

◀ Excessive anxiety may be a feature of mental subnormality

◀ Mentally handicapped patients may have associated sensory defects such as deafness, which must be considered in management

Dermatological diseases

15

Diseases of the skin are common and are often obvious to the dentist; some disorders have particular importance because of oral manifestations.

Infections of the skin may be a primary event or secondary to another lesion, the usual infecting organism being *Staphylococcus* which is present in the nostrils and body creases in 10-50% of healthy individuals.

A boil is an acute, painful infection of a hair follicle by *Staphylococcus pyogenes*. A conglomerated mass of boils is called a *carbuncle*, occurring particularly in diabetics and those with a heavy alcohol consumption. *Folliculitis* constitutes multiple small pustular lesions centred on hair follicles affecting the beard area and other parts of the body. Recurrent boils are often associated with generalized itching and neurotic excoriation.

Impetigo is a skin infection, also caused by *S. aureus*, occurring mainly in children and characterized by superficial thin-roofed blisters that rupture, releasing a yellow exudate that dries to form a golden crust.

◀ Recurrent boils occur in patients with diabetes mellitus and those who carry staphylococci in the nose, axilla and groin

Table 15.1.   Some terms used to describe skin lesions

Macule — small flat area of discoloration of the skin
Papule — small raised area
Vesicle — small blister
Bulla — large blister
Pustule — a papule that contains pus
Erythema — redness due to increased blood supply of the skin

Lesions occur particularly on the face, hands and buttocks. It may be a primary infection in children but, more commonly, is superimposed on another skin disease, such as eczema or scabies. The treatment for impetigo is topical or, if the lesions are extensive, systemic antibiotics.

Streptococcal infections of the skin are less common than those due to *Staph. aureus. Erysipelas* is characterized by a sharply demarcated scarlet edge, with small vesicles and a tendency to spread via lymphatics. Lesions can occur on the face or any part of the body. Glomerulonephritis, but not rheumatic fever, may be a late complication of infection with certain types of streptococci (*see* Chapter 10).

Fungal infections of the skin are common, particularly the superficial mycoses, which also affect the hair and nails. Deep mycoses occur during corticosteroid and immunosuppressive therapy, with lymphomas, and following cardiac or gynaecological operations.

Superficial mycoses are usually due to *Candida* or *ringworm (tinea)*. Diagnosis is made by microscopy of scrapings from the lesions, nails or hair.

Ringworm of the scalp (tinea capitis) occurs mainly in children before puberty, manifesting as a bald patch, with scaling and broken-off hairs; it is easily distinguished from bald patches caused by rubbing. Tinea in the beard region is less common but may be mistaken for folliculitis. It can occur in non-hairy skin and may sometimes be mistaken for acne. Nails are sometimes infected by ringworm causing distortion of normal architecture. Ringworm infections respond to griseofulvin, an oral antifungal agent.

Candidiasis may affect the skin of the nail fold (paronychia) and intertriginous areas where there is maceration. The infection may be acute or chronic (usually in the nail folds). Generalized forms occur in association with candidiasis of the mucous membranes.

◀ Predisposing factors for candidiasis include diabetes mellitus, immunosuppression, use of broad-spectrum antibacterials and some patients with iron deficiency

Dermatitis and eczema

Dermatitis is the inflammatory reaction that develops in the skin when the normal protective layers (keratin) have broken down. The cause is usually injury by a recognizable agent. However reaction may follow relatively mild stimuli, as the result of constitutional or inherent vulnerability, a condition called *eczema*. Epidermis and dermis are affected, with vesicle formation, as well as cracks through the cornified layers.

Atopic eczema is a constitutional inflammation of the skin occurring particularly in infancy and early childhood, the face and flexures (elbow and knee) being the principal sites affected. There is a low itch threshold, and in non-excoriated areas the skin is dry. Some patients respond to certain foods (cow's milk and egg white) and to house dust with immediate itching and swelling of tissues.

Contact dermatitis is a skin reaction following application of a particular substance to which there has been previous exposure and sensitization, often over the course of many years. The condition can occur on the face, related to use of cosmetics, on the neck from jewellery and on the hands, due to wearing rubber gloves, use of instruments or resins. Application of the suspected substance under a plaster patch provokes reaction and confirms the diagnosis.

Seborrhoeic dermatitis is characterized by the excessive scaling of the scalp (dandruff) and hair loss. There is scaling of the eyebrows; scaling and redness of the nasolabial folds and other areas (chest, armpits and groin). Two factors play a part in causing the condition: the inherent tendency of the patient's skin and low grade infection.

◀ Dentists and their assistants may become sensitized to instruments and resins causing eczema of the hands

The dermatoses

Rosacea is a disorder of middle age, more common in women, causing papules in the blush areas on the face, neck and upper chest. There may be associated thickening of the skin and greasiness. The condition is made worse by heat, emotion and spicy or warm foods.

Psoriasis is a disease of accelerated epidermal turnover producing salmon-pink lesions in white-skinned races, which may be associated with sterile pustules. The lesions scale and show pin-point haemorrhages when scraped. They are usually the size of rain

◀ The face is an uncommon site for psoriasis but many forms of dermatitis can affect the perioral region associated with scaling and pustules

drops or coins but coalesce to form larger lesions which occur in the flexures. The nails can be involved. Psoriasis frequently involves the scalp but rarely the face. Some patients develop a seronegative arthritis, indistinguishable from rheumatoid disease, or present a picture similar to ankylosing spondylitis (*see* Chapter 12).

Lichen planus is a condition that usually occurs in early and middle adult life characterized by small, shiny macules, appearing lilac against the background of white skin. Lesions occur on the forearms, back, lower legs and the buccal mucosa. As the skin lesions fade, over a period of weeks or months, they leave a brown stain. The buccal mucosal lesions consist of either tiny, milky-white papules, or thin thread-like streaks, which also occur on the tongue and lips. The oral lesions may be painful and pre-malignant.

◀ The mouth is commonly affected by lichen planus causing white streaks, with a network pattern, opposite the pre-molars and on the tongue

The cause of lichen planus is not known but anti-malarial drugs and gold compounds cause similar lesions.

Urticaria is usually an acute disorder, occasionally chronic, consisting of raised spots which coalesce to form weals, accompanied by itching and pricking sensations. Most patients do not have systemic disease although occasionally urticaria is due to small vessel disease (vasculitis) complicating SLE and periarteritis nodosa (*see* Chapter 12). The commonest causes are allergy to sea food, drugs, (e.g. penicillin, sulphon-amides, cephalosporins), heat and cold, parasites (fleas and lice) and inhalants (house dust and feathers). *Angio-oedema* is a similar condition, but at a deeper level, affecting eyelids and lips and, sometimes, the larynx.

◀ Urticaria is usually due to specific food, food additive or drug, although sometimes a cause cannot be found

Diseases of hair

Localized loss of hair (*alopecia areata*) is the most common hair disease. There is often a family history of the condition, or it can be related to stress. There is genetic linkage in some patients with vitiligo, thyroid disease or pernicious anaemia. The areas sometimes coalesce, causing loss of all scalp hair (*alopecia totalis*) and, rarely, all body hair.

Diffuse hair loss can occur with a variety of disorders but in most cases no cause is found. Acute physical and mental stress can be a cause, as may iron deficiency, endocrine disorders (thyroid, adrenal and pituitary hypofunction) and drugs (cyclophosphamide; anti-thyroid and anticoagulant drugs). Hair loss can also occur in the female postpartum, when taking oral contraceptives or after the menopause.

Abnormalities of pigmentation

The commonest cause of *loss of skin pigmentation* is vitiligo which can be associated with pernicious anaemia, diabetes and autoimmune thyroid or adrenal disease. The condition is inherited as a dominant, although variable penetrance makes it difficult to predict. There is complete lack of melanin in affected areas which burn easily on exposure to the sun, a factor that provokes new lesions, as does stress. The hands, eyelids and axilla are the sites commonly affected.

◄ Vitiligo is a common form of depigmentation and may be an indicator of autoimmune disorders as well as being of cosmetic importance

Depigmentation also occurs with tinea infections, inflammatory lesions and congenital disorders such as albinism (accompanied by white eyebrows, pale blue irides and red pupils). Generalized loss of skin melanin also occurs with hypopituitarism.

Increased pigmentation may consist of circumscribed brown areas; some are like giant freckles (*café-au-lait* spots) which may be associated with multiple nerve tumours — neurofibromatosis). Others occur on non-exposed areas, being darker than the freckle (lentigo), and are sometimes associated with polyposis of the small bowel. The pigmentation of the face in pregnancy (chloasma) may be simulated by the contraceptive pill and anticonvulsant therapy. *Acanthosis nigricans* consists of increased pigmentation and thickness of the skin flexures in the neck, often causing itch, and sometimes associated with oral lesions; it may be a marker of internal malignancy.

◄ A profusion of lentigines around the mouth may be associated with polyposis of the small bowel, Peutz–Jeghers syndrome

Generalized brown pigmentation with accentuation over pressure points, skin creases and flexures occurs with porphyria (on the face), Addison's disease (gingiva), vitamin B_{12} deficiency (hands) and scleroderma. Chronic liver disease, endocrine disorders (hyperthyroidism and Cushing's syndrome), malnutrition, drugs (busulphan, ACTH and arsenic) and a rare small bowel disease with malabsorption (Whipple's syndrome) cause generalized hyperpigmentation, occasionally with mucous membrane changes.

Generalized, slate-grey hyperpigmentation of skin, oral cavity and nail bed occurs with long-term phenothiazine treatment. Similar pigmentation, due to melanin in the dermis as opposed to epidermis, occurs with haemochromatosis (a disorder of iron storage) and gold poisoning.

◀ The commonest cause of generalized hyperpigmentation is racial

Blistering skin diseases

Blistering may be due to physical damage (friction, pressure, and burns), light sensitivity or contact with chemicals. Where there is no obvious explanation the likely causes are dermatitis herpetiformis, bullous pemphigoid and pemphigus vulgaris.

◀ Blistering of the skin is usually due to physical causes (friction or pressure), light sensitivity (which may be drug-induced), chemicals and, rarely, pemphigus or pemphigoid

Dermatitis herpetiformis is an uncommon condition, occurring mainly in young adults, presenting as small, itching, fluid-filled vesicles arising from red areas of skin on the upper back, sacral area and buttocks. Occasionally the face, scalp and buccal mucous membrane are affected. The scratched skin may become pigmented. Many patients have malabsorption of varying degree, small bowel biopsy showing changes of coeliac disease (*see* Chapter 6).

Bullous pemphigoid is a disease of older people with subepidermal, non-itching tense blisters that occur in any part of the body and, occasionally, the mouth. The condition responds dramatically to short courses of corticosteroids.

Pemphigus vulgaris is another rare condition characterized by intra-epidermal blisters, affecting the mouth first, bursting and leaving painful erosions. Corticosteroids — sometimes in massive doses — may be life-saving.

◀ Pemphigus vulgaris usually begins with mucous membrane ulceration

Drug-induced skin disease

Most drugs can cause skin eruptions. It is unusual for a

drug eruption to develop earlier than 10 days after initial exposure, unless there has been previous therapy with this or a chemically similar drug (cephalosporins and penicillin). The longer the patient has taken a drug the less likely it is to be the cause of the rash. Most eruptions improve within a few days of stopping the drug and, if new lesions appear more than 10 days later, another cause is likely.

A variety of patterns of skin change occur; none is exclusive to a particular compound. Urticaria is an immediate response to drugs such as penicillin, aspirin, and barbiturates. The commonest rash is that which resembles measles, a deep red-to-bluish macular appearance; small weals may develop. Ampicillin, phenylbutazone, sulphonamides and phenothiazines

◄ Few drugs cause skin eruption within 10 days of starting treatment, unless there has been previous use of the agent, an important exception being co-trimoxazole

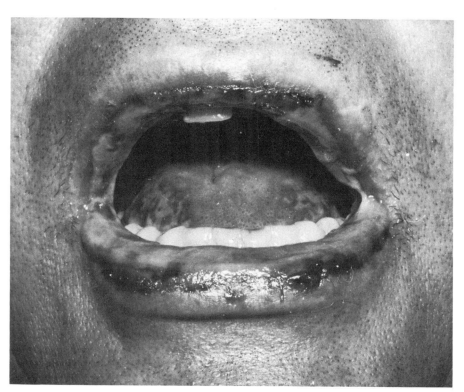

Fig. 15.1. Mucocutaneous syndrome. Extensive lip and oral ulceration complicating antibacterial (co-trimoxazole) treatment for acute bronchitis.

cause morbilliform reactions. Stevens–Johnson syndrome, consisting of fixed, urticaria-like, target lesions, can develop with sulphonamides and barbiturates, accompanied by extensive oral ulceration.

Purpura due to capillary fragility can develop with barbiturates, and small vessel disease, with blood blisters and necrotic ulceration of the skin, can occur with methyldopa and thiazide diuretics.

Small, annular patches of red skin which itch, swell and sometimes blister, occurring in any site of the body (fixed drug eruptions) may complicate treatment with tetracyclines and chlordiazepoxide. Some drugs make the skin sensitive to sunlight, the exposed area often showing blisters. Drugs that cause photosensitivity include phenothiazines, tetracyclines and sulphonamides or related compounds, such as thiazides and sulphonylureas (antidiabetic agents).

Some drugs can cause a multisystem disease resembling systemic lupus, although kidney damage is unusual and the illness improves when the drug is withdrawn. Hydrallazine, procainamide and phenytoin can cause lupus (*see* Chapter 12).

Lichen planus-like eruptions may follow gold and antimalarial therapy; methyldopa causes similar lesions as well as isolated ulceration of the tongue which is slow to heal.

There is no test, *in vitro* or *in vivo*, that confirms the diagnosis of drug allergy other than drug challenge, but this may not be safe except with fixed eruptions.

◀ Lichen-planus-like lesions of the mucous membrane with chronic ulceration may occur with antimalarial drugs and methyldopa

Skin tumours

There are many *benign skin tumours*, as would be expected of an organ with such complex structure. The benign lesion usually enlarges gradually, does not infiltrate surrounding structures and does not metastasize. Although some tumours can be identified by specific features others require biopsy. Solitary secondary tumours from carcinoma of bronchus or breast can occur.

Warty skin lesions are most often due to virus infections and usually occur on the sole of the foot (verruca) and in non-pressure areas such as the hands and neck. Seborrhoeic warts occur mainly in older patients on the back and chest and are often pigmented, the colour ranging from fawn to black.

Cystic skin lesions can arise from the hair follicles and associated glands (sebaceous cysts) or may be of developmental origin (dermoid cysts). The former may become infected and discharge foul-smelling material through the punctum which can be seen overlying the cyst.

There are three important *primary malignant skin tumours*, the basal cell (rodent ulcer) epithelioma, squamous cell carcinoma and some melanoma. *Rodent ulcer* occurs on the face and neck as a persistent, crusted sore that fails to heal. Although it may grow in size it does not metastasize and is treated by local excision or radiotherapy.

◀ A persistent crusted sore on the face of older patients is suspicious of rodent ulcer (basal cell carcinoma)

Squamous carcinoma is less common but does metastasize. Tumours occur in sun-damaged skin on the face, lips, ears and other exposed areas or at the site of scars and irritation. The characteristic lesion is indurated, has rolled edges, may ulcerate or show cauliflower-like proliferative changes. Early treatment by excision and radiotherapy is curative.

Malignant melanoma usually arises *de novo* as a pigmented spot which rapidly enlarges; some arise from a benign naevus, malignant change in which should be suspected by rapid enlargement, spontaneous bleeding or itching. Malignant melanoma is treated by wide excision and block dissection of the regional lymph nodes. Perfusion of the arteries supplying the region with cytotoxic drugs is also employed.

A *naevus (or mole)* is a circumscribed developmental anomaly that is a tumour of cells of neuroectodermal origin, appearing as a raised lesion, varying in colour with the degree of melanin pigmentation. Lesions may develop at any age, but are usually present at birth, enlarging during puberty and pregnancy. They can occur anywhere on the body, may be flat or raised, hairy or hairless, and are largely of cosmetic importance, rarely becoming malignant. Occasionally naevi that are present at birth become warty and more conspicuous with age. These lesions need to be excised because of the risk of malignancy.

◀ A pigmented lesion that enlarges, becomes darker, ulcerates or bleeds spontaneously could be a malignant melanoma

Tumours may arise from an abnormal proliferation of skin blood vessels, called *angiomas*. There are several categories of these tumours, principally the 'port-wine stain' and the 'strawberry naevus'. The former is a *capillary haemangioma* caused by minimal increase in capillaries in the upper dermis, is present at birth and does not fade. Some patients with 'port-wine stain' on the face have associated vascular malformation of the brain and a tendency to epilepsy.

The strawberry naevus appears shortly after birth as a small red spot, which rapidly enlarges to reach its maximum over a few weeks, followed by whitish discoloration preceding spontaneous resolution and disappearance by the time of adolescence. In a few patients with large lesions there may be sequestration of platelets in the angioma causing widespread bruising.

◄ Port-wine stains may be associated with vascular malformations of the meninges and an epileptic tendency

The strawberry naevus resolves spontaneously over a period of years

Drug-induced diseases and metabolic disease 16

Drug therapy may result in oral lesions affecting the hard or soft tissues of the oral cavity and the oral flora; additionally, other side effects of drug therapy, such as haematological complications, may cause important problems for the dentist. Some of the drugs that dentists can prescribe have, in a few patients, important interactions with concurrent therapy or may precipitate serious disorders (e.g. barbiturates and acute porphyria).

Drug-induced oral lesions and salivary gland disorders

Several drugs may cause *abnormalities of taste*; some may cause loss of, others abnormal, taste. Penicillamine, a drug used to suppress the disease process in rheumatoid arthritis, causes loss of taste in many patients after approximately 6 weeks' therapy, often transient, whether or not the drug is discontinued. Other drugs cause abnormal taste, often described as 'metallic', associated in the patient's mind with dental fillings (e.g. ethionamide, an antituberculous drug). A large number of drugs is reported by patients as interfering with the normal taste of food, the most frequently blamed being lithium salts (used for manic/depressive psychosis), griseofulvin (for fungal infections of the skin and nails) and metronidazole (an antimicrobial used for anaerobic bacterial infections and protozoan infections). Adrenergic neurone blocking agents used for the treatment of raised blood pressure (e.g. guanethidine) cause nasal stuffiness and

Table 16.1. Drug-induced oral and salivary gland disorders

Oral ulceration
    cytotoxic drugs
    any drug that causes agranulocytosis
    indomethacin
    pancreatin
    blistering diseases of skin caused by drugs (Stevens–
        Johnson syndrome)
Disorders of taste
    penicillamine
    griseofulvin
    metronidazole
    lithium salts
Salivary disorders
    excess salivation — neostigmine, pyridostigmine
    dry mouth — antidepressants, antiparkinsonian drugs,
        hypotensives (clonidine)
    painful swelling of glands — clonidine
Gingival hypertrophy
    phenytoin
Mucosal pigmentation
    phenothiazines

loss of smell, which may be misinterpreted by patients as loss of taste.

Oral ulceration can also complicate drug treatment, notably the cytotoxic drugs and any drug that induces agranulocytosis. Among the drugs reported as causing oral ulceration are indomethacin (an antirheumatic), pancreatin (an enzyme mixture used for treating chronic pancreatitis and cystic fibrosis), which also causes irritation around the mouth, and phenylbutazone (a non-steroidal anti-inflammatory drug). Whilst a patient is being treated with cytotoxic drugs for malignant disease, and immunosuppressants following transplantation or for collagen disease, it is important to maintain good oral hygiene and control caries and periodontal disease.

Some blistering diseases of the skin, due to an immunological reaction induced by drugs, can also cause oral lesions, often extensive coalescent ulceration, with pyrexia, involvement of the eyes and genitalia (Stevens–Johnson syndrome). Barbiturates, sulphonamides, phenylbutazone, phenytoin and some antibiotics (penicillin and clindamycin) have been reported as causing erythema multiforme.

Gingival hyperplasia occurs in a large number of epileptics treated with phenytoin. *Pigmentation of the mucosa* may occur with phenothiazine therapy and intrinsic pigmentation of the *teeth* can be seen in patients who have taken tetracyclines during tooth formation, associated with dental hypoplasia. *Staining of the teeth* may occur with long-term ingestion of liquid iron preparations.

Excessive salivation can be caused by some drugs, including iodides and anticholinesterase (neostigmine and pyridostigmine), used in the treatment of myasthenia gravis. *Dryness of the mouth* (xerostomia) is a more frequent drug-induced disorder, predisposing to candidiasis and salivary gland infections. Tricyclic antidepressants, antihistamines and anti-Parkinsonism drugs cause varying degrees of xerostomia. Clonidine (a centrally acting hypotensive drug), ganglion-blocking drugs (used to treat hypertension) and monoamine oxidase inhibitors (MAOI) also cause xerostomia.

Swelling of, and pain in, the salivary glands can occur during treatment with clonidine and iodides. Guanethidine may also cause salivary gland pain.

◄ Tetracyclines given to the mother can cross the placenta, causing staining of the deciduous teeth of the fetus and are taken up by developing bone

Effects of antibacterial therapy

Adverse reactions to antibacterial agents are common, particularly the hypersensitivity reactions that occur with penicillin and cephalosporin therapy. The adverse reactions that occur are either related to the particular agent, or increased patient susceptibility or interactions with other drugs. Some of these side-effects can be trivial (diarrhoea) but some are fatal (chloramphenicol-induced bone-marrow aplasia).

Sulphonamides and the pencillins are the antibacterials that commonly cause hypersensitivity reactions varying from mild urticaria (hives) to the Stevens–Johnson syndrome, with ulceration of all mucosal surfaces. Hypersensitivity can occur in organs other than the skin (e.g. cholestatic jaundice due to the estolate salt of erythromycin).

Oral candidiasis causing thrush and stomatitis are a

◄ Antibacterials, particularly sulphonamides and the penicillins, are the most common drugs to cause hypersensitivity reactions

frequent sequel of injudicious and prolonged use of antibacterials and withdrawal usually leads to resolution. Systemic candidosis is unusual but invasion via the gastrointestinal tract, having spread from the oral cavity, can occur in some patients on prolonged antibiotic therapy and those who have drug- or disease-induced immunosuppression. Candida overgrows in the oral cavity and gut because commensal bacteria are destroyed by broad-spectrum antibacterials, a predisposition increased by dentures and systemic disorders, such as diabetes mellitus and malignant disease.

Antibacterials can induce blood disorders, usually bone-marrow hypoplasia with anaemia, neutropenia and thrombocytopenia. Chloramphenicol, in particu-

Table 16.2.   Adverse reactions to antibacterial agents

	Major	Minor
Co-trimoxazole	Stevens–Johnson Agranulocytosis Interactions Kidney impairment	Allergic rashes
Tetracyclines	Liver damage (intravenous therapy) Renal damage (worsening of existing disorder) Tooth staining (children under 7 years)	Diarrhoea (up to 50%) *Candida* overgrowth Photosensitivity
Penicillins	Immediate hypersensitivity (IgE mediated) Delayed hypersensitivity Haemolytic anaemia (rare)	Rashes Diarrhoea (up to 20%)
Cephalosporins	Renal damage Hypersensitivity (5% cross reaction with penicillin hypersensitive subjects)	*Candida* overgrowth
Erythromycin	Cholestasis (estolate salt only)	Rarely skin reactions
Clindamycin Lincomycin	Pseudomembranous colitis	Skin rashes
Chloramphenicol	Aplastic anaemia Dose-related neutropenia	Diarrhoea (rare)

Table 16.3.   Drug interaction: major mechanisms

Hepatic enzyme induction — reduces pharmacological
activity
danger of withdrawal — toxicity
Hepatic enzyme inhibition — increased pharmacological
effect
danger of toxicity during
combination
Synergism — additive effect
centrally acting drugs enhanced by alcohol
Competitive antagonism — drugs competing for same
receptor site
Displacement from protein-binding sites
Competition for renal excretion mechanism
Altered rate of drug absorption from gut

lar, along with sulphonamides, penicillins, tetracyclines
and rifampicin can cause blood dyscrasias, which are
not always related to the total dose given. Haemolytic
anaemia can occur with antibacterial therapy either
because of red cell enzyme deficiencies (sulphonamides
and chloramphenicol), or the development of IgG
antibodies to penicillin-coated red cells.

Diarrhoea associated with antibiotic therapy is
common but the mechanism is not known. It is rarely
due to staphylococcal infection and only neomycin
interferes with intestinal function. Most antibacterials
have been reported as causing pseudomembranous
colitis, due to colonization of the gut by *Clostridium
difficile*.

Specific organ damage can follow antibacterial
treatment, including renal damage, with sulphonamides and the cephalosporins, and damage to the
organ of Corti and vestibular apparatus by aminoglycosides (streptomycin and gentamicin).

Penicillins and cephalosporins are the safest antibacterials to use in pregnancy. Tetracyclines are best
avoided, since they are taken up by developing bone;
and sulphonamides, in late pregnancy, can cross
the placental barrier causing jaundice in the neonate.

Antibacterials given with other drugs, particularly those with a narrow therapeutic range (anticoagulants, anticonvulsants, antihypertensives and antidepressants) may result in toxicity or loss of therapeutic effect, thus interfering with treatment of a serious disease. Interaction may occur because of induction or inhibition of enzymes responsible for drug metabolism; competition for protein binding sites or renal excretion mechanisms; and competitive antagonism or synergism. Examples of drug interactions involving antibacterials likely to be used by the dentist are:

◀ When two or more drugs are given at the same time they may exert their effects independently or they may interact

Ampicillin	— interferes with steroid breakdown in gut resulting in failure of oral contraception
Cephalosporins	— given with frusemide (a diuretic) increases renal toxicity by an unknown mechanism
Erythromycin	— by enzyme induction causes toxic effects of concurrently administered theophylline
Sulphonamides	— enzyme inhibition will cause potentiation of anticoagulant effects of warfarin, hypoglycaemia in the diabetic on tolbutamide and phenytoin toxicity in epileptics
Tetracyclines	— by forming insoluble complexes in the gut cause failure of treatment with iron salts and antacids

Prescription of antibiotics by the dentist should therefore take account of the patient, the presumed organism, the concurrent use of other drugs for serious medical disease, and known hypersensitivity.

Drug interactions and anaesthesia

Before any patient is anaesthetized current and recent drug therapy should be reviewed and the choice of anaesthetic technique considered. It is rarely necessary to stop drugs before dental operations but possible interactions can be avoided, particularly with some hypotensives and monoamine oxidase inhibitors (used for treating depression), by withdrawal of treatment.

Resistance to the effect of intravenous barbiturates and benzo-diazepines is often seen in patients who regularly take large amounts of alcohol, tranquillizers and sedative drugs. The mechanism is probably a reduced responsiveness of cerebral cells.

Virtually all drugs used to induce general anaesthesia lower blood pressure and so care is needed in inducing anaesthesia in any patient on hypotensive therapy. Since the fall in blood pressure will be greatest if the patient is seated, anaesthesia should be induced with the patient lying flat. Rebound hypertension may occur if some hypotensive drugs are withdrawn (clonidine) and drug therapy for raised blood pressure should be continued unless otherwise advised by the anaesthetist.

Tricyclic antidepressant drugs interfere with the intake of noradrenaline at the noradrenergic nerve endings. Exogenous adrenaline and noradrenaline cannot be taken up and therefore their effects are enhanced. Adrenaline should also be avoided in the diabetic patient since it causes hyperglycaemia.

MAOIs interact with pethidine causing a rise in blood pressure, which may occur during anaesthesia irrespective of specific drug interaction. These drugs should be stopped about 3 weeks before non-urgent surgery.

The patient who has recently drunk a large quantity of alcohol will be very sensitive to any CNS sedative drug because of inhibition of drug oxidation. On the other hand, chronic alcoholism is associated with decreased sensitivity, so that larger doses of intravenous barbiturates may be needed. A reduced response can also be expected if a benzodiazepine is used.

◀ Patients taking tranquillizers and sedative drugs, or regular quantities of alcohol, may show resistance to the effects of intravenous barbiturates and benzodiazepines

◀ Drugs used to treat hypertension, chlorpromazine and beta-adrenoreceptor blocking drugs may interact with anaesthetic agents causing potentiation of hypotensive effects

◀ The recent consumption of a large quantity of alcohol may cause an increase in sensitivity to any CNS sedative, and smaller doses of intravenous barbiturates may be needed to achieve light level anaesthesia

Drugs causing metabolic disorders

Drug therapy is the commonest precipitating factor for acute porphyria. Barbiturates, for example, may aggravate attacks and lead to respiratory paralysis. In addition to barbiturates other drugs that the dentist may prescribe — carbamazepine, chloramphenicol, pentazocine, and sulphonamides — can interfere with haem synthesis.

Table 16.4. Drugs that can be prescribed by dentists that may precipitate porphyria

Barbiturates
Chloramphenicol
Alcohol
Pentazocine
Sulphamides

Caution is also needed in prescribing for the diabetic patient taking oral hypoglycaemic agents. Sulphonamides interact with chlorpropamide to cause hypoglycaemia and chloramphenicol can also interfere with the action of tolbutamide by the mechanism of enzyme inhibition.

◀ Sulphonamides should be prescribed with caution in diabetic patients on oral antidiabetic therapy with sulphonylureas because of the risk of hypoglycaemia

Prevention of adverse reaction to drugs

Almost any drug may produce unwanted or unexpected adverse reactions, some of which may be a hazard to life. Prevention is possible if drugs are only prescribed when there is a good indication; by asking if there have been previous allergic reactions; ensuring that there will not be any interaction with other drugs that the patient is already taking; taking account of age, hepatic and renal disease; prescribing as few drugs as possible; and using drugs that are familiar to the prescriber.

Inborn errors of metabolism

The inborn errors of metabolism are a group of inherited disorders involving genetically determined abnormalities in metabolic pathways or structural proteins, leading to a typical and specific picture. Most are uncommon but a few, sickle cell anaemia and gout, are seen quite often. Diagnosis depends on the clinical picture and demonstration of specific enzyme defect in blood cells, skin or other affected organ that can be biopsied.

It is not possible to give a full account of all the inborn

◀ An inborn error of metabolism may be diagnosed by demonstration of a specific enzyme defect which can, in some instances, be detected prenatally as part of the management of families at risk of having an affected child

errors of metabolism but two, homocystinuria and porphyria, are of some importance to dentists.

Homocystinuria is a disorder of amino acid (methionine) metabolism, transmitted as an autosomal recessive and presenting with skeletal, cardiovascular and cerebral involvement. It is similar to Marfan's which is, however, inherited as a dominant, is not associated with mental retardation and the causal defect is not known (*see* Chapter 9).

There is kyphoscoliosis, long fingers and increased height in spite of the spinal deformity. Cardiac problems including myocardial ischaemia and venous thrombosis occur. Mental retardation and epilepsy are frequent but some are of normal intelligence. Ocular problems due to dislocation of the lens occur in most patients.

Diagnosis of homocystinuria is made by screening tests on the urine and confirmed by column chromatography of the plasma. One variant is responsive to pyridoxine, the other is not. Early detection and strict dietary measures seem to prevent the serious complications. Heterozygotes can be diagnosed by biochemical techniques and by culturing of skin fibroblasts.

◀ Marfan's syndrome can be distinguished from homocystinuria by absence of mental retardation and the ocular changes

The *porphyrias* are a group of disorders affecting haem synthesis resulting in accumulation of porphyrin in certain tissues and increased excretion. Diagnosis depends on determining the specific porphyrins in urine, blood and faeces. Some variants are inherited as autosomal dominant traits (hepatic porphyria).

The hepatic porphyrias usually present with acute episodes of abdominal pain, peripheral neuropathy (mainly motor weakness), or acute psychosis. The episodes are usually provoked by drugs and alcohol. Attacks may be fatal and can be prevented by avoidance of alcohol and the drugs concerned. The urine may become transiently red, 'like port wine', in the episodes.

◀ The hepatic porphyrias present with acute abdominal pain provoked by drugs or alcohol

The non-acute porphyrias are mainly autosomal recessives and present with photosensitive skin eruptions which may result in gross scarring and disfigurement. Some forms have an associated haemolytic anaemia, others hepatic disorder and gallstones. Porphyrins may accumulate in the teeth causing reddish discoloration and red fluorescence.

◀ The non-acute porphyrias present with photosensitive rashes on the face and exposed areas and have reddish discoloration of the teeth

Immunological disorders

There is a constant interaction between man and micro-organisms which has, at present, reached a balance between man's resistance to and ability to surmount infection and the capacity of bacteria and viruses to overcome these defences. The mechanisms range from simple mechanical barriers to highly specialized defences that have evolved over many years, having their origins in lower animals.

Mechanical barriers

Skin provides an effective layer against infection and micro-organisms do not normally invade the body via this route except when large areas have been damaged by burns or following insect bites (malaria), animal bites (rabies) and injections (hepatitis B).

◄ The skin and mucosal surfaces provide an effective protective layer against infection

The mucosal surfaces are also open to the external environment and particulate matter is trapped in the

Table 17.1. Mechanical barriers to infection

Skin
Mucosa — mucus and flow of fluids (e.g. saliva), ciliated
              epithelium and lysozymes in secretions
Gastric juice — pH
             — proteolytic enzymes
             — mucus
Renal tract — flushing action of urine
Normal flora — affected by antibiotics

mucus that covers the upper gastrointestinal and respiratory tract. Ciliated epithelium in the respiratory tract maintains a flow of mucus towards the mouth where it can be expectorated or swallowed. Defects in the mucociliary lining, such as cystic fibrosis and chronic bronchitis, result in an increased susceptibility to infections. Some micro-organisms interact with defence mechanisms: for example, the influenza virus destroys ciliary epithelium, leaving the patient susceptible to bacterial infection.

Other physiological barriers to infection are the pH of body fluids, such as the gastric acid and vaginal secretions. Some organisms, such as poliomyelitis virus, have inherent resistance to the effects of gastric pH. Enzymes, including lysozymes, present in tears and saliva, also have a protective effect.

Any bacterial pathogen must compete with established normal flora but when the latter is reduced, for example by broad-spectrum antibacterials, much smaller infecting doses of pathogens are required. *Candida* infection in the oral cavity is a good example of the effect of external agents on susceptibility to infection.

Flow of fluids, such as saliva or urine, is a further effective mechanism against infection. Where the flushing action is impaired, as with salivary calculus or disease of the glands (e.g. Sjögren's syndrome), there is increased susceptibility to infection (*see* Chapter 12). Urinary stasis predisposes to infection (*see* Chapter 10).

Phagocytic cells

Phagocytes respond to invasion by ingestion and digestion of organisms. Macrophages occur in the subepithelial layers of the skin, intestine and respiratory tract acting as the initial response to invasion by organisms. The second line of defence by phagocytic cells are the monocytes, which become macrophages on leaving the circulation, and the polymorph.

Some organisms, staphylococci and streptococci, have evolved so as to become resistant to the phagocytic cell system and viruses, even when ingested, actually replicate in macrophages as they do in other cells.

◄ Staphylococci, streptococci and viruses are resistant to the phagocytic cell system

The macrophage has an early place in the immune response by processing antigens and presenting them in a form which either stimulates lymphocytes or induces tolerance. Particulate antigens and immune complexes are ingested by the phagocytic cells.

The immune response

The lymphoid immune system has evolved in man and the vertebrates so that it can adapt and respond to a large range of foreign proteins or other antigens. It produces T cells, thymus-dependent lymphocytes, which can bind the antigen and represent the cell mediated immune response, and B cells, precursors of the plasma cell, which secrete antibody and express the humoral immune response. In addition to T and B cells, a third category of mononuclear cells can be identified, which are capable of lysing antibody coated cells, and are known as 'Killer' cells.

◀ There are two major types of lymphocytes: B cells, that produce antibody, and T cells, associated with cell-mediated immunity

Of the four main classes of immunoglobulin (IgA, IgG, IgD, IgE) which are involved in the immune response it is IgA which is chiefly involved in surface protection, contributing an 'antiseptic' effect to mucous secretions of the mouth, respiratory and gastrointestinal tracts. IgA is produced by plasma cells in the mucosa-associated lymphoid tissue (MALT). MALT is distributed widely in Peyer's patches in the gut and localized lymphoid collections in the bronchial mucosa, lacrimal and salivary glands, breasts and genito-urinary system.

◀ IgA immunoglobulin is chiefly involved in surface protection and is produced by plasma cells in the mucosa-associated lymphoid tissue

Table 17.2.   Main classes of immunoglobulin

IgA — serum — does not have the same function as secretory form
    — secretions — resistance to alimentary tract infection, short response
IgE — reaginic antibody, submucous tissues, antibody response for immediate allergic and anaphylactic reactions
IgG — secondary response to infection, longest lasting antibody after antigenic stimulus
IgM — initial antibody in primary response, short life

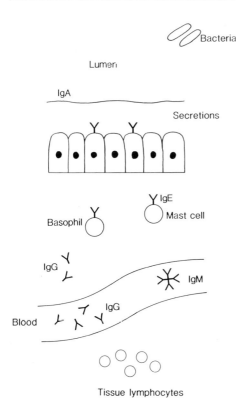

Fig. 17.1. Mechanisms of the immune response. IgA provides surface protection. IgE, bound to basophils and mast cells, is the antibody response for immediate allergic reactions. IgG can diffuse into interstitial fluid but IgM remains in the blood vessel. Both combine with antigen to activate complement to produce inflammation, cell damage and coagulation. Lymphocytes produce a specific response when triggered by antigen.

Once the barrier of the skin or mucous membrane has been breeched other mechanisms operate, notably IgE which is concentrated in submucous tissues and which is the major antibody response for immediate allergic anaphylactic reaction.

IgG is the major plasma immunoglobulin but can diffuse into the interstitial tissues where combination with antibody provides the stimulus to activation of complement and a series of enzyme reactions, causing inflammation, cell damage, coagulation and the attraction of other lymphocytes to the site.

Immunologically mediated disease

At normal levels of exposure to antigens the IgE antibody response does not lead to serious disorder but when the dose is high in tissues, such as the skin and lung, reactions such as urticaria and asthma occur. The most extreme systemic reaction is acute anaphylaxis, in which there is massive release of histamine and other mediators from the mast cell. This occurs on injection or ingestion of a substance to which the subject has become sensitized to produce IgE antibody. One example is the occasional severe reaction in penicillin allergy.

A familial tendency (atopy) to produce high levels of IgE antibody against one or more common antigen causes clinical disorders such as allergic asthma, hay fever and cow's-milk allergy in infants. Other factors, in addition to the familial trait, predispose to atopy, including deficient IgA production, lack of T cells that suppress IgE production and mucosal defects, such as cystic fibrosis.

Antigenic determinants may form part of the cell membrane or may be absorbed there, as is the case with some drugs, and when combined with antibody there is complement fixation and cell lysis. Drugs absorbed onto the surface of red cells, white cells and platelets may, in this way, cause haemolysis, agranulocytosis and thrombocytopenia. The membrane is not always damaged by antibodies however, the combination with surface antigen sometimes causing stimulation of cell function, as in Graves' disease.

The combination of antibody with antigen to form immune complexes, to which enzymes of the complement series become attached, generates substances that attract leucocytes, increase vascular permeability and stimulate clotting. Phagocytes digest the complexes and thus control the inflammatory mechanism. Acute serum sickness is a typical example of the production of disease by immune complexes. For example, fever, skin rash, proteinuria and joint inflammation may

◀ Acute anaphylaxis follows injection or ingestion of a substance to which a subject has become highly sensitized to produce IgE antibody

◀ Predisposing factors to atopy include a familial trait, immunoglobulin deficiencies and mucosal defects such as cystic fibrosis

follow meningococcal meningitis and treatment with penicillin.

Chronic immune complex disease may follow persistence of the antigen such as a bacterial or viral infection — when the antigen is a dietary constituent; arises from a growing tumour; and when a normal tissue antigen has not been recognized as self and elicited an antibody response. If the complexes are produced in excess of phagocytic activity deposition occurs in various sites including the joints, skin, blood vessels and kidneys. Examples of chronic immune complex disease are SLE, rheumatoid arthritis, drug-induced diseases that resemble 'serum sickness', dietary antigen-induced disease (gluten sensitivity) and the arthropathy associated with hepatitis B.

Adaptive immunity depends on both the stimulating process and regulating mechanisms, which taper off the response once the foreign antigen has been eliminated, thus preventing damaging autoimmune responses to self-antigens. This mechanism is used in the prevention of rhesus isoimmunization, small doses of antibody administered to the mother stimulating, by a complex process, elimination of fetal red cells which leak through the placenta into the maternal circulation.

Failure of control of the immune response accounts for lack of antibody response to self-antigens like thyroglobulin and the tolerance of tissue grafts between different strains. Sometimes self-antigens share determinants with foreign antigens (for example heart muscle with group A haemolytic streptococci) and activated T cells co-operate with B cells to allow auto-antibody production.

Immune deficiency

In some cases of infection evidence of absolute or relative failure of the immune response can be demonstrated. This is especially true of malnutrition, may occur with certain antibiotics (penicillin, co-trimoxazole, chloramphenicol and rifampicin), and in immuno-compromised individuals such as those with lymphoma, myeloma, leukaemias (non-lymphocytic) and the transplant patient.

Table 17.3. Impaired immune response in disease

Acute myelocytic leukaemia — CMI and impaired granulo-
cyte function
Lymphoma — CMI, granulocyte function and humoral
Myeloma — humoral, granulocyte function
Carcinoma and other tumours — CMI, granulocyte function
(CMI: Cell mediated immunity)

Non-specific defence mechanisms may be impaired in all
because of disrupted barriers (e.g. skin, mucosal ulceration)
and impaired nutrition

Deficiencies may occur in any or all of the immune
processes. There may be abnormalities of the mechanical barrier (skin — as in burns; mucociliary lining —
as in cystic fibrosis), of the phagocytic cells (neutropenia), of antibody formation (hypogammaglobulin-
aemia) and of cell-mediated immunity. In the
immuno-compromised host there may be deficiency in
more than one mechanism, due to either the underlying
condition or its treatment, such that organisms with
little virulence become, in these patients, life-
threatening pathogens.

Immunoglobulin deficiency is associated with persistent, recurrent, severe and, sometimes, unusual bacterial infections. The course of viral illnesses such as
measles, and the response to smallpox vaccination, is

Table 17.4. Deficiencies in immune mechanisms

Mechanism	Condition	Infections to which subject is susceptible
Barriers Skin	Burns, intravenous sites, wounds	Staphylococci, streptococci, pseudomonas
Mucociliary lining	Cystic fibrosis	Staphylococci, pseudomonas
Phagocytes	Neutropenia	Gram +ve and −ve, Candida
Antibody	Agammaglobulin-aemia, myeloma, lymphoma	Streptococci, haemophilus, staphylococci, entero-viruses (CNS)
Cell-mediated immunity	Leukaemia chemotherapy	Measles, viruses, mycobacteria and Candida

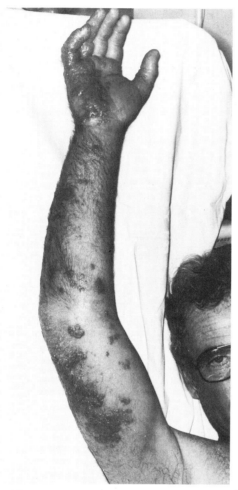

Fig. 17.2. Extensive herpes zoster of R. arm in
an immunocompromised patient receiving treatment
for lymphoma.

usually normal. IgA deficiency is the most common,
but the classic form is IgG deficiency, which is usually a
sex-linked recessive occurring only in boys. IgG
deficiency in an adult is often associated with multiple
myeloma. Circulating B cells are usually reduced in
number and the type of immunodeficiency syndrome
can be accurately characterized by study of the
immunoglobulin on the surface membrane.

Cell-mediated immune deficiency results in recurrent, protracted fungal, viral and unusual opportunistic infections. Measles virus, for example, may progress to give a giant cell pneumonia and vaccination against smallpox results in progressive vaccinia, in which the local lesions enlarge and spread through the soft tissues of the upper arm. Chronic mucocutaneous candidosis also occurs in these patients and there is an increased susceptibility to mycobacterial infections. T cell function is depressed in these patients and the delayed hypersensitivity skin reactions to injected antigens, such as *Candida* or tuberculin, are impaired.

A recently recognized syndrome of acquired immune deficiency has been described in homosexual men and to a lesser extent in drug addicts, haemophiliacs and Haitians. AIDS usually presents with fever, weight loss, diarrhoea and lymph node enlargement; later features are opportunistic infections including cytomegalovirus, mycobacteria and pneumocystis. A previously rare tumour (Kaposi's sarcoma) is common in AIDS patients. There is profound deficiency of cellular immunity, but humoral response is normal. There appears to be association with viruses of the type that may be the cause of T-cell lymphoma leukaemia. Necrotic gingivitis and oro-oesphageal candidiasis can occur in patients with AIDS.

Immunization

Specific immunity to micro-organisms may occur naturally, following infection during life, or artificially, by deliberate exposure to antigenic stimulus before natural exposure has occurred. Natural and artificial immunity may be either passive, by transferring preformed antibody from one species to another or from mother to fetus, or it may be active, when either live or dead organisms, their subunits or their toxins are given, or the patient acquires the infection naturally.

Active immunity induced by artificial means may employ non-pathogenic toxins, such as those of diphtheria and tetanus which have been treated with formalin so as to retain their antigenicity. Active immunity may also employ live vaccines, such as BCG, measles and poliomyelitis. Although there is a trend to

◀ 'Immunization' is the term applied to the means by which specific immunity to micro-organisms is acquired

◀ Specific immuno-globulins are available to prevent viral hepatitis B, chickenpox and smallpox vaccination by the process of passive immunity

the use of live vaccines, because small doses of organisms, which subsequently multiply, have to be given, some killed vaccines (typhoid, influenza and pertussis) are still used although they are less successful.

Antibody persistence after vaccines is unexplained but lifelong immunity does occur, although it tends to wane and booster doses are necessary. Mass immunization programmes are used to control endemic diseases but can also be used selectively in relation to importation of disease (smallpox) or when individuals from non-endemic areas travel to endemic ones (yellow fever). Post-exposure vaccination is not commonly employed, but can be of value in virus diseases with long incubation periods, such as rabies.

◀ One object of immunization is to induce immunity prior to infection, either to control endemic disease or to prevent importation into non-endemic areas

Autoimmune disease

In a variety of diseases circulating organ-specific antibodies can be detected, although they may not necessarily be causing the disease. Auto-antibodies increase with age and in some non-immunological inflammatory diseases such as cirrhosis of the liver. High titres of auto-antibodies are found in diseases limited to one target organ, such as autoimmune thyroiditis, pernicious anaemia and some forms of acquired haemolytic anaemia. Cell-mediated immune mechanisms may also be operative in these diseases.

Table 17.5.   Association of auto-antibodies

Auto-antibody to	Associated disease
Thyroglobulin	Autoimmune thyroiditis
Gastric parietal cell; intrinsic factor	Pernicious anaemia
Skin basement membrane	Pemphigoid
Intercellular cement substance	Pemphigus
Acetylcholine receptor	Myasthenia gravis

Non-organ-specific auto-antibodies are found in RA, SLE, Sjögren's syndrome, scleroderma, some forms of liver disease

Non-organ-specific antibodies (rheumatoid factor and antinuclear factor) are found in the so-called 'connective tissue diseases', such as rheumatoid arthritis, SLE, scleroderma and chronic active hepatitis.

Biopsy of organs damaged by autoimmune antibodies may help to confirm that immunoglobulin is the mediator of the disease, antibodies being demonstrated by immunofluorescent techniques. This is particularly useful in those diseases with basement membrane antibodies, such as pemphigus and pemphigoid.

HLA antigens

Genetic predisposition to autoimmune and some other disorders can be ascertained from HLA typing. HLA antigens occur in leucocytes and all other human cells that have been investigated. The genetic information for the HLA system is found on the short arm of chromosome 6. The major histo-compatibility complex, of which HLA is a part, plays an important and complex role in transplant rejection and contains genes that may determine susceptibility to disease.

A locus is a site on a chromosome where alternative forms of a gene (alleles) may be found and four have been identified for the HLA system (HLA-A, -B, -C and -D). Many diseases have been reported as being associated with different HLA combinations (genotypes) but the exact relationship is complex and imperfectly understood.

Amongst the HLA-associated diseases is ankylosing spondylitis, nearly all the patients have an uncommon antigen, HLA-B27, found in only 8% of healthy

◄ Many diseases have been reported as being associated with different HLA combinations but the exact relationship is complex and not fully understood

Table 17.6.   Disorders which may be HLA-associated

Ankylosing spondylitis	HLA-B27
Myasthenia gravis	
Graves' disease	HLA-DR3
SLE	
Insulin dependent diabetes mellitus	HLA-DR3 and DR4
Behçet's disease	HLA-B5

Europeans (*see* Chapter 12). There is also an increased incidence of this antigen in Reiter's syndrome and seronegative arthritis. Insulin-dependent diabetes mellitus is another disorder associated with HLA-DR3 and DR4 antigens. With the exception of ankylosing spondylitis, however, none of the HLA and disease associations is strong enough to be used for diagnostic purposes.

The major histocompatibility complex is closely related to the defences of the individual against some virus infections, lymphocytes being restricted in their ability to kill only those virus infected cells which share HLA antigens with the host. The large number of different HLA types could result in some individuals being resistant to any virus.

Malignant disease 18

Malignant disease, commonly referred to as 'cancer', is the second commonest cause of death in the United Kingdom. Although there is a tendency to talk of 'cancer' as if it were a single disease entity there are many cancers which differ widely in their behaviour and prognosis. To understand what constitutes a cancer it is necessary to review basic cell biology.

Basic cell biology

All tissues of the body consist of cells. Growth occurs by cell division but once the adult size is achieved growth stops. At this time certain highly specialized tissues lose the capacity for cell division. In other cases, division continues, but only at the rate necessary to replace cells lost. In these tissues there is a constant turnover of cells. An obvious example is the epithelium of the gastrointestinal tract which is completely renewed in three days. The mechanisms which control this process of renewal are ill understood. In particular, it is not known why cell division stops when the normal size of the organ is achieved.

The process of cell division is known as 'mitosis' and is a part of the 'cell cycle'. The cell cycle is divided into phases labelled G_1 (resting), S (synthesis), G_2 (resting) and division. At any given time a proportion of cells in any tissue are in the cycle. The majority are inactive and are said to be in 'G_0'.

During S phase reduplication of DNA is occurring allowing pairing of the chromosomes during G_2 prior to mitosis occurring.

The cell cycle takes 24–36 hours. A more important concept is tissue (or tumour) doubling time. This in part relates to the cell cycle time but also is affected by the percentage of cells undergoing the cycle at any time and the number of those cells that will survive. This latter figure is known as the 'tumour growth fraction'. Tumour cells are genetically defective and as few as 5% will survive. This seems a very low figure but it should be realized that the effective growth fraction for normal tissue is 0%.

If the doubling time of cells in normal tissue is calculated it will be found to be around 40 days (but doubling does not occur *in vivo* because the cell division exactly balances cell loss). Cancers, contrary to what is commonly assumed, have a longer doubling time than normal tissue. The problem with cancer is not that it grows more quickly than normal tissue but that it does not stop growing when it should.

Cells can be grown in tissue culture as monolayer sheets. When normal cell monolayers meet one another division stops. When the monolayers consist of cancer cells, division continues and the cells pile up on one another. They are said to have lost 'contact inhibition'. This is considered to be one of the basic defects in malignancy but the reason for it is not known.

There is also a loss of adherence of cancer cells. Again this is most easily seen in tissue culture where the cancer cells can be easily displaced from the surface on which they are growing. This same lack of adherence occurs between cells and allows cells to split off from one another *in vivo*. This is partly the reason why cancer cells metastasize from the primary tumour to distant parts of the body. Lack of adherence and lack of contact inhibition probably also explain the other major characteristic of cancer which is its ability to invade surrounding tissues, penetrating between normal cells.

◀ Cancer is a result of failure of control of growth of cells. The major defects are loss of adherence and loss of contact inhibition

Types of malignant disease

Malignant disease may be diffuse or solid.

Solid cancers are divided into two main types according to the type of cell from which they arose. Carcinomas arise from the epithelial germ layers, and sarcomas arise from mesodermal structures. Epithelial

Table 18.1.   Carcinoma

Type	Cell of origin	Common sites	Response to radiotherapy
Squamous cell (epithelioma)	Squamous epithelium	Skin, buccal cavity, oesophagus	+ +
Adenocarcinoma	Glandular epithelium	Breast, gastro-intestinal tract, salivary glands, thyroid	±
Transitional cell	Transitional epithelium	Bladder	+
Basal cell carcinoma (rodent ulcer)	Basal cell layer of epithelium	Face	+ +
Melanoma	Melanocytes	Skin — lower leg, trunk, face	—

tissues being much more active than mesodermal, carcinomas are very much more common than sarcomas. A third rare type of solid tumour is the teratoma which arises from pluripotential cells in the genitalia and contains cell types from all three germ layers, endoderm, ectoderm and mesoderm.

Carnicomas can be further subdivided according to the type of cell from which they arose. This division is

Table 18.2.   Diffuse malignancies

Arising from blood cells
Lymphocytes and precursors
    Acute lymphoblastic leukaemia
    Chronic lymphoblastic leukaemia
Polymorphonuclear leucocytes and precursors
    Acute myeloid leukaemia
    Chronic myeloid leukaemia
Plasma cells
    Myeloma

Arising from reticuloendothelial (lymphatic) tissue
Hodgkin's lymphoma
Non-Hodgkin's lymphoma

These groups can be further subdivided. The full classification is beyond the scope of this book.

of some value in predicting likely response to treatment (*Table* 18.1).

Sarcomas are named by prefixing the name of the tissue of origin to the word sarcoma, e.g. 'osteo-sarcoma' (from bone), 'fibro-sarcoma' (from fibrous tissue) and 'rhabdomyosarcoma' (from muscle). They are rare tumours and all those arising from the soft tissue behave in much the same way as one another.

The diffuse cancers can be divided into the blood dyscrasias and the reticuloses, although the distinction between the two can be blurred.

The blood dyscrasias arise from the cells in the bone marrow which give rise to blood cells (*Table* 18.2). The reticuloses arise in the cells of the reticulo-endothelial system which are mainly found in the lymph nodes, liver and spleen, but also are scattered throughout the gastrointestinal tract.

Spread of cancer

Carcinomas tend to metastasize via the lymphatics whereas sarcomas tend to metastasize through the bloodstream. This is a generalization and many carcinomas have blood-borne metastases.

The site of metastasis depends on the site of the primary tumour. Lymphatic spread is initially in the line of normal drainage to the regional lymph nodes. Thus a carcinoma of the anterior third of the tongue will metastasize initially to the submental and subman-dibular nodes, while a carcinoma of the posterior third of the tongue will metastasize to the jugular lymph node. A knowledge of the normal routes of lymphatic drainage is, therefore, of importance in planning treatment.

Blood-borne metastases tend to grow only in some sites. The common sites for secondary tumours are lung, liver, bone and brain. Gastrointestinal tumours metastasize to liver because the gastrointestinal tract is drained by the portal venous system directly through the liver. Prostatic carcinoma shows a predilection for bone.

Some apparently blood-borne metastases may occur by lymphatic spread. It is thought that liver involve-

◀ The spread of cancer is by lymphatics, by the bloodstream or trans-coelomically. This process is known as 'metastasis

ment in the case of breast cancer may be because of retrograde lymphatic spread.

A third specialized type of spread occurs with tumours involving the body cavities, especially the peritoneum. The cancer may spread directly across the peritoneum — so called 'transcoelomic spread'. This may give rise to multiple deposits of tumour on the peritoneal surface, often referred to as 'peritoneal seedlings', or may result in secondary tumours in other organs. The classic example of this is the so-called Krukenberg tumour which is a secondary in an ovary arising from a primary gastric carcinoma.

Effects of cancer

The effects of cancer may be local or generalized. Local effects are easy to understand.

Ulceration may occur because the malignant tissue is close to the surface and withstands trauma less well than normal tissue. The ulcer frequently becomes infected and the resultant unpleasant smell may be the patient's main complaint. This is particularly common in surface cancers such as squamous carcinoma of the lip or adenocarcinoma of the breast. The ulceration may give rise to bleeding.

When the cancer occurs in a hollow organ such as the stomach it may block the tube and give rise to an obstruction. A tumour in the lungs may present as breathlessness.

Cancers may give rise to symptoms because their bulk causes pressure on surrounding structures. This is especially the case in brain tumour where the rigid enclosing skull exacerbates the rise in pressure as the tumour grows.

Generalized effects may be due to specific actions of the given tumour or an effect of cancer in general. The latter depends partly on the bulk of the tumour. It is not known why patients with cancer should have generalized ill health progressing through marked cachexia to death. The obvious solution — that the tumour uses nutrients for the body and therefore effectively starves the body — is probably not true.

◀ Advanced cancer is characterized by wasting of the patient. The cause for this is not known

However, it is known that, even in the absence of any localized complications from cancer, when the bulk of malignant cells present in the body reaches 1 kg the patient inevitably dies.

A closely associated phenomenon is the marked anorexia that cancer patients develop. This is easy to understand if the cancer is in the upper gastrointestinal tract but it occurs even with non-gastrointestinal tumour. The mechanism is entirely unknown. It is postulated that the tumour secretes a substance which acts on the appetite centres of the brain to produce a feeling of satiety.

Some tumours produce hormone-like substances which mediate systemic effects. In some cases this hormone may be identifiable with certainty — for example some bronchogenic carcinomas may produce anti-diuretic hormone. In other cases, the 'hormone' has not been identified although its effects are obvious. In 1867 Trousseau described a flitting phlebitis, thrombophlebitis migrans, which was associated with an intra-abdominal carcinoma. Other skin changes may occur such as acanthosis migrans.

Tumours that bleed may produce anaemia. This is a common presentation for gastric and caecal carcinomas without any other symptoms. For this reason patients with iron deficiency anaemia must be carefully investigated until a cause is found.

◀ Anaemia is a common presentation for cancer. It should be investigated thoroughly

Contrary to popular opinion, cancer does not give rise to pain unless it invades bone or nerve. When such invasion does occur, however, the pain is progressive and unremitting. Such persistent pain has a deleterious effect on the patient's general health. An associated depression is common and may aggravate the situation as the pain may seem worse to a depressed person and this may make them more depressed, setting up a vicious circle. A profound fear of cancer exists in society at large. This engenders anxiety in the patient, and may lead to interpersonal conflict between the patient and his friends and family. The influence of the psyche on cancer is ill-understood. Biological scientists are reluctant to abscribe power to the mind over something as tangible and organic as a carcinoma but evidence does exist that a patient's attitude to his disease influences his survival.

Staging of cancer

Before deciding that the cancer requires local or systemic treatment it is necessary to stage the cancer. Essentially this means determining the extent of spread of the disease. The staging is frequently expressed in coded form as this is more easily handled, when comparing the results of different forms of treatment, than is an individual description of a given tumour. Initially there was a separate staging system for each tumour type but increasingly use is made of the TNM classification produced by the Union International contre Cancer (UICC). T refers to the characteristics of the tumour, N to the nodal involvement and M to distant metastases. Such an internationally agreed code allows comparisons to be made between treatments for tumours in different centres. It is important to realize that the staging code expresses in shorthand those factors which have influenced the decision to adopt a course of treatment. The code does not dictate the treatment although we sometimes talk loosely as if it did.

Investigations

In order to stage patients accurately a number of investigations may be employed. The art of the onocologist is knowing which of the many available investigations will give useful information — that is information which will affect the management of the patient — most cheaply and efficiently.

The most important investigation is biopsy of the lesion to obtain confirmation of the diagnosis. This may be carried out by fine needle aspiration to obtain cells for cytological diagnosis. A special biopsy needle can obtain a core of tissue for histology. A similar core is obtained by drill biopsy. Biopsy forceps may be used

◄ Biopsy of the lesion to confirm the diagnosis must be performed before treatment is started

through endoscopic instruments. These are all sampling methods and a negative result must be confirmed by formal surgical excision of the lesion. Positive histology must be obtained before treatment is instituted.

With the diagnosis established other investigations are undertaken to assess the degree of spread. Knowledge of the likely spread of the tumour guides the investigations to be undertaken.

◄ Full investigation is necessary to determine the extent of spread. The mode of treatment is influenced by the extent of spread

Blood tests

The simplest (and cheapest) tests are routine blood tests. The full blood count will detect anaemia and abnormalities of the blood cells suggesting marrow involvement. Biochemical profiles are also carried out. Raised levels of alkaline phosphatase may indicate liver involvement or bone involvement. In prostatic carcinoma the acid phosphatase level gives an indication of metastatic disease. Efforts have been made to find other blood markers of the presence of tumour, but these have not been successful except for certain very rare tumours.

Radiology

The simplest radiological investigation is the chest X-ray. All patients with cancer should undergo chest X-ray to exclude lung metastases. Computerized tomography (CT scanning; CAT scanning) is the newest form of imaging technique. Multiple radiographs are taken of the patient and stored electronically. A computer then interprets the data and displays them. It is especially useful in assessing mediastinal and intra-abdominal lymph node involvement.

If CT scanning is not available, lymphangiography may be required to delineate the nodes. This is a tricky technique which involves cannulating a suitable lymph vessel and injecting radio-opaque contrast medium. Nodes containing tumour either do not appear or else have missing areas within them.

Many tumours are not visible because they involve internal organs. Radiology has been the traditional method for detecting these. Contrast medium is introduced to outline the organ under investigation. For example, barium may be drunk to outline the stomach (barium meal) or introduced by a rectal tube to outline the colon (barium enema). An iodine-containing compound injected intravenously is excreted by the kidneys and can be used to outline the urinary tract (intravenous urogram). Such methods can only suggest the presence of tumour and not confirm it.

Isotope studies

Radioactive labels can be attached to molecules which will be taken up by different cells. The radioactivity can then be detected using a gamma camera and a map of the organ of interest can be obtained.

The most useful scans in oncological practice are bone scans and liver scans.

In a bone scan the ^{99}Te label is taken up by the metastases more than by the normal bone. The metastasis, therefore, shows up as an area of increased activity (a 'hot' spot).

In contrast, the isotope is not taken up by metastases in the liver which show on the scan as areas of low activity ('cold' spots).

Ultrasound

An ultrasound scanner may be used to image any organ. It is particularly accurate in detecting liver metastases. Because it is non-invasive and safe, ultrasound can be used serially to measure changes in lesions with time, for example in assessing response to treatment.

Endoscopy

Lesions of internal organs can be viewed (and biopsied) using endoscopic instruments. The longest established procedure of this nature is cystoscopy, used to view the urinary bladder.

The invention of the flexible fibreoptic endoscope in the 1960s has extended the range of lesions that can be directly viewed. The oesophagus, stomach and duodenum can be easily and quickly examined in the conscious patient. Colonoscopy is routine as is bronchoscopy. Endoscopy is now considered an essential investigation in patients with upper gastrointestinal symptoms and in cases of doubt in the lower gastrointestinal tract.

Treatment of cancer

The treatment of cancer can be considered under two headings:(a) the treatment of localized disease and (b) the treatment of generalized disease. Under both headings the treatment may attempt to be curative or may be merely palliative.

1. Localized disease

There are two major modalities used in the treatment of local disease: surgery and radiotherapy. Both modalities may be curative or palliative. The decision to accept palliation rather than cure is based on the patients' general condition (they may be unfit to withstand a curative procedure) and on technical considerations (the lesion may be too advanced for any local measure to be potentially curative).

Surgery

Arguments rage as to the extent of tissues to be excised in any given tumour. It is clear in all cases that a margin of normal tissue must be removed to ensure clearance of the cancer itself. It is a good rule in cancer surgery that the method of reconstruction (e.g. closing the skin defect or reanastomosing the gut) should not be considered until after the excision has been completed, in order to obviate the risk that a less than adequate excision will be carried out so that closure will be obtained. In some centres for head and neck surgery in the U.S.A. this is carried to the point of having separate teams of surgeons for the two phases of the operation.

The surgery may be extended to include the lymph nodes draining the area of the tumour. Fears that removing the lymph nodes may remove one of the body's defences against the tumour are offset by the knowledge that often the lymph nodes contain tumour at the time of primary treatment. In clinical practice, the evidence is largely in favour of treating the lymph nodes. The aim of curative surgery is to remove all the involved tissue.

◄ The aim of treatment must be decided before treatment starts. Palliative measures are aimed at relieving symptoms and should not be too uncomfortable or dangerous. Curative measures may be more drastic

◄ Radiotherapy and surgery are treatments for localized disease

Palliative surgery is commonly practised even when it is known that metastases are present. The aim is to ensure relief of the patient's symptoms or the prevention of symptoms developing. A good example of this is found in colonic tumours which are developing obstruction. Even if there are widespread metastases in the liver it is beneficial to the patient to remove the tumour and relieve the obstruction. In addition, removal of the primary tumour may prevent future local infiltration which can give rise to intractable pain.

Radiotherapy
Radiotherapy may be administered by external beam or by the implantation of radioactive needles. External beams may be generated by high voltage X-ray machines or by a radioactive source such as Cobalt 60. More recently photon generators and electron generators have been used, and most recently the use of neutrons generated in a cyclotron has been investigated. Whichever method is applied the broad general principles remain. All tissue is damaged by radiation but normal tissue regenerates itself more rapidly. By dividing up the dose of radiation given and spreading it over a period of days or weeks it is possible to give a dose that is lethal to the tumour but causes minimal longterm damage to normal tissue. Some skin reaction is almost inevitable but provided that the skin remains dry this will amount to no more than a severe 'sunburn'. With modern techniques, provided the gastrointestinal tract is not directly involved, there should be little nausea and systemic upset.

Radiotherapy in an appropriate tumour is as curative as surgery. It is less effective in a large tumour where the hypoxic centre is less responsive to radiotherapy. A combined modality of approach where surgery is used to debulk a large tumour and radiotherapy is used to sterilize the surrounding area (removing the necessity for a wide surgical excision) is often worth considering. This approach to breast cancer allows it to be treated without mastectomy. This is one of the current controversies in oncology and is being actively studied in the U.K. and Europe.

Palliative radiotherapy is most useful in relieving pain, particularly from bony metastases. A single dose of treatment is often sufficient to eliminate pain although not causing healing of the lesion. The exact mechanism involved is unknown.

2. Generalized disease

When disease has spread then systemic therapy is necessary. Two major modalities of systemic therapy are used: hormonal therapy and chemotherapy. Of the two, hormonal therapy has the lower incidence of side effects, but chemotherapy is applicable to a wider variety of tumours.

a. Hormonal therapy

Only a limited number of types of tumours will respond to hormonal manipulation. Fortunately, these are among the commonest of tumours. The two classic examples are breast cancer in the female and prostatic cancer in the male. Treatment may be by removing a hormonal stimulus from the tumour or adding an abnormal hormone stimulus to the tumour. Both methods are employed.

The earliest hormonal treatment of a tumour was undertaken in 1896 by Beatson who carried out an oophorectomy for advanced breast cancer. Removal of hormone-producing glands remained a mainstay in the treatment of breast cancer for many years. Recently drugs which block the action of hormones on the tumour have been used instead. The most common of these is tamoxifen, which blocks the action of oestrogen.

Paradoxically, tumours which respond to the removal of oestrogens will also respond to added oestrogen. Stilboestrol has been used in the past to treat breast cancer and is still used to treat prostatic cancer.

Hormone therapy causes little upset to the patients. Unfortunately, even among those types of cancer which are said to be hormone-dependent only a proportion of tumours will actually respond. Efforts are being made to identify which tumours can be treated with hormone therapy by measurement of oestrogen receptors and other markers within the tumours. Tumours which do not respond must be treated by chemotherapy.

◄ Hormonal treatment is systemic. It is of limited application as only few tumours are endocrine controlled

b. Chemotherapy

Chemotherapy, in the context of oncology, means the

use of cytotoxic drugs. These substances damage all cells. As in the case of radiotherapy normal cells repair themselves more rapidly than malignant cells. Chemotherapy is best given, therefore, in pulsed doses with time for normal cells to recover between each treatment.

Because the treatment is systemic the whole body is affected, but since only dividing cells are damaged the effects are seen in those tissues with rapidly dividing cells — the bone-marrow, gastrointestinal tract and the hair follicles. Typical side effects are bone-marrow suppression with leucopenia and thrombocytopenia, nausea and diarrhoea, and alopecia.

◀ Chemotherapy is systemic. The severe side effects must be weighed against any potential benefit

Chemotherapy is now a specialty in its own right and for each tumour there are several different appropriate regimens, the selection of which depends on factors relating to the tumour and to the patient. In general, a combination of drugs has been found to be more effective than single drugs.

Diffuse malignancies, such as the blood dyscrasias, respond better to chemotherapy than do solid tumours, and in childhood leukaemia cures have been achieved. Some solid tumours do respond well and the use of cis-platinum has resulted in cure of tumours arising from the ovary or testis. In other solid tumours, however, the best that can be hoped for is palliation and the side effects of the treatment must be balanced against the potential benefits that are expected. Good palliation of symptoms can be achieved and patients with advanced cancer should be considered by an expert oncologist for chemotherapy before it is decided that nothing more can be done.

When the primary tumour has been removed surgically it is obvious that undetectable metastases are already present or else recurrences would not occur. For this reason, it has been suggested that chemotherapy should be given as an adjuvant to surgery to eliminate such micrometastases. To date it has been found to be generally ineffective although certain special groups of patients may benefit. This approach is still under investigation.

At the other end of the spectrum, a large tumour which is too big to be dealt with by surgery or radiotherapy may be reduced in size by chemotherapy and after shrinking can be treated by a localized treatment to finally eliminate it.

Management of the patient

So far we have considered the technical aspects of cancer. It must not be forgotten that cancer carries very strong emotional and psychological connotations for the patient. Despite efforts to educate people into seeing cancer as just another disease it is still perceived by many as an inevitably fatal, untreatable and extremely painful condition. Tact and patience are necessary in dealing with cancer patients but it is now becoming more widely recognized that honesty is essential, as trust between doctor and patient can only be built on honesty. Within the context of honesty, a positive approach to the problem must be maintained and the patient encouraged always to hope. Honesty does not mean telling the patient he is incurable and nothing can be done. Always some treatment can be offered to eliminate symptoms if nothing else and at the very worst a patient with terminal cancer should be free from pain, free from distressing symptoms such as vomiting and free to communicate with his or her family and friends. The care of the terminally ill patient is increasingly being undertaken by specialists in this field but anyone undertaking the care of patients with cancer should have a working knowledge of advances in this area.

Having said that, it is important to remember that many cancers can be cured and the patient presenting with early cancer should be made aware of this. The plan of treatment and the likely problems should be discussed fully with the patient. Any questions the patient raises should be answered carefully and as fully as possible. The family should be kept informed and at all times the doctor should be prepared to go back over what has already been discussed perhaps several times before. In this way, the patient and the family can be helped to come to terms with the situation and to understand the need for and the benefit from some of the more severe forms of treatment proposed.

The important thing to remember is that patients with cancer are people and must be treated as such.

◀ Cancer occurs in people. Sympathetic communication is an essential part of management

Trauma

Trauma is the commonest cause of death in the population under 50 years of age. Accidents may happen in the home, at work or with increasing frequency on the roads. While from an epidemiological point of view and in an effort at prevention these different groups merit separate study, their effects on the organism are the same. Treatment does not therefore depend on what produced the injury but on what is the damage sustained. We need to consider two factors prior to discussing the management of injury. The first is the immediate effect of injury on the body and the second is the healing process on which we are dependent to achieve recovery.

Immediate effects

There is a complex physiological response to trauma but there is little that can be done to modify this response; indeed, we are not certain which modifications would be of benefit to the patient. The most notable effect is a greatly increased production of hormones, particularly ACTH, from the pituitary. This in turn stimulates the production of the corticosteroids from the adrenal gland. The adrenal gland also produces large quantities of the catecholamines adrenaline and noradrenaline. As a result of these changes the body becomes 'insulin resistant' and the blood sugar rises. Glycosuria not infrequently occurs and is not a sign either that the patient is a latent diabetic or that treatment for an elevated blood glucose is needed, although it may happen that the blood sugar does become so high that treatment with insulin must be started. Of greater longterm significance is that protein breakdown begins. This results in the loss of muscle bulk and in the depletion of serum albumin and important enzyme systems in the liver and kidneys. If not reversed these losses can lead to death from organ failure as all the enzymes are used up. This risk increases with the severity of the injury and is the major reason for introducing nutritional support (by the parenteral route if necessary) at an early stage in the injured patient.

Of more immediate practical importance is the shock syndrome which may develop in response to injury. This is fully dealt with in the Appendix.

Healing

The healing process is fundamental to recovery from injury. All efforts on the part of the clinician are directed to making the natural healing process proceed smoothly. There is little we can do at present to speed up or otherwise modify healing. All tissues heal by a similar process and, except for bone which heals by new bone formation, all tissues heal by scarring, that is the laying down of fibrous tissue. We will consider more closely the healing of a skin wound.

Skin wounds can be divided into incised wounds and those in which there has been tissue loss. The fundamental healing processes are the same but the nature of the wound alters the apparent response.

After wounding the first event is the formation of a haematoma by the clotting of blood. An inflammatory response then appears with the ingress of white blood cells of the neutrophil polymorph type. These are followed by chronic inflammatory cells called 'macrophages' which seem to have two functions. First they begin to demolish the blood clot by phagocytosis and then they act as chemotactic agents attracting the fibroblasts, which are the definitive repair cells, into the area. Along with the fibroblasts come capillary blood vessels. The mixture of blood vessels, fibroblasts and inflammatory cells is known as 'granulation tissue'.

In an incised wound this is of very small volume and lies between the edges of the wound. In a wound where tissue has been lost and approximation of the edges has not been possible, granulation tissue is a predominant feature and the wound is often referred to as a 'granulating' wound. The fibroblasts begin to lay down the fibrous protein collagen. At first this is laid down at random but as time goes on remodelling occurs and the collagen comes to lie in regular bundles along the lines of stress in the wound. The initial phase of ingrowth of cells and vessels lasts about three days and is known as the 'proliferative' phase. During this period there is no increase in the measurable strength of the wound. Over the next 3–4 weeks the collagen is being formed and the wound's strength slowly increases. However, at 3 weeks after injury the wound has only regained about 20% of its former strength. The phase of remodelling takes up to 6 months and leaves the wound with about 60% of the normal tissue strength. The change in the wound is clinically visible with the wound being hyperaemic and active-looking until the end of the remodelling phase, when many of the capillary vessels will disappear. The patient should be told that the wound is going to be red and itchy for up to 6 months to prevent worry that something is going wrong when the wound appears slow to settle.

◄ Wounds are slow to regain strength. Remodelling occurs for at least 6 months

While the deep layers of the wound are healing in the manner described the epithelium at the edge of the wound begins to divide actively and migrates across the surface of the wound. Decrease in the area of the wound is aided by the process of contraction which depends on muscle type fibres in the fibroblasts.

Healing in bone follows much the same initial course as healing in soft tissue. However, the ingrowth of fibroblasts is supplemented by the ingrowth of osteo-blasts (bone-forming cells) from the periosteum and endosteum. Fibrils grow out from the osteoblasts and become embedded in a homogeneous matrix. Calcium salts are then laid down to form an irregular bony area known as 'callus'. At one time it was thought desirable that healing should take place with minimal callus formation, but it is now felt that good callus is an important step in the healing process. After the callus is formed weight bearing can take place. This results in remodelling of the bone around the fracture site until the normal configuration is attained. During this process the irregular woven bone gradually assumes the normal laminated bony structure.

Many factors may delay healing. The most important, in that it is susceptible to control, is infection. Every effort must be made to avoid infection in the wound. This means careful excision of all contaminated and necrotic tissue prior to suturing of the wound.

◀ Infection inhibits healing

Poor nutrition and the presence of malignant disease also inhibit healing.

Management

It is crucial to establish priorities in dealing with the injured patient. It is self-evident that keeping the patient alive is the most important aim.

Faced with the injured patient the first concern is the airway. Occlusion of the airway is a common cause of death especially after injuries to the head and neck. In the unconscious patient this obstruction can be due to the patient's tongue.

The first manœuvre is to clear debris such as teeth, dentures, blood and vomit from the mouth and throat. The patient must then be positioned in the semi-prone position. Fear of worsening the patient's injuries by moving him are offset by the knowledge that he is likely to choke if he is not moved.

If clearing the airway does not result in adequate respiration it is necessary to start assisted respiration. In the first aid situation this usually takes the form of mouth-to-mouth or mouth-to-nose respiration, but as soon as possible the airway should be intubated with an endotracheal tube which has an occlusive cuff which protects the airway from the inhalation of foreign material and allows the use of mechanical aids in providing ventilation.

◀ The first priority is to keep the patient alive. Therefore, attention to airway and respiration takes precedence over everything else

With the patient's breathing under control the next most urgent matter is the control of any overt bleeding. It should be noted, however, that it is unusual for active external bleeding to be a major problem. Control can almost always be achieved by direct pressure on the bleeding point. A tourniquet is rarely necessary and is only to be recommended when the patient with severe bleeding from a limb is to be transported some distance before formal medical treatment can be undertaken.

It is more likely that the bleeding is concealed. Two litres can easily be lost into the thigh in a case of fractured femur. Abdominal injuries may also produce a marked loss of circulating blood volume. Such patients suffer from hypovolaemic shock and require urgent fluid replacement. Priority is, therefore, the assessment of the degree of shock and the setting up of an intravenous infusion. The treatment of shock is considered in the Appendix. If severe shock is present control of fluid replacement needs a central venous pressure (CVP) line. This measures the pressure in the superior vena cava just above the heart and is an indicator of the amount of circulating blood and of the efficiency of the heart. In very difficult cases a more accurate estimate of these parameters can be obtained by using a Schwann–Ganz catheter to measure the wedge pressure in the pulmonary artery.

◀ Blood loss must be treated by replacement

Oxygen should be administered to all shocked patients.

Assessment

After the initial stabilization it is essential that a full assessment is made. The patient should be examined systematically and all injuries recorded. Clinical findings may suggest the need for further investigations to confirm the full extent of the injuries. Often, however, the required management is obvious without resort to special investigations and in these circumstances not only is it wasteful of resources to carry out such tests but it may be detrimental to the patient, as delay is inevitable. Full assessment includes as good a history as can be obtained, as there may be factors in the patient's medical history which will influence treatment. For example, a patient who is taking steroids for asthma will need extra steroids to cover the period of injury and may well prove refractory to resuscitation if steroids are not given.

◀ A full and careful assessment of the patient must be carried out in order to plan treatment

Radiology

The most common special investigations ordered are radiographs.

It is universal practice to order skull radiographs in the case of head injuries. The police and the courts place great emphasis on the results of these radiographs. In practice facial radiographs are more important as they allow assessment of facial fractures, which is necessary in the planning of treatment. A clinical suspicion of a fracture will lead to a closer scrutiny of the radiograph and increases the likelihood of spotting the abnormality.

Chest radiography should be carried out whenever the chest has been involved. Fractured ribs may be seen (although special oblique views may be necessary to confirm the finding). More serious findings are pneumothorax (air in the pleural cavity) or haemothorax (blood in the pleural cavity). These may be accompanied by collapse of the lung or shift of the mediastinum. The chest radiograph may also reveal abnormalities of the diaphragm or air under the diaphragm (indicating a perforated viscus).

Straight X-ray of the abdomen is rarely helpful in trauma cases but if a renal injury is suspected an intravenous urogram is mandatory. This will not necessarily show the injury but in treating renal injuries it is important to know that both kidneys are present and functioning. It is, to say the least, embarrassing to remove the only working kidney that a patient possesses. In addition, previously unsuspected abnormalities may be revealed as the abnormal kidney is more likely to suffer damage from a given amount of trauma than a normal organ.

The commonest use of radiography is in the assessment of fractures. It must be remembered that while fractures may be the most dramatic part of the picture of the injured patient they are rarely fatal and, therefore, have a low priority in the initial post-injury management of the patient. Radiographs of the fractures are of more help if they are of good quality. There are good reasons for delaying the X-raying of limbs until the patient is otherwise stable. If fracture of the spine (particularly the cervical spine) is suspected either from the examination or from a knowledge of the type of injury involved then radiographs should be obtained at an early stage, as an unstable spinal fracture will demand special care in the moving of the patient.

More esoteric investigations are now available. Computerized axial tomography (CAT scan) of the brain now has an established place in the management of head injuries. Whereas the skull radiograph gives little useful information, the CAT scan may materially alter the management of a patient. In particular failure to show a space-occupying haematoma on the scan will prevent unnecessary surgical exploration of the brain. Whole body CAT scanning has a less certain role. In some centres in the U.S.A. it has become a routine. For most centres in Europe there is insufficient provision of machine time to allow immediate screening of all injured patients. No good evidence exists that the provision of such facilities would improve the outcome for trauma victims.

In the absence of CAT scanning some centres resort to arteriography in cases of abdominal injury. Again, it is important that no delay should result from the application of such special investigations and it has yet to be shown that the patient benefits substantially from such manœuvres. In cases of vascular injury, of course, arteriography may be very helpful.

A useful investigation in cases of abdominal injury is peritoneal lavage. Saline is introduced into the peritoneal cavity through a catheter inserted through the abdominal wall. After 10 minutes the saline is allowed to run out. If there is any intra-peritoneal injury the fluid will be blood-stained or contain bile or faeces. This then is clear indication for immediate laparotomy. It is particularly useful when the usual clinical signs are not available: for example, in an unconscious patient who will be lacking in the pain responses which normally indicate intra-abdominal mischief. If the fluid returns clear it is unlikely that a major injury is present and a further period of observation can be embarked upon.

Once the extent of the injuries has been decided and the patient's general condition has been stabilized a treatment plan must be formulated. As in the resuscitation phase an order of priorities must be clearly established. Again the most life-threatening injury must be treated first. It is difficult to lay down rules that cover all situations but in general any lesion which is resulting in blood loss is the first priority for definitive treatment. Injuries that will cause loss of function are next to be treated and only then, do cosmetic factors enter the equation. For this reason abdominal injuries are normally dealt with first, then orthopaedic injuries, then facio-maxillary. Occasionally a rapidly expanding intracranial haematoma will require immediate decompression and this will take priority over everything else. The important thing is that the patient survives the treatment plan. Six hours of plastic surgery to facial lacerations is of little value if the patient subsequently died of bleeding from a ruptured liver.

Head injuries

The mark of a serious head injury is that the patient has had a period of unconsciousness, and for practical purposes the severity of the head injury is related to the length of the period of unconsciousness. When a patient is admitted following a head injury the level of consciousness is noted. Standard criteria exist for estimating consciousness levels (*Table* 19.1). Recovery of consciousness is a good sign while deepening unconsciousness is a bad sign. Special attention must be paid to the patient who having been unconscious regains consciousness and then becomes unconscious again. This occurrence of the so-called 'lucid interval' suggests the diagnosis of an extra-dural haemorrhage. This lesion is usually related to the middle meningeal blood vessels in the region of the temple. It is rapidly expanding and leads to an increase in intracranial pressure. If not relieved by surgery death ensues

◀ Conscious level is the single most important sign in head injury

Table 19.1.   Criteria for consciousness

Level 1 — Patient apparently normal. Able to answer questions. Orientated
Level 2 — Patient rousable
Level 3 — Unconscious but responds in purposeful manner to painful stimulus
Level 4 — Unconscious but responds, in non-purposeful manner, to very painful stimuli
Level 5 — Unresponsive to stimuli

rapidly. The diagnosis is confirmed by CAT scanning and burr-holes are drilled to allow evacuation of the clot and control of the bleeding vessel. If sophisticated investigations are not available exploratory burr-holes may have to be drilled for diagnostic purposes on clinical suspicion alone.

Less dramatic changes in intracranial pressure are much more common. These are heralded by a gradual deterioration in the conscious level. Other useful signs of increasing pressure are dilatation of the pupil and a slowing of the pulse rate with a widening of the pulse pressure, that is an increasing systolic blood pressure with a falling diastolic pressure. If the patient is conscious increasing intracranial pressure may present as increasing headache or vomiting. Visual disturbance may also be reported such as double vision or blurring of the vision. Such signs may be due to diffuse intracerebral · oedema or intracranial haemorrhage, particularly subdural haematoma. More severe head injuries in which the patient never recovers consciousness may produce haemorrhages in the brain substance either in the cerebral hemispheres or in the brainstem. Brainstem injuries may affect the specialized control centres located in this region of the brain and manifest themselves as disturbances of the autonomic nervous system. A common example of this is the hyper-pyrexia which develops in cases of injury in the pontine region of the brainstem. Diagnosis is again best confirmed using a CAT scanner.

If a space-occupying lesion is present then craniotomy is indicated. Often, however, the scan reveals diffuse oedema and then there is no effective surgical measure that will relieve the symptoms. Dexamethasone, a potent corticosteroid, is often used to reduce the cerebral oedema and reduce the pressure. Other surgeons use urea or mannitol, which are osmotic diuretics and reduce the swelling by withdrawing water from the brain substance.

The presence of a skull fracture does not materially affect the treatment unless it is compound, that is the fracture is in communication with the atmosphere. It should be remembered that fractures that enter the paranasal sinuses are technically compound and as such carry a high risk of intracranial infection developing. Compound skull fractures should be treated with

◀ Compound skull fractures should be treated with antibiotics

prophylactic antibiotics to avoid the development of meningitis. The usual combination chosen is sulpha-dimidine and penicillin. Fractures of the vault of the skull will be seen to be compound because they are overlain by an open wound. Those of the base of the skull will present as a discharge of cerebrospinal fluid from the nose or ear. This fluid can be identified by the use of a standard reagent strip (such as is used for urinalysis on the ward) which will reveal the presence of a high concentration of glucose.

The majority of patients with head injuries are suffering from concussion, which is a temporary derangement of the function of the neurones without any longterm structural damage. This may be associated with obvious abnormalities of function, such as the presence of amnesia for a variable period related to the accident. Amnesia for the actual event is very common but other patients may be unable to remember events leading up to the accident (retrograde amnesia) while others are unable to recall events following the accident (post-traumatic amnesia). The presence of amnesia suggests a severe concussion. No active treatment is required for concussion but rest is advised until the patient is symptom-free. Too early a resumption of activity may lead to the development of the postconcussional syndrome, with persistent headache, loss of concentration and a variety of other neurological symptoms. This syndrome may be exacerbated if there is a question of compensation for the accident involved.

It is common practice to admit patients with concussion to hospital for observation as exclusion of a severe intracranial lesion can only be done in retrospect.

Following a severe head injury intensive rehabilitation is often necessary. This involves physiotherapy, occupational therapy and speech therapy, with sometimes the help of psychologists. This is best carried out in specialist units but unfortunately there are not enough such units to cope with all the severely head injured patients in the country.

Chest trauma

Chest injuries can be divided into two categories:

closed injuries (usually the result of blunt trauma such as a road traffic accident) and penetrating injuries such as stabbing or gunshot wound.

Closed injuries rarely require formal surgical exploration, whereas it is commonly necessary in penetrating injuries.

The mildest blunt injury which we will consider is the fractured rib. The history is usually of a direct blow to the ribs although the fracture may result from an indirect injury, such as a bout of coughing. A single fractured rib is of little consequence other than the fact that it is painful. It is treated by reassurance and simple analgesics. There is no indication for strapping or other attempts at immobilization, which are either ineffective but harmless or else they immobilize the chest wall and lead to collapse and pneumonia in the underlying lung. Multiple rib fractures may cause significant interference with breathing especially in the patient who already suffers from a bad chest. In such patients it may be necessary to administer oxygen. Good relief from pain with consequent improvement in respiratory function can be obtained by injecting long-acting local anaesthetic into the intercostal nerves. Active breathing exercises supervised by a physiotherapist are of great benefit in preventing deterioration of lung function.

A more serious situation arises if multiple rib fractures occur in such a distribution that a segment of the chest wall becomes free to move independently of the rest of the chest. Such a 'flail segment' results from the impact of a steering wheel on the chest with two rows of parallel fractures being produced. This flail segment will be sucked into the chest cavity during inspiration and will therefore interfere with adequate filling of the lungs. Respiratory difficulties ensue. The usual treatment for this type of lesion is to pass an endotracheal tube and maintain the patient's respiration with intermittent positive pressure ventilation. This results in the pressure rising in the chest during the filling phase of the lungs so that the flail segment is blown out at the same time as the rest of the chest wall. This effectively splints the flail segment into its natural position in relation to the other ribs and allows healing to take place. If this is not successful it is sometimes necessary to wire the fractured ribs back into place.

Blunt injury may produce intrathoracic trauma without any fractures of the ribs. The applied force may tear the lung, producing either a haemothorax or a pneumothorax. The latter is probably the more dangerous especially when the lesion is of such a nature that a valvular mechanism is produced in the lung surface which allows air to escape from the lung but not to be reabsorbed. In this circumstance pressure builds up in the chest cavity displacing the lung and collapsing it. As the pressure continues to increase the opposite lung also becomes compromised and the patient becomes grossly dyspnoeic. In addition the displacement may affect the action of the heart. Such a rapidly progressive situation is known as a 'tension pneumothorax'. Urgent treatment is essential if the patient is not to die rapidly. A chest drain must be inserted.

◀ Respiratory difficulty in a patient with a history of injury to the chest may be due to an expanding pneumothorax or haemothorax. In either case urgent drainage is necessary

Because the pleural space is at a negative pressure compared to the atmosphere some valvular system is needed to prevent air being sucked in through the drain, making further collapse of the lung inevitable. Special portable valves exist, but for long-term use it is still customary to use underwater seal drains as the valve. Drainage continues for a number of days until all evidence of the pneumothorax has disappeared on X-ray. The tube is then clamped to ensure that the pneumothorax does not reaccumulate before the drain is removed.

Haemothorax is also treated by insertion of a chest drain. Continued loss of blood from the drain or continued bubbling of air in the case of a pneumothorax indicates the need for a thoracotomy with repair of the lesion.

Penetrating injuries give rise to 'sucking wounds' of the chest. The puncturing of the chest wall leads to a loss of the negative pressure which is responsible for keeping the lung expanded and as a result the lung collapses. The situation is not quite so critical as with a tension pneumothorax but rapid treatment is necessary. The wound must be occluded by an impermeable dressing as a first aid measure and then repaired as soon as possible. A chest drain is necessary in the case of a closed injury. Extensive intrathoracic trauma may require formal exploration and surgical repair. This will usually be injury to the lung but injury to the heart and great vessels is survivable and can be surgically corrected.

Abdominal injury

As with chest trauma, abdominal trauma may be blunt or penetrating, with the former being many times more common. Road traffic accidents are the commonest source of injury. The commonest lesion is a ruptured spleen. Traditionally the treatment for this condition has been splenectomy, but more recently concern has been expressed at the increased incidence of serious pneumococcal sepsis in patients who have undergone splenectomy in the past. This certainly occurs in children who have had their spleen removed but the case is less certain in adults. Because of these worries many surgeons now attempt to repair the spleen rather than to remove it. This takes much longer and should, therefore, only be carried out if there is no associated injury.

The liver also may be injured but it is rarely necessary to remove part of the liver. The bleeding can usually be controlled by a combination of suturing and the use of haemostatic gauze. If this is inadequate then partial hepatectomy may have to be undertaken. Total removal of the liver is incompatible with life.

When the bowel is injured it is usually best to resect the damaged segment. In the small bowel it is possible to reanastomose the bowel immediately but in the large bowel it is often better to form a temporary colostomy with a view to later anastomosis.

Renal damage rarely needs surgical intervention but if operation is needed then an intravenous urogram must be carried out to ensure that the other kidney is working before the injured kidney is removed. If unexpected renal injury is found at laparotomy an intravenous urogram should be carried out on the table.

◄ Intravenous urogram should be carried out in patients with renal damage

Fractures

There are three principles involved in the treatment of fractures: (1) restoration of anatomical alignment, (2) immobilization and (3) return of function by rehabilitation.

Fractures are classified in a number of ways. The first classification concerns the damage to the bone itself. *Greenstick fractures* occur mainly in children. Only part of the cortex is disrupted so that slight angulation is the only deformity possible. When a *complete fracture* occurs the break may be *transverse* or *spiral*. In either case the fracture may be *undisplaced, angulated* or *over-riding*. Often there may be more than one fracture at the site of injury, giving rise to multiple fragments of bone at the fracture site. The fracture is then said to be *comminuted*.

The second classification depends on the involvement of other tissues in the injury. A *simple* fracture involves the bone only. It must be noted that the bony injury may be extremely complex with multiple fragments and gross displacement, but if no other tissue is affected the fracture is still said to be simple. If the fracture is exposed to the air because of an overlying soft tissue wound the fracture is said to be *compound*. A fracture is *complicated* when other structures such as nerves or blood vessels are also damaged. A combination of terms may be used to describe a fracture, for example a 'compound, comminuted spiral fracture of the femoral shaft with angulation'.

The restoration of anatomical alignment at the fracture site is known as 'reduction' of the fracture. Some form of anaesthesia is always required before this is undertaken. It is usually possible to reduce the fracture by manipulation without the need for an operation. This is referred to as 'closed reduction'. Sometimes muscle becomes interposed between the broken ends of the bone. It is then impossible to reduce the fracture by closed manipulation and in these cases operative reduction must be carried out. The fracture is exposed by a suitable incision and the offending muscle can be removed from the bone ends and the reduction achieved.

◀ Operative reduction of fractures may be necessary if closed reduction fails

Immobilization or fixation of the fracture is usually achieved by the use of external splintage. Everyone is familiar with the plaster-of-Paris cast which is normally employed. This is retained until healing has taken place, which is anything from 6 to 12 weeks in most cases. Femoral fractures are very difficult to hold in an external cast although a square-topped cast has recently been found to be useful by some surgeons. The alternative form of external fixation is traction. In children this can be applied by attaching weights to the leg with sticky tape. The pull needed to overcome an adult's muscles is too great for this method of attachment and a pin must be drilled through the tibia to take the attachment of the weights. If it is decided to treat the fracture by traction the patient will be confined to bed until healing takes place, which in the case of the femur will be 12 weeks at least. To avoid this problem it is common to treat some fractures by internal fixation. Internal fixation is also used when a stable reduction cannot be obtained with external methods. This often happens in fractures around the ankle joint.

Bones may be fixed by screws, by wires, by intermedullary nails or by plates. The latter is the most widely used method. Having exposed the site of the fracture and reduced it the surgeon applies a metal plate across the fracture site which is fixed to the bone with multiple screws. Three types of plate exist. The original plates were made of alloy steel and were rigid. A Swiss group of workers decided that the fixation produced by such plates was not sufficiently stable and they devised a system of plates, which is now in widespread use (the AO system), which produces compression of the bone ends together. This provides a very rigid immobilization.

More recently some surgeons have felt that while the AO system gives a very stable reduction, allowing the patient to mobilize very early after the accident, it actually delays healing of the fracture as stimulation of callus formation depends on some movement at the bone ends. They have, therefore, developed a plate made of carbon fibre which is as strong as the steel plates in use but is sufficiently flexible to allow enough movement to stimulate profuse callus formation. It is, nevertheless, sufficiently strong to allow the patient to mobilize as early as with the steel plates. Early trials of these plates are encouraging.

If a fracture is compound there is a high risk of infection, which is a marked inhibitor of bone healing. Careful surgical debridement of the wound must be undertaken and skin cover obtained. If there has been tissue loss in the injury it may be necessary to use a skin flap to cover the bone. Antibiotics are usually given prophylactically to patients with compound fractures. Internal fixation is best avoided in the initial stages of the treatment of a compound fracture. A reasonable

◄ Compound fractures are at high risk of infection. Surgical cleansing and antibiotics are necessary

position of the fracture is held by either a plaster cast or traction until the soft tissue injury has healed. If it is then necessary, a formal operation can be performed to internally fix the fracture without risk of infection.

Complications such as vascular injury demand immediate surgery for correction. When there is an associated vascular injury it is common practice to fix the fracture internally because it is absolutely critical that there should be no movement which would disrupt the fragile vascular repair.

◀ If associated injuries are present internal fixation may be needed

Rehabilitation starts as soon as possible after operation. Even while the limb is in plaster the patient must be encouraged to make as much use of it as is possible. For instance, a patient with a fractured tibia should be up and about on crutches as soon as the plaster is dry. Within 2 weeks it should be possible to put a rubber heel on the plaster and the patient should be able to weight-bear. A patient with an upper limb injury should be encouraged to use the hand as far as they are able while the plaster is in place. Activity will be very restricted but a wrist in plaster does not prevent the patient from holding a pint glass.

◀ Active rehabilitation is essential

Once the fracture has healed and the plaster has been removed active and passive physiotherapy are of benefit. The joints are put through a full range of movement and exercises are devised to strengthen the muscles which will have become partially atrophied through disuse.

Dislocations

Dislocations are a less serious injury than fractures in that the bone remains intact. They may, however, give rise to greater morbidity as any significant dislocation means disruption of the ligaments which support the joint affected. Ligaments do not heal well. Once the dislocation has been reduced the joint must be immobilized as for a fracture to allow the ligaments to heal. Failure to do so results in a permanently unstable joint which will dislocate under minimal trauma. Operation may be undertaken in some cases of disrupted ligaments to formally repair the ligament. Carbon fibre has been used for this purpose.

Sprains

In a sprain there is damage to a ligament not resulting in disruption of the ligament. Long-term serious morbidity does not occur but if the part is not rested there may be persistent pain in the region of the joint.

Burns

Two problems exist with burns. The first is general. Because of the loss of fluid from the burnt surface the patient develops shock (q.v.). The severity of this depends on the area of the burn and this is usually calculated as a percentage of the total body area using a simple diagram which gives a rough estimate of the body surface area. Fluid replacement is managed as in any shocked patient but various formulas exist which give a rough guide to the likely amount of fluid required. The major fluid loss is plasma and it is usual to give plasma proteins as part of the fluid replacement.

◄ Mortality from burns depends on area of involvement. Morbidity from burns depends on depth of injury

The second problem is local and this depends on the depth of the burn. Three categories are recognized. Superficial burns are characterized by erythema (reddening of the skin) and affect the epidermis only. These heal within 7–10 days without residual damage. Partial-thickness burns are characterized by blistering. These blisters affect the upper layers of the dermis but because there is epidermis within the hair follicles and sweat glands which grows out over the surface they heal fairly rapidly. The healing time is around 3 weeks. Scarring is minimal.

Full-thickness burns destroy all layers of the skin and often deep tissue as well. They are characterized by loss of sensation in the burnt area. Healing is slow and scarring is a major problem.

First aid treatment consists of cooling the area rapidly (in cold water), to relieve pain and prevent extension of the burn. Superficial and partial-thickness burns may either be treated by exposure or with an occlusive dressing. The decision is governed mainly by the site of the burn. Facial burns are difficult to dress and are therefore exposed. Burns on the trunk are best dressed. Burns on the hand are treated by enclosure in

◄ The first aid treatment for burns is immediate cooling

plastic bags. Silver sulphadiazine cream is often applied to burns but it is by no means essential.

Full-thickness burns often require grafting. Some surgeons excise the burnt area immediately but others wait until the areas of partial-thickness burn have healed, thus revealing those areas that will require surgery.

Burns are serious injuries. If possible they should be treated in a specialized unit.

Cardiac arrest

Sudden circulatory failure caused by abrupt failure of the heart to pump the blood may happen suddenly in the dental chair, although it is often possible to predict the patient at risk — those who have had a recent myocardial infarction or a history of disturbances of rhythm. The underlying disturbance is either cessation of cardiac contraction (asystole) or ineffectual activity (ventricular fibrillation). Very rapid heart rates (usually ventricular tachycardia) or extreme slowing (bradycardia or complete heart block) may also cause circulatory arrest.

Immediate steps must be taken to maintain respiration and the circulation, since irreversible brain damage occurs within 3–4 minutes of cessation of cerebral blood flow. The diagnosis is confirmed by the history of sudden collapse, loss of consciousness and absent carotid pulses. Apnoea is usual but not constant, as is central cyanosis and dilatation of the pupils. It is important to distinguish cardiac arrest from other causes of collapse such as Stokes–Adams attacks (*see* Chapter 3), vasovagal attack, acute haemorrhage and postural hypotension, as may occur in patients receiving treatment for hypertension (*see* Chapter 3).

It is important to get the patient on to a firm surface. A firm blow with the fist over the lower sternum may be sufficient to restart the heart in asystole. If this is unsuccessful the lower third of the sternum is compressed with the heel of one hand, the other hand on top. In this way the heart is compressed against the vertebral column 60 times a minute. After four or five compressions the procedure is stopped to allow lung inflation, and then restarted.

355

It is important to clear the airway and remove or suck out blood, vomit, and other objects. The neck is extended, the chin lifted up and the jaw pulled forwards. The tongue must not be allowed to fall back into the pharynx to cause airway obstruction.

Mouth-to-mouth artificial respiration is performed by extending the patient's head fully, pinching his nose and holding the jaw forwards; after a deep breath the operator's mouth is placed over the patient's and expired air forced into the patient's mouth. The patient exhales passively. A Brook airway is equally effective in achieving artificial ventilation, but the most efficient method is to pass an anaesthetic airway over the tongue and, with a face mask, inflate the lungs with air or 100% oxygen.

When circulatory arrest occurs in general dental practice one member of staff should be told to contact emergency services. Ambulancemen and other para-medically trained persons are trained in external cardiac massage and some are trained to pass endotracheal tubes; they will be able to continue resuscitation, if needed, during transfer of the patient to hospital.

It is important to inform the patient's next-of-kin and general medical practitioner of the emergency.

Choking

Foreign body obstruction of the airway usually occurs when the patient is eating but may also occur during oral surgery, particularly under general anaesthesia or in the sedated patient.

If the patient is conscious he is unable to speak but clasps his throat; he becomes pale and then increasingly cyanosed, finally collapsing and losing consciousness. In the anaesthetized patient airway obstruction is recognized by stridor and increasing cyanosis with cardiac slowing.

The obstructing object can be removed by a series of thrusts with the clenched fist in the upper abdomen (Heimlich manoeuvre). If the patient is seated his waist is encircled with the arms from behind, the hands are positioned just below the xiphisternum and above the umbilicus and a clenched fist is pressed into the epigastrium, with a quick upward thrust, up to six times. Resumption of breathing and return of normal colour indicate that the obstruction has been moved; the object is sometimes expelled with force. If the patient is supine the operator's hands are placed one on top of the other, in the same site, and several quick upward thrusts made.

It is important to avoid lateral pressure over the lower thorax since this may cause rib fractures. Vomiting may follow the Heimlich manœuvre; the patient should be laid flat with the head down and turned to one side, if this occurs. The mouth should be sucked out and the tongue pulled forwards.

Shock

A wide variety of conditions can cause circulatory insufficiency resulting in reduced perfusion of many organs, including the brain and kidneys. Anaphylactic and hypovolaemic (haemorrhage) shock may be encountered in dental practice; bacteraemic and cardiogenic shock are two other forms.

Anaphylactic shock is usually a manifestation of drug or food allergy; it may also follow insect bites. The initial features are generalized itching, particularly on the soles and palms, followed by generalized flushing (hyperaemia) and swelling of the face and neck, due to rapid oedema formation, which may extend into the pharynx causing upper respiratory obstruction. The sudden loss of intravascular fluid causes hypovolaemia and reduced perfusion of various organs.

Acute anaphylaxis is caused by a massive release of histamine and other mediator substances as part of systemic reaginic reaction (*see* Chapter 17). An example is that of penicillin allergy when there has been previous exposure to the drug, with or without a maculopapular rash.

Hydrocortisone sodium succinate in doses of 100–300 mg, intravenously is life-saving in anaphylaxis; adrenaline (0·5–1 mg) given by slow intravenous injection may also be helpful.

Hypovolaemic shock is the result of reduced

circulating blood volume from haemorrhage, trauma or severe burns. Vomiting, diarrhoea, diabetic keto-acidosis and Addisonian crisis (*see* Chapter 9) may also cause hypovolaemia by depletion of extracellular fluid.

Shock can complicate coagulation disorder, such as haemophilia, or it may follow trauma, surgery and gastrointestinal bleeding from oesophageal varices, complicating portal hypertension, or from peptic ulcer. The clinical features are pallor, sweating in spite of cold peripheries, shivering, faintness on standing or sitting and syncope. Respiration may be sighing, the pulse is rapid and difficult to palpate because of reduced blood pressure. Bleeding may be obvious but in haemophilia or blood loss from the bowel the diagnosis depends on recognition of the clinical picture, since the source of haemorrhage may not be immediately obvious.

The urgent treatment of hypovolaemic shock is to restore blood volume with intravenous plasma or a synthetic substitute. Blood lost is replaced by trans-fusion as soon as it can be cross matched but in the case of torrential bleeding it may be necessary to give unmatched (blood group O, Rhesus negative). Once the patient has been resuscitated the underlying cause is treated and any coagulation disorder is reversed.

Prolonged hypotension and reduced kidney per-fusion may cause acute renal failure; it is important to observe urinary output and blood urea following severe blood loss although dialysis is rarely necessary.

Bacteraemic shock may complicate pneumonia, urinary tract infection, peritonitis and osteomyelitis with Gram-positive or, particularly, Gram-negative organisms. The mechanism is not known but is thought to be vasodilatation caused by bacterial toxins which results in a reduction in 'effective' circulating blood volume. The clinical features are those of tachycardia, hypotension, peripheral and central cyanosis, tachy-pnoea and wheezing. The problem may be compounded by heavy, spontaneous bleeding due to a disturbance of coagulation as a result of infection (diffuse intra-vascular coagulation).

Treatment of bacteraemic shock consists of intra-venous fluids and plasma expanders to overcome the effective reduction in plasma volume. Vasoconstrictors may be used with variable success and heparin is given in patients with coagulation defects. Antibiotics are given intravenously according to the sensitivities of the organism.

Cardiogenic shock can complicate myocardial infarction or follow circulatory arrest due to disturbances of cardiac rhythm. The clinical features are hypotension, cold, pale peripheries, evidence of reduced organ perfusion, reduced urine volume and mental clouding or confusion due to cerebral ischaemia. In some patients the cause is hypovolaemia and myocardial depression caused by drugs but, having excluded these possibilities, the explanation is impaired cardiac pump function.

There is no satisfactory treatment for cardiogenic shock although some sympathomimetic drugs (dopamine and dobutamine) may increase contractility of heart muscle, with little effect on rate, and can be of benefit. Sympathomimetics causing vasoconstriction are not beneficial and may be harmful.

Index

Thyroid
  diffuse enlargement, 163
  ectopic, 284
  nodule, 163
  retrosternal, 284
  swelling, 162–4
Thyroidectomy, 166
Thyrotoxicosis, 164–6
Tics, 11, 213
Tidal volume, 74
Tinea, 293
Tinnitus, 263
Tolerance, immune, 316
Tonsillar disease, 268–70
  exudates and, 273
  inflammation, acute, 268–9 (*Table* 13.4)
  tumours, 269, 278–9
Transitional cell carcinoma, 325
Transplantation, renal, 191–2
Trauma
  abdominal, 342, 343, 349
  assessment of, 341
  management of, 340–1
  metabolic effects, 337–8
  thoracic, 342, 346–8
Tremor, 24, 212
  benign essential, 220
Trigeminal neuralgia, 225–6
Trismus, 275
TSH, 167
Tuberculosis
  adult, 91
  cervical lymph noded, 283
  haematogenous spread, miliary, 91
  laryngeal, 270–1
  notification of, 91
  primary, 90–1
  risks of dental treatment, 91, 92, 97
Tuberous sclerosis, 102
Tumours of
  bone, 255–7
  intracranial, 233–4 (*Table* 11.12)
  jaw, 279 (*Table* 13.8)
  larynx, 271
  lip, 278
  lung, 87 (*Table* 5.8)
  mouth, 26 (*Table* 2.9), 275
  palate, 278
  pharynx, 271
  pituitary, 233, 234
  skin, 299–301
  stomach, 108–9
  tongue, 278
  tonsil, 269, 278–9
  vascular, 324

Tumour growth, 324

Ulcer
  corneal, 11
  drug-induced oral, 303
  oral, 25, 26 (*Table* 2.10)
  peptic, 106–8
  rodent, 14, 300
Ulcerative colitis, 112–4
Ultrasound, 331
Urinary calculi, 193–4
Urinary tract
  infection, 194–5 (*Table* 10.6)
  obstruction, 195–6 (*Table* 10.7)
Urticaria, 295

Vascular disease, peripheral
  acute, 62
  chronic, 61
  investigation of, 63
  treatment, 64–8
Ventricular
  extrasystole, 37
  failure, left, 35
  tachycardia, 37
Vitiligo, 210 (*Table* 11.3), 263 (*Table* 13.2),
    296
Verucca, 299
Vesicle, 292
Vital capacity (forced), 69
Vitamin
  B_6, 25
  B_{12}, 25, 110, 140
  D, 110, 122, 130, 168, 250, 252
  D_3, 252
  K, 109, 131, 157
Vocal cord paralysis, 271
Von Willebrand's disease, 157

Wheeze, 8, 71, 74
White blood cells, 135–6
Wilson's disease, 129, 130
Wound healing, 338–9

Xanthelasma, 14
Xerostomia, 27 (*Table* 2.11), 304
X-ray therapy, *see* Radiotherapy